1882
7267

D0948763

VISUAL PROSTHESIS

The Interdisciplinary Dialogue

ACM MONOGRAPH SERIES

*Published under the auspices of the Association for
Computing Machinery Inc.*

Editor ROBERT L. ASHENHURST   *The University of Chicago*

A. FINERMAN (Ed.)   University Education in Computing Science, 1968
A. GINZBURG   Algebraic Theory of Automata, 1968
E. F. CODD   Cellular Automata, 1968
G. ERNST AND A. NEWELL   GPS: A Case Study in Generality and Problem Solving, 1969
M. A. GAVRILOV AND A. D. ZAKREVSKII (Eds.) LYaPAS: A Programming Language for Logic and Coding Algorithms, 1969
THEODOR D. STERLING, EDGAR A. BERING, JR., SEYMOUR V. POLLACK, AND HERBERT VAUGHAN, JR. (Eds.) Visual Prosthesis: The Interdisciplinary Dialogue, 1971

In preparation
JOHN R. RICE (Ed.) Mathematical Software

*Previously published and available from The Macmillan Company,
New York City*
G. SEBESTYN   Decision Making Processes in Pattern Recognition, 1963
M. YOVITS (Ed.)   Large Capacity Memory Techniques for Computing Systems, 1962
V. KRYLOV   Approximate Calculation of Integrals (Translated by A. H. Stroud), 1962

VISUAL PROSTHESIS
THE INTERDISCIPLINARY DIALOGUE

Edited by

T. D. STERLING   *E. A. BERING, JR.*

S. V. POLLACK   *H. G. VAUGHAN, JR.*

*Proceedings of The Second Conference
on Visual Prosthesis*

ACADEMIC PRESS   New York and London   1971

WW 358
C76V
1971

LIBRARY
CORNELL UNIVERSITY
MEDICAL COLLEGE
NEW YORK CITY

JUN 2 1 1971

COPYRIGHT © 1971, BY ACADEMIC PRESS, INC.
ALL RIGHTS RESERVED
NO PART OF THIS BOOK MAY BE REPRODUCED IN ANY FORM,
BY PHOTOSTAT, MICROFILM, RETRIEVAL SYSTEM, OR ANY
OTHER MEANS, WITHOUT WRITTEN PERMISSION FROM
THE PUBLISHERS.

ACADEMIC PRESS, INC.
111 Fifth Avenue, New York, New York 10003

United Kingdom Edition published by
ACADEMIC PRESS, INC. (LONDON) LTD.
Berkeley Square House, London W1X 6BA

LIBRARY OF CONGRESS CATALOG CARD NUMBER: 74-137600

PRINTED IN THE UNITED STATES OF AMERICA

CONTENTS

v

I.3   Brain Stimulation

I.4   Preprocessing of Visual Information

I.5   *System Design*

Part II.   **Other Possibilities**

Part III.   **Thoughts on Prosthetic Experiments on Humans**

Part IV.   Why or Why Not a Visual Prosthesis?

LIST OF CONTRIBUTORS

Numbers in parentheses indicate the pages on which the authors' contributions begin.

J. E. ADAMS (49), Department of Surgery, University of California, San Francisco, California

P. BACH-Y-RITA (281), The Institute of Medical Sciences, Pacific Medical Center, San Francisco, California

E. A. BERING, JR. (371), National Institute of Neurological Diseases and Stroke, National Institutes of Health, Bethesda, Maryland

J. BLISS (259), Engineering Sciences Laboratory, Stanford Research Institute, Menlo Park, California

H. BOMZE (253), Department of Bioengineering, Irene Johnson Rehabilitation Institute, St. Louis, Missouri

G. S. BRINDLEY (23, 41, 43), Department of Physiology, Institute of Psychiatry, London, England

W. M. BRODEY (199), Environmental Ecology Laboratory, Boston, Massachusetts

J. CARR III (169), The Moore School of Electrical Engineering, University of Pennsylvania, Philadelphia, Pennsylvania

C. C. COLLINS (267), The Institute of Medical Sciences, Pacific Medical Center, San Francisco, California

A. DEL CAMPO (129), Av. Revolucion No. 1734, Mexico, D.F.

R. W. Doty (81), Center for Brain Research, River Campus Station, University of Rochester, Rochester, New York

C. E. Hallenbeck (327), Department of Psychology, University of Kansas, Lawrence, Kansas

K. Ingham (305), Research Laboratory of Electronics, Massachusetts Institute of Technology, Cambridge, Massachusetts

A. R. Johnson (199), Environmental Ecology Laboratory, Boston, Massachusetts

K. C. Knowlton (157), Bell Telephone Laboratories, Murray Hill, New Jersey

W. Kuprianowicz (295), Pomorska Akademia Medyczna, Klinika Okulistyczna, Szczecin, Poland

W. S. Lewin (23), Physiological Laboratory, University of Cambridge, Cambridge, England

R. W. Mann (301), Department of Mechanical Engineering, Sensory Aids Center, Massachusetts Institute of Technology, Cambridge, Massachusetts

E. Marg (241), School of Optometry, University of California, Berkeley, California

M. Minsky (315), Department of Electrical Engineering, Massachusetts Institute of Technology, Cambridge, Massachusetts

E. F. Murphy (309), Research and Development Division, Prosthetic and Sensory Aids Service, Veterans Administration, New York, New York

G. Nagy (193), IBM Watson Research Center, Yorktown Heights, New York

F. Petruczenko (295), Pomorska Akademia Medyczna Klinika Okulistyczna, Szczecin, Poland

L. R. Pinneo (109), Neurophysiology Program, Stanford Research Institute, Menlo Park, California

B. B. Rutkin (49), Department of Surgery, University of California, San Francisco, California

H. Schimmel (65, 215), Department of Neurology, Albert Einstein College of Medicine, Bronx, New York

W. STARKIEWICZ (295), Pomorska Akademia Medyczna, Klinika Okulistyczna, Szczecin, Poland

T. D. STERLING (1, 145, 253), Department of Applied Mathematics and Computer Science, Washington University, St. Louis, Missouri

T. G. STOCKHAM, JR. (173), Department of Computer Science, University of Utah, Salt Lake City, Utah

L. L. SUTRO (249), Instrumentation Laboratory, Department of Aeronautics and Astronautics, Massachusetts Institute of Technology, Cambridge, Massachusetts

K. TROUERN-TREND (371), Medical Systems Division, Travelers Research Center, Hartford, Connecticut

H. G. VAUGHAN, JR. (1, 65, 215), Department of Neurology, Albert Einstein College of Medicine, Bronx, New York

J. J. WEINKAM (145), Department of Applied Mathematics and Computer Sciences, Washington University, St. Louis, Missouri

PROLOGUE

During the period of June 2–4, 1969, some fifty active investigators in neurophysiology, neurosurgery, engineering, and computer science met at the University of Chicago and considered ways and means by which a visual prosthesis could be produced. This book is a record of that conference. It preserves the formal presentation by its participants as well as the exchange of their views.

In retrospect it seems incredible that three days of the most intense intellectual excitement may be summarized in a few dry and brittle sentences. Being scrutinized were methods for the fulfillment of what may turn out to be one of the most creative acts in human scientific history. For, to replace vision, even in the primitive form we contemplated there, represents a triumph of man's knowledge and abilities, of his science and technology and, above all, of his humanity and determination over the brutish forces which govern many of his actions as a biological organism. A good deal of the excitement originated with the purpose of the Conference. Much more, however, stemmed from the unique contributions of the participants—all of them knowledgeable in their fields (encompassing a wide range of disciplines) and most of them working on one or more of the many aspects that make artificial vision a possibility. Their contributions lay not only in the knowledge they brought to the conference; important new insight also emerged because of the searching and incisive dialogue through which problems, obstacles, and opportunities were carefully examined and illuminated.

The challenges and pressures in editing these proceedings were greatly intensified because the most important business took place during discussions and not during presentation of prepared position papers. The free exchange of views that took place after a brief discussion of prepared

materials (these papers had been previously circulated among all participants) was often wittty, sometimes sharp, on occasion even hostile, but
always to the point. It brought out and put in proper perspective what
was scientifically important and humanistically relevant. Thus, in organizing the material of these proceedings we sought to put together in a
logical order informative and didactic papers and discussions pertaining
to them. We deemphasized extraneous material so that the reader could
partake of some of the enjoyment and stimulation of the Conference. The
substance of the Conference has been divided into a number of sections,
each self-explanatory and each with some editorial comment to serve as a
guidepost. Each section consists of a series of position papers and subsequent discussions. Again we remind the reader that the richest concentration of information is contained in the discussions. The most striking
example of this is the conversation with Giles Brindley—an event that is
unrivaled for sheer scientific excitement.

A Few Historical Remarks

The first and the second conferences on visual prosthesis were held
under the sponsorship of the Association for Computing Machinery. This
is neither strange nor wondrous to those of us who participate in the
development of creative new artifacts and concepts, because computers
have transformed our world of sensing devices and machines into a new
technology.

This new technology provides more than jumbo jets and miniature
radios. It is an intricate way of linking sensing and working devices by
means of digital logic. The resulting complex has creative capabilities
that are in many ways entirely new to man's experience. Of direct concern here is that this intricate combination of electronics and logic can
sense attributes of the environment and take appropriate actions as a consequence, thus making it potentially possible to scan the environment
with camera devices, reduce the output of these camera devices to a
formatted "picture," and present it to an array of electrodes embedded
directly in the visual cortex. The result of this peculiar combination would
be an illusion of vision—an illusion because it does not originate with
input through the eye into the nervous system, but a visual experience,
nevertheless, since it takes advantage of an existing neurophysiological
apparatus to interpret images.

Accordingly, work on a prosthesis requires the close collaboration of
individuals, predominantly in four areas—visual physiology, neurosurgery,
engineering, and computer science. As is usual in such cases of intense

interdisciplinary cooperation, a common language needs to be created and a dialogue pursued for some time to ensure a proper understanding of what the major problems are and how they can be resolved. A number of years must pass during which contacts among the four fields could be established and permitted to flourish to the point where they may produce fruitful and imaginative approaches. It also required willing, nay, eager cooperation among all collaborating disciplines. This, alas, has not been easy to accomplish.

The visual prosthesis is based on a phenomenon which in the past has been considered more of a curiosity than a useful observation by most neurophysiologists. An illusion of a point or of a surface of light is created when cells in the visual cortex are stimulated. (These sensations are called *phosphenes*.) By implanting multiple electrodes onto the visual cortex, it is possible to create arrays of these "lights." When combined with a clever system that arranges to turn some on and others not, this may be used to present images in a literal sense. However, such an enterprise almost completely bypasses the traditional visual scientist who has been deeply concerned with what is happening in the retina and how complex stimulations from the retina are passed on, worked over, modified, formatted, and finally sent to and interpreted by the higher nervous structures. The fact that visual illusions can be created by direct stimulation of higher nervous structures has been noticed, to be sure, but not assigned much importance. Perhaps this is because they could only be observed and reported by human subjects during the rare opportunities for brain stimulation provided by therapeutic surgery in the occipital region. Phosphenes may well be of little importance to the understanding of vision; instead, their immense consequences might be for the creation of a practical visual prosthetic device. Whatever the reasons, the community of clinical specialists or physiologists, with some notable exceptions, has lacked enthusiasm for investigating how phosphenes may be employed for sensory substitution. Neither did many of the engineers whose jobs were defined by prevailing needs and attitudes toward blindness feel favorably inclined to give up their ongoing work on visual aids for the uncertainties of an untried sensory modality. As a consequence, the development in thinking and work in visual prosthesis has taken place against a somewhat bewildering background of passive indifference (and even occasional active hostility) in which a few physiologists, engineers, physicians, and computer scientists, with the personal encouragement and support of a small number of concerned administrators and friends, pursued the opportunity to build what is clearly a realistic prospect of a visual prosthesis.

The first conference had been held at MIT's Endicott House during the winter of 1966. That conference clarified and articulated the opposition to the ideas on which a visual prosthesis could be based. The firm conviction expressed by most visual scientists present—that a stable phosphene could not be created by an implanted electrode, that this phosphene would disappear with time, that the material inserted would poison the wearer, that the threshold would rise with time to the point where not enough current could safely be generated to stimulate the electrode—all these contentions were nullified by the daring experiment of Giles Brindley and Walpole Lewin. Brindley, who, incidentally, was to have been a participant, was at the time of the first conference busy implanting a group of 80 electrodes onto the visual cortex of a recently blinded nurse to test some of the basic contentions which were at issue. When Brindley's results became known in February, 1968, the then National Institute of Neurological Diseases and Blindness (now renamed the National Institute of Neurological Diseases and Stroke) encouraged me to bring together the same individuals and others to reconsider the outlook for a visual prosthesis. This book tells the story of the Conference. It also describes the present state of visual prosthesis and what has to be done to produce it as a workable reality.

What no book can recount, however, is the immense effort that has been necessary to endow the discussion of a visual prosthesis with what scientific respectability it enjoys today. In 1964, when Edgar Bering,[1] John Dupress,[2] Herbert Vaughan [3] and I first considered a general discussion on this topic, we met like conspirators, plotting how we could bring together a group of astute yet openminded colleagues. We were very much of the opinion that whatever the outcome, no reasonable discussion of visual prosthesis could take place or work on such a device ensue unless and until the taboo surrounding this subject was openly violated. After initial disappointments and after many refusals, we settled for the confidential format of the first conference at MIT's Endicott House in which we assured participants that no public records of our meeting would be preserved. (The confidential summary of the first conference, produced with the help of Jim Bliss [4] and Edgar Bering, is included here as an appendix.)

The scant records of this conference hardly reflect its subsequent im-

---

[1] Special Assistant to the Director, National Institute of Neurological Diseases and Stroke/DHEW.

[2] Former Head, Sensory Aids Development and Evaluation Center, Massachusetts Institute of Technology (Deceased).

[3] Department of Neurology, Albert Einstein College of Medicine.

[4] Chief, Engineering Sciences Laboratory, Stanford Research Institute.

portance. It served as a valuable sounding board for all the good reasons why a useful artificial visual device could not be built. Having thus aired all rusty thoughts on this subject, it made possible a realistic assessment of prospects of encouraging work that ultimately would lead to direct cortical stimulation. Indeed, it was this conference that made it openly possible for work on a visual prosthesis to begin. It made possible such actions as the release of some seed money by the National Institute of Neurological Diseases and Blindness for the support of a few exploratory planning studies—largely through the persuasiveness of Edgar Bering, its then associate director. There began the collection and review of information on some of the crucial experimentation that was taking place in this country in which electrodes were directly implanted into the nervous system for a variety of purposes and left there for long periods of time. Perhaps it would not have been possible for Brindley's experiment to obtain the credibility and response that it did had it not been for the preparation laid by the first conference. And, indeed, it was its purpose to provide for such a climate and to make scientifically respectable what had been a taboo topic among visual scientists. Alas, direct experimentation of the sort Brindley undertook was still not possible in the United States (and, in fact, has yet to be repeated here as of this writing). To Giles Brindley goes the credit of cutting through the clouds of doubt, skepticism, and proscrastination and, with one bold experiment, demonstrating the feasibility of the direct implant. In retrospect, there does not appear to be a single finding resulting from Brindley's work that was not predictable from earlier experiences. The signficance of Brindley's experiment was not in producing a startling discovery but in affirming the ascendancy of scientific procedures and creative acumen over dogma and prejudice—even, and especially, in science.

This second conference was again sponsored by the Association for Computing Machinery, specifically by its Committee on Professional Activities of the Blind, of which I had served as the chairman since its inception. Having provided the forum for the first conference at a time when to do so took some intestinal fortitude, it appeared to me that ACM might well be entitled to the credit that results from backing a good show. Fortunately, we did not lack for funds for this round. Besides a grant from NINDS, we received additional financial support from the Vocational Rehabilitation Agency and the American Foundation for the Blind. Nevertheless, a large amount of the funds needed to get both conferences underway came from friends. I am eternally grateful for the help given so freely by Robert Kehoe [1] and David Hardy. Many thanks, too, belong

[1] Former Director, Kettering Laboratory, University of Cincinnati.

to Leslie L. Clark [1] for giving us his valuable encouragement and helping us to get additional financial support from the American Foundation for the Blind for the second (as well as the first) conference. Acknowledgements are due to the former Vocational Rehabilitation Administration which began support of visual prosthesis research as early as 1965. This support derived in great measure through the interest of Mary Switzer,[2] William Usdane,[3] and Douglas MacFarland.[4] As important as the financial support (without which no wheel in science turns) was the kind encouragement the conspirators received from a few persons, especially Leslie L. Clark, Robert C. Drews,[5] Robert Kehoe, Sy Pollack, and William Shinn. My personal gratitude goes to Edgar Bering, John Dupress and Herbert Vaughan for all the work and effort and toleration of divergent views. Let us hope it has been a good cause.

St. Louis, 1970   THEODOR D. STERLING

[1] International Research Information Service, American Foundation for the Blind.

[2] Administrator, Social and Rehabilitation Service/DHEW.

[3] Chief, Division of Research and Demonstration Grants, Social and Rehabilitation Service/DHEW.

[4] Director, Division of Services for the Blind, Rehabilitation Services Administration, SRS/DHEW.

[5] Department of Ophthalmology, Washington University School of Medicine.

AN OVERVIEW:

What Makes a Visual Prosthesis Possible

T. D. Sterling and H. G. Vaughan, Jr.

When the portions of the brain which receive and disseminate visual impulses are electrically excited, a visual sensation is elicited. This visual sensation is referred to as a *phosphene*. Phosphenes have been reported as sharp dots, either round or elongated in form, as larger nebular lights, or in a variety of different shapes and colors. The existence of such phenomena has been known for some time. In 1953 Krieg first suggested that artificial visual perception in blind persons could be achieved through direct electrical stimulation of central visual structures. He pointed out that a spatial map of the external field of vision is projected onto the visual cortex of the brain in such a way as to permit a crude type of form perception by patterned electrical stimulation of the cortical surface. This possibility was questioned through the years by physiologists who felt that the complexity of the neural mechanisms of vision precluded any attempt at artificial vision through cortical stimulation.

A crude preliminary attempt to utilize the phosphene phenomenon in the development of a visual prosthesis for the blind was reported by Button and Putnam in 1962. In this much criticized experiment, they inserted wires into the occipital lobe through burr holes in three blind volunteers. When stimulated electrically, all of the subjects reported phosphenes, and in one instance, two distinct light flashes were seen when two electrodes were activated concurrently. By using a photosensitive element to actuate the stimulator, the subjects were able to locate the position of discrete light sources. However, this primitive device could not serve the subjects in any practical way in their everyday lives. Yet the investigators expressed the hope that further studies, employing more sophisticated instrumentation, would result in a useful prosthesis. Due to the theoretical objections to a prosthesis employing phosphenes, the enormous technical problems facing a sophisticated system and, perhaps most importantly, objections based on ethical considerations, further progress along these lines was halted for several years.

Despite the apparent difficulties of building a prosthesis based on the phosphene phenomenon, its attractive features have maintained interest among some investigators. There is one unique feature in the use of phosphenes as a basis of visual prosthesis which is lacking in other approaches based on some sort of sensory substitution. By the use of phosphenes, it is possible to provide a spatial display having the essential characteristics of a visual experience. In addition, this display is presented to the portion of the nervous system that specializes in analyzing spatial configurations. While such stimulation may result in a relatively crude visual presentation of space and objects in it, it would substantially increase the ability of the blind person to move about in his environment. Any other kind of prosthesis would have to rely upon alternative sensory channels such as audition or touch, achieving only a limited amount of freedom and mobility. The extent to which mobility would be made possible through a crude visual representation of space depends, of course, upon the density of phosphene points in the screen. However, even a relatively sparse number of phosphenes could be instrumental in allowing direct perception of written and printed materials, thus eliminating the major barrier to free participation of blind persons in many areas of employment and, in fact, in many activities of daily life. Thus, even with the limitations that appear to be inherent in the punctate phosphene screen, a successful visual prosthesis could free the blind user from dependence on several forms of human technical assistance required now, even by those who have achieved a reasonably successful adaptation to their loss of vision.

Just how good a cortical prosthesis may be in terms of the quality of visual experience it permits depends on a number of factors. It is clear that such a prosthesis cannot recreate normal vision. Since the entire visual cortex is not accessible to surface stimulation, an incomplete spatial map is all that can be expected from this technique. Furthermore, it seems unlikely that technical and physiological factors will permit more than a few thousand stimulating points to be effectively utilized in creating a phosphene screen.

There are two quite distinct factors which may prove of major value in improving the quality of the visual information achieved from a stimulus matrix providing far fewer inputs than the normal visual system. The first of these is the remarkable ability of the brain to adapt to distorted visual inputs and to form gestalts from quite limited information. It is well known that even gross gaps in the field of vision produced by temporary or fixed lesions of the visual pathways are eliminated from the percept by some brain mechanism which must operate on the output from the primary visual cortex. The efficacy of these processes in reducing some of the imperfections of the visual scene obtained by cortical stimulation can only be evaluated through actual human experience with appropriate experimental prosthetic devices.

The construction of a usable electrode array depends on a number of factors. None of them can be considered constant for every human subject. The size of an array of electrodes that may be implanted is limited by the amount of heat developed by the electrodes and associated circuitry, the spatial response of the nervous system to the implanted electrodes, and considerations of bulk and amount of circuitry. Even under the best of conditions, the number of electrodes which can be implanted will be small compared with normal visual input. It is at this point that our new computer technology holds out the promise of a real breakthrough. By pre-processing an image and reformatting it in such a way that optimal use can be made of available punctate phosphene screens, it is possible to present a relatively rich information content based on a small number of points for transmission of information.

Preprocessing: The Central Concept for Prosthesis

Modern technology offers many effective approaches to the construction of different sensory aids for blind persons. Imaginative approaches have been used to present information through the skin, by auditory signals, and lately, by direct stimulation of the visual cortex. Multiple features of the environment can be represented from a wide choice of sources. However, little work has been done so far on one approach that could appreciably increase the effectiveness of most sensory substitutes— *adaptation of signals to the information processing capabilities of a perceptual system* to permit better discrimination and greater ease of learning the stimulus patterns.

The information gathered by a variety of sensing devices is still presented to blind persons more or less as *raw* impulses with the hope that the nervous system will be able to organize these impulses and learn to respond to them. The effectiveness of an "aid" has always depended to a large extent on the ability of the handicapped user to learn the meaning of the developed signal. Only recently, with the development of digital logic, has it become feasible to process the raw signal and adapt it to the unique response characteristics of a particular perceptual system. Development of these capabilities will produce a dramatic expansion in the possibilities for conveying information about the environment. Optimal display techniques can then be constructed to provide an improved perception of the surround.

The uses of sensory aids depend on thorough training by which the blind person learns the meaning of the various signals emitted by the instrument and how variations in these signals relate to specific environmental features. The success of a particular aid depends largely upon the ability of the nervous system to make sense out of its signals. One example of a successful aid has been the cane—an example of a less successful aid, the optophone. The combination of auditory and tactual stimuli obtained from proper use of the cane make a meaningful pattern about many features of the environment and, on the other hand, the sounds and warbles emitted by the optophone in response to print are difficult to learn and only few blind people have obtained passable reading skills using this instrument.

With the development of digital logic devices (i.e., computers), it is possible to modify a signal and present it in such a way that the nervous system can learn to understand its meaning faster and more reliably. A signal can be transformed in shape or in time and its sensory target can be changed. For instance, it is distinctly possible to translate the image of a printed page into a variety of patterns of presentations such as sound (either by spelling out the words letter by letter or by pronouncing many of these words through computer generated speech), by touch (presenting the words as a constant flow of understandable signals to the skin), or as "visual" images (using a punctate phosphene screen as in Brindley's patient, combined with scanning techniques to permit a relatively poor and irregularly arranged punctate phosphene screen to give a more usable picture). There is no reason why signals could not be presented to more than one sense modality at the same time. The combination of tactual and auditory display might lead to faster and more efficient reading than the use of either touch or sound separately.

Simulation experiments by Sterling and Weinkam as well as by Knowlton (shown at this Conference) have demonstrated that a sparse and irregular screen consisting of no more than 30 points can be utilized for reading, that reading becomes simple for a punctate screen consisting of no more than 80–120 points, and that simple pictures of obstacles can be recognized easily on screens consisting of fewer than 200 points. It is true that these experiments were done using sighted individuals. However, there are good reasons to suppose that the experiences of sighted individuals under controlled conditions mimic the experiences of blind individuals whose visual fields are filled with phosphenes rather than with points of light transmitted through the eyes.

What can computer-controlled preprocessing and formatting do?

There are two methods by which a punctate display screen made up of phosphenes can be exploited. First, the rich and variegated visual scene can be summarized and coded into a symbol or symbol percept. Thus, a man might become a combination of lines and circles (resembling perhaps a stick man), and an obstacle such as a fireplug might appear as an upright bar. Stairs can be simplified by schematically indicating either an upward or downward obstacle.

Secondly, computer preprocessing can be used to filter an image. Here the preprocessing may eliminate interfering noise, present the outlines of obstacles, and compensate for shadows and other sources of interference. Both methods can be used together and a final prosthesis will take advantage of preprocessing involving formatting as well as filtering.

The image itself, whether a coded representation of a complex view or its filtered simplification, need not be presented as a static display. A much more complex picture may be perceived when it apparently moves over an array of points rather than when the picture is stationary. This dynamic presentation of images works because of a principle with which most of us are familiar and which may be called the "picket fence" phenomenon. When walking by a picket fence, a complete view of the scene behind the fence appears which is ordinarily hidden to the stationary observer. This is due to the rapid succession of views presented through small openings which, because of the ability of the human nervous system to put rapidly appearing images together, fuse into a comprehensive view of what is behind the fence. In a similar way, the collection of phosphene points may be used to scan an image. Rather than the viewer moving by the phosphene points, a computer, controlling the impulses to the implanted electrodes, creates the phosphene points as if they were holes in a screen moving by an image. The speed of movement as well as the shape of the image, of course, are all controlled by a program and the result is very much the same as that experienced by a moving observer passing a fence with holes in it. A more complex picture may be presented and perceived as a unified information complex by repeated scanning of the image back and forth, up and down, or however the subject may find it more easy to understand.

Strategy for the Development of a Visual Prosthesis

These first and second conferences on visual prosthesis reached no formal consensus on how a usable device should be developed. In view of the extraordinarily complex interaction among the physiological, technical, and human aspects of prosthesis development, definition of an optimal strategy poses problems of virtually unprecedented difficulty in the field of biomedical development. Beyond the basic question of physiological feasibility—which has largely been laid to rest by the Brindley demonstration— there remain a number of specific unanswered questions concerning the proper methods of cortical stimulation to provide safe and reliable phosphene production. A carefully designed program of animal and human investigation will be needed to resolve these issues. Since further preliminary experiments in human subjects will be necessary before a final prosthesis design is possible, questions of an ethical nature arise in the formulation of this program. As some have suggested, should all questions of stimulation methods be resolved in experimental animals prior to any further human studies? Or at the other extreme, should all potential opportunities provided by neurosurgical practice to stimulate the human brain be utilized to answer some of the critical questions on stimulus parameters? It is clear that we must seek a path of development which minimizes any physical or psychological risk to human participants, but at the same time advances the goal of a workable and effective prosthesis at the fastest possible pace.

While these physiological issues are being resolved, the exacting technical demands of a prosthetic system must be met. There are essentially two main areas requiring special technical effort: Development of an implanted stimulating module meeting stringent requirements for safety and reliability, and provision of a stimulus programming system possessing the flexibility needed for experimentally defining the optimal patterns of stimulation and effective modes of preprocessing.

Preparatory Experiments

Since direct studies of the perceptual effects of patterned cortical stimulation will be required to develop the final system designs for a generally useful prosthesis, the safety of these studies for the human participants is a *sine qua non*. It goes without saying that the stimulating system must not produce damage to the brain and it must not cause discomfort. Furthermore, it must be capable of continuous and prolonged operation without inducing deleterious effects, such as seizures or neural fatigue. Since no implanted electrode design can be expected to have an indefinite life, it may be necessary to replace the implant when failure occurs. This much be accomplished without cortical damage.

These requirements must be evaluated in a series of studies in experimental animals. It will be necessary to design and fabricate electrodes of nontoxic and biologically stable materials which can be implanted chronically and to test the limits of safe electrical stimulation, delivered continuously over periods of several months or more. The critical information to be derived from these tests is the earliest physiological sign of irreversible functional or structural changes in the stimulated brain tissue. Such effects cannot be detected with adequate sensitivity by changes in behavior of the animal or by histological examination of the stimulated tissue. This will require monitoring of the electrical brain responses to stimulation during the course of the experiment. Initially, single electrodes and groups of electrodes must be stimulated to define the levels of current which can be delivered without producing unacceptable short-term effects such as heating and gas production. These studies will be required to test specific electrode dimensions and materials planned for the human system. Once the acceptable limits of stimulation have been checked in acute experiments, prolonged monitoring of the electrophysiological response of the stimulated brain will be required to evaluate the possible development of pathological responses after chronic stimulation. Although some evidence on this point has been obtained by investigators using chronic brain stimulation in animals for other purposes, the conditions of stimulation and the sensitivity of the criteria for detrimental effects have not been sufficient for the prosthesis application. It is quite critical that the physiological responses of the stimulated brain remain stable indefinitely. Brindley's observations in experimental animals and in his single human patient indicate that this is possible, but the general stability of the cortical responses clearly requires further confirmation in experimental animals before further chronic human prosthesis implantations are made. Following prolonged stimulation, histological examination of underlying brain tissue will be required. Even more importantly, removal of the original implant and successful placement of a satisfactorily functioning replacement electrode must be accomplished.

Behavioral Experiments in Animals?

Beyond the evaluation of biological compatibility of electrode materials and criteria for safe cortical stimulation, it is unlikely that experiments intended to test the behavioral responses of animals to cortical stimulation will be useful. Although monkeys can be trained to discriminate between electrical stimulation of two adjacent points of visual cortex, the very limited amount of information that can be unambiguously obtained from further behavioral studies would require an extraordinarily laborious program of investigation lasting many years. It is possible to determine the threshold for detectable electrical stimulation and, by inference, the perceptual threshold for each electrode in a stimulating matrix. However, definition of brightness as a function of stimulating current, tests of form discrimination, and other complex aspects of phosphene pattern perception would demand animal studies which become prohibitively elaborate. The notion that a camera-actuated prosthetic system could be properly tested in animals is patently absurd, but has been advocated by some otherwise responsible scientists prior to further studies of cortical stimulation in man. At this second Conference there was general agreement, among those who had carefully considered the problem, that a few days of tests with a human recipient implanted with a suitable multielectrode system would provide vastly more useful information concerning stimulus parameters than years of laborious and ambiguous animal studies. For the analyses of perceptual responses to complex phosphene patterns which are necessary for development and evaluation of preprocessing strategies, human reports of perceptual effects are essential. In the light of Brindley's unequivocal demonstration of the feasibility of setting up a stable spatial array of phosphenes, it is difficult to see how animal experiments could provide any stronger case for the basic feasibility of a cortical visual prosthesis.

Electrode Design for Initial Human Implantation

A cortical prosthetic system would comprise three main components: a camera, a stimulus encoder, and a cortical electrode matrix. The functions of each component are straightforward. The camera will translate a matrix of light values sensed from the external environment. The number of sensed values may greatly exceed the number of points available for cortical stimulation, and will provide more data than the prosthetic system could directly transmit to a cortical matrix. Some form of data reduction or preprocessing will be required to produce an optimal transformation of the sensed picture to a spatiotemporal pattern of electrical impulses for cortical stimulation. In the final system, this job will be accomplished by the encoder, which will consist of digital circuitry. This component will be essentially a special purpose computer. Before a suitable encoder can be designed for an ultimate prosthetic system, it will be necessary to perform extensive tests of stimulus parameters on each electrode to define its dynamic stimulating characteristic and then to evaluate the effects of stimulating electrodes in groups. Various strategies for preprocessing, including such simple manipulations as microscanning and edge enhancement, must be developed and assessed. It is evident that these exploratory analyses will comprise a critical aspect of prosthetic system development and will require the use of general purpose computers for the required flexibility of stimulus presentation. The final component, the cortical electrode matrix, is a difficult and critical component of the system, since it must be constructed in such a manner as to provide safe, long-term stimulation of a sufficient number of cortical points to provide a useful phosphene screen.

The design of a satisfactory cortical electrode presents a significant challenge, since several difficult requirements must be met concurrently. Past experience indicates that the noble metals (gold and platinum) will prove suitable for the stimulating electrodes themselves, since they are relatively inert and thus present comparatively little hazard of toxicity or electrochemical dissolution. Similarly, biologically inactive insulating materials such as Teflon, Silastic, and certain new organic polymers are now available as substrates for the stimulating electrode matrix. Of course, the biological properties of these materials will be reassessed during the preliminary animal safety experiments. Due to the convolution of visual cortex, it is difficult to maintain close electrode contact with the brain surface over the entire area of the electrode matrix. Thus, alternative constructions in the form of a highly flexible film electrode, a set of small chips, or possibly even an electrode custom molded to the cortex of each individual recipient need to be considered.

Perhaps the most critical question for prosthetic design concerns the feasible number of functioning cortical contacts. The actual density of the phosphene screen will be limited by technical and physiological factors related to the stimulating interface. There is no definitive answer to the question of maximum electrode density and total number. The most conservative estimate, based upon Brindley's experience with electrode spacings no less than 2.5 mm apart and a success rate of 50%, would limit the phosphene screen perhaps to 200 points or so. However, by improving the proportion of functioning points and reducing spacing to 1 mm, a tenfold increase in number of points could be achieved. Further increases in density might be possible, but would have to be assessed by actual experimental testing in human recipients. Regardless of the matrix size actually selected for the first additional studies, provision must be made to determine the maximum usable density by including at least a subset of closely spaced electrodes. On physiological grounds it is not likely that spacings of less than 300 μ will elicit phosphenes which are discriminable from one another, but guesses based on physiological data have been wrong in the past—as exemplified by the disagreements prior to Brindley's experiment. This question must be submitted to empirical test.

Another, perhaps more serious, limitation of electrode density is presented by the problem of heating of the brain by the stimulating current. Since current density increases with diminishing electrode size for a given value of total current, reduction of electrode spacing and size cannot be carried below some as yet undertermined limit. If each electrode requires a comparable average power delivery, total power requirements could become excessive with large high-density matrices. This limit will again be defined by tests of required levels of stimulating current for specific electrode configurations. Theoretical calculations and the limited experience from cortical stimulation studies provide only a crude guide. However, this problem can be resolved to a large extent in advance of human studies.

It is clear that the choice of matrix size for further human studies will critically affect the strategy for prosthesis development. Here there are two divergent schools of thought. On the one hand, by presenting a more or less direct transformation of the sensed patterns of light and dark to a cortical electrode matrix comprising the maximal number of feasible contacts, perhaps 4000 or so, it is considered possible by some that brain mechanisms will permit a sufficient ordering of whatever discontinuities and irregularities of the spatial phosphene array which are sure to be present. It is not likely, however, that such effects can be fully relied upon for producing an optimal perceptual effect even with maximal arrays, and it is certain that some form of encoding will be necessary if arrays of a few hundred contacts are to be effective.

An additional important feature of a cortical prosthesis system will be provision for transmitting the stimulating pattern of electrical pulses through the intact skin from the encoder to the implanted stimulating electrodes. This feature is necessary to eliminate wiring connections through the skin which would provide a possible pathway for infection. This potential hazard was avoided in Brindley's experiment by the use of radio frequency transmission of stimulus pulses across the scalp. Future systems will transmit much higher rates of information and will require more sophisticated approaches involving inductive, capacitive, or even photoelectric transmission of stimulus code and power to actuate the stimulating electrodes.

Evaluation of Prototype Prosthetic Systems in Human Participants

Since the perception of phosphene patterns which forms the basis for the visual prosthesis can properly be studies only in man, it will be necessary to obtain the participation of blind volunteers in this highly demanding and complex phase of prosthesis development. The amount of information which must be obtained from the earliest recipients is truly enormous. Due to limitations in available stimulating equipment and lacking means to program a flexible pattern of stimulation, Brindley was able to evaluate only the results of stimulating single electrodes and a few instances of simultaneous activation. In order to define properly the perceptual properties of a large phosphene matrix and to explore the possible techniques for preprocessing of the visual information sensed by a camera, it will be necessary to provide convenient and flexible methods for stimulation of the entire electrode matrix or any selected part of it.

The first aspect of these studies will be to test the optimal parameters of stimulation for each of the electrodes in the matrix and to define their spatial position in the field of vision. At this point it may be desirable to eliminate some electrodes or perhaps to rearrange the pattern of electrode activation so as to improve the topography of the phosphene screen. These tests could be performed using specially designed stimulating hardware, but a computer controlled stimulating system would offer major advantages even for these relatively simple studies.

Once the characteristics of each individual electrode have been assessed, the effects of increasingly complex stimulus patterns must be studied to determine the sort of preprocessing circuitry which will lead to the most efficient perception of the environment. This will require a computer directed stimulating system. This system must be set up to provide flexibility of stimulation and to permit the convenient and rapid presentation of patterns. It may be desirable for it to be directed in an interactive way by the blind recipient himself. Provision must be made for this by development of an appropriate language which would allow the user to instruct the computer how to manipulate the parameters of pattern stimulaion.

As the evaluation of the prototype prosthesis proceeds, it will be possible to specify more precisely the hardware options which must be retained in later implants and some of the circuit features that will be demanded of a camera actuated encoder. It will not be possible to specify the details of encoder design until the evaluation phase is completed, although even now educated guesses can be made about its probable characteristics. If all of these guesses are correct, the encoder design and fabrication could be relatively simple and inexpensive. However, this is not likely, since we must anticipate the possibility of substantial differences in functional characteristics of the phosphene screens of different individuals. These will have to be accumulated by "custom tailoring" the encoder to each user. Although this is not at all beyond feasibility—both technically and economically—the features of each phosphene matrix will have to be tested by a flexible programming arrangement directed by a computer.

Capabilities for flexible test stimulation will also be required for further development of more sophisticated systems, such as those which would link the sensing camera to the muscles that move the eyes. The servosystem which integrates information related to the head and eye movements with visual input must be mimicked in such a prosthetic system. These interactions introduce another order of complexity into the situation.

A final application of computer directed pattern generation is in the simulation of various preprocessing strategies by tests in sighted persons before actual cortical systems are available for use by blind individuals. In sighted subjects we cannot precisely mimic the situation with cortical stimulation, but the evidence derived from Brindley's studies indicates some of the main features of the cortical phosphene matrix. This information permits reasonable simulation of the percepts which could be obtained by the blind. Using these techniques it has been demonstrated that a discriminable presentation of alphanumeric information might be feasible through the use of moving patterns, employing a phosphene screen as sparse and unfavorably shaped as that obtained in Brindley's patient. It is essential that computer facilities be available to evaluate the efficacy of such preprocessing strategies.

Some Necessary Remarks about Hardware and Software

The preparation of the initial facilities necessary to evaluate the prototype visual prosthesis and design its encoding, preprocessing, and sensing components demands considerable technical development on its own. Unless sufficient attention is paid to these needs, human experiments will not be able to exploit the conditions of discrimination potentially created by implanting stimulation devices.

Computer simulation of an environment is done by a relatively large program consisting basically of two parts—a scene and a camera. The scene is a collection of objects which have location, size, dimension, and a variety of other attributes such as the ability to reflect light, heat, or sound. A camera provides a mapping operation which transforms any point in the scene within the camera field into a particular type of signal. For example, our currently operating simulating language, PROSIS (see "Preprocessing of Sensed Information for Analysis and Display" in these Proceedings) creates a scene which is fundamentally like a photograph having either white or black shades and a camera that converts shades of gray into signals. The scene which the final simulation program needs to create should endow objects with many more properties than just flat, black outlines—it should give them three dimensions and supply them with temperature information or echoes.

Each type of simulated camera can have its own properties and response characteristics which in a unique way describe a particular attribute or collection of attributes of objects in the scene. The response of the camera may also differ depending on a number of other parameters such as the angle of incidence, the light or temperature levels present in the environment, presence of other signal emissions with competing frequencies, and so on.

This program has to be implemented on a computer-instrumented complex, consisting of four basic parts. First will be the central processor with sufficient storage to permit easy program assembly and implementation and additional disk space to store a sufficient number of programs for actual experimentation. The system should have multiprogramming and multiprocessing hardware so that more than one subject (sighted or blind) may work with a display simultaneously while other users do program debugging. Secondly, an interface between digital and analog components has to be built to energize the transmitting coils situated under the subject's scalp. Thirdly, the system must have visual display consoles to provide access for sighted subjects and programmers. Finally, analog-to-digital conversion hardware has to be designed to permit attachment of various "camera" devices which subjects can manipulate.

There are many demands on software design. The primary need is for a programming language permitting investigators to achieve ultimate flexibilities in simulation. This would be a (compiler) language in which one can specify with relative ease figures and shapes of arbitrarily complex structures, present figures to the punctate phosphene screen in a desired size of intensity of stimulation, and move these figures as the situation dictates. A protoype language to do that (with the acronym of PROSIS) has been described and demonstrated by Sterling and Weinkam and could serve as a model. However, the construction of such a compiler solves only one of the many software problems created by the simulating hardware. Others require the construction of a dedicated timesharing system to permit simultaneous access by subjects and programmers.

The Human Side of Prosthesis Development

It would be a mistake to view the development of a cortical visual prosthesis primarily as a technological marvel. We must not lose sight of the fact that the purpose of this device is to enhance the ability of blind users to live a more normal life. By enriching the content of information directly available to them, they can be freed from their present extensive reliance upon specially prepared artifacts such as Braille and recorded materials, as well as upon direct human assistance in guidance and interpretation of the visual environment. Such enrichment appears to be a unique possibility of a visual prosthesis, despite the existence of a number of ingenious aids employing alternate sensory modalities of touch and hearing. These methods have demanded extensive training in their use and have not achieved general acceptance. The cane, with its readily interpretable pattern of auditory and kinesthetic information, remains the most effective aid to mobility for the blind. Even aids of proven effectiveness, such as Braille, are presently effectively utilized by but a minority of the blind. The difficulties encountered by the blind in using most sensory aids derive from the need to learn unfamiliar and unnatural sensory codes. Additional factors which have limited acceptance of some aids, including the cane, are related to psychological reactions of the blind concerning their self-image and reactions of others to their handicap. In the view of a number of professional workers, both blind and sighted, the usefulness of sensory aids in a truly practical sense has often been slighted by technological preoccupations. There is a serious danger that such a situation might be repeated in the development of a visual prosthesis, which presents such broad and exacting technological demands. To those who have compared the potential value of a visual prosthesis with sensory aids employing alternative sensory channels, its superiority seems so obvious as to require little defense. As clearly demonstrated in the discussions during the conference, this belief was not shared by a number of blind professionals and others working in the sensory aids field. The reasons for this disagreement are worth examining with care.

Perhaps the most dramatic aspect of the visual prosthesis is its status as the first attempt at a direct input of information to the human brain, bypassing the normal sensory apparatus. Many of the psychological reactions surrounding this situation are embodied in what was aptly designated during the conference as the "skull taboo"—a resistance to or outright rejection of procedures involving direct brain stimulation. These reactions must not be dismissed lightly as such feelings, which contain a mixture of rational doubts and irrational fears, can form the basis for strong opposition both to development and application of a system with great potential benefits and minimal risks to the user.

Another source of resistance by blind professionals arises from achievement of a personally adequate adjustment to their handicap. They literally do not "need" a visual prosthesis, despite the objective gains they might make in access to the environment. This, and the even more subtle problem that they would face were a visual prosthesis to be both successful and widely utilized, forms an important consideration in evaluating the human problems associated with prosthesis development.

Notwithstanding this opposition to visual prosthesis development, there is among the blind a large amount of interest and acceptance of this possibility for improving their contact wtih the environment despite the need for a surgical implantation and the uncertainties that accompany any novel approach. For these individuals questions must be answered concerning physical and psychological safety, cosmetic acceptability, convenience of use, and, most important, the functional results that may be anticipated from initial prosthetic devices. The questions of safety will be dealt with largely by careful preliminary animal experimentation. The initial recipients, upon whom rests a large burden of participating in demanding and prolonged experimental observation, will be selected with great care and particular attention to their ability to withstand the psychological stress of their exacting role. Although cosmetic aspects and convenience will necessarily be subsidiary conditions in the prototype studies, the existence of miniature cameras and integrated microcircuitry has brought the hardware required for a functioning prosthesis well within the size for convenient head mounting.

A critical question in further experimental studies of visual prosthesis is the degree of sophistication required of the system prior to further study in human volunteers. Here, there may be differences of opinion. At the time of Brindley's experiment it had become clear to all who were seriously thinking about prosthesis development that a crucial demonstration of the feasibility of cortical stimulation for generating a stable phosphene pattern was essential to further progress. This was so not only because of considerable skepticism among physiologists concerning this point, but also because of the need for specific information about the nature of the electrical stimuli which would prove effective in stimulation of the human visual cortex. Brindley partially accomplished both of these objectives. Now there is a need for defining effective means for achieving pattern vision, as well as for obtaining additional details of optimal stimulus parameters. These questions can only be answered by further human studies. There is presently no clear consensus as to whether these studies should be carried out in a "stepwise" fashion, employing at first relatively small electrode matrices under computer control, or whether human studies should await the fabrication of an "optimal" prototype prosthesis system, comprising a high-density cortical electrode matrix capable of being driven by a camera actuated encoding system.

In favor of the first approach is the possibility of providing a useful prosthesis with a relatively small cortical matrix by employing an efficient preprocessing strategy. This would place relatively modest demands upon new technical development for the implanted portions of the system and would utilize a highly flexible computer for testing of preprocessing techniques. The main disadvantage to the implantation of a small electrode matrix is the limit on direct presentation of form information, especially that required for moving through the environment. The recipient would not be able to benefit from later improvements in encoding of camera generated information without replacement of the initial implant. If technological problems of electrode development do not unduly delay the progress of prosthesis evaluation when the other components become available, it would seem desirable to provide even the first participants with an implanted electrode which could make use of refinements in external system components. The present state of materials technology suggests that fabrication of an electrode containing several thousand points may be no more difficult and only slightly more expensive than one containing a few hundred electrodes.

But even a minimal prosthesis implanted experimentally would answer almost immediately a number of questions about the kinds of discriminations possible by the use of phosphenes. Many crucial questions could be answered by the insertion of just a few electrodes in a human volunteer. Certainly most problems concerning the discriminability of objects by the use of phosphenes could be resolved by the implantation of 150 to 200 electrodes—an act well within present capabilities. It is not enough, of course, to plead lack of serious risk and demand human experimentation because it would be more convenient to work with humans than with animals. There are risks—albeit minimal—and some understanding of visual phosphene phenomena could be gained through animal experiments. There are always serious questions about the use of human beings for exploratory studies—especially for studies which may not benefit the subjects and in fact may even prevent them later on from enjoying the benefits of their daring.

Perhaps this last consideration is the most relevant of them all. After all, the human volunteer, who is willing to undergo risks of unknown magnitude by becoming a subject in this type of experiment, ought not to cut off for himself the option of enjoying the consequence of his brave and bold action. It is indeed possible that precisely because they are experimental, the first prosthetic devices will create enough damage on the visual cortex of the first subjects so that they may be prevented in the long run from utilizing a successful device once it has been developed. We do not know how to deal with these problems except to inform human volunteers precisely and fully of the possible consequences of their actions.

One more consequence of this very pressing ethical issue is the need to ensure that appropriate preparations are made to exploit the human experiment. There is a real danger that by focusing on the physiological problems, investigators may overlook the equally complex preparations necessary to explore the human implant experiment to the fullest. Unless computer and visual scientists work hand-in-hand from the very beginning of this effort, there is a good likelihood that early human experimentation will fall short of its objectives.

Would it be possible to perfect a visual prosthesis without human experimentation? The answer must be "no." Certainly well-designed preliminary animal studies, carefully pretested electrodes, the development of early warning systems, cautious step-by-step progressions, and responsible limits on experimental procedures all will combine to increase safety for the human volunteer. Nevertheless, there still remains the act of daring and self-sacrifice for a human to volunteer to undertake for such a series of experiments. It is fortunate, indeed, that there are those in our society who would welcome the opportunity to offer their person for the good of others.

Part I

PROSPECTS FOR ARTIFICIAL VISION

I.1 OBSERVATIONS OF
PHOSPHENES IN HUMAN SUBJECTS

INTENTIONALLY INDUCED PHOSPHENES IN MAN

The most significant landmark in prosthetic development is the recent successful implantation of multiple cortical electrodes in a blind subject. This event resolved one of the major points at issue at the first conference. Stable phosphenes can be safely produced—at least within the limits of carefully conducted laboratory-like procedures. The experiments of Brindley and Lewin in Cambridge and of Adams in San Francisco have furnished the recent basis for charting the direction of consequent efforts.

Because of the pivotal importance of the classic paper by Brindley and Lewin, it is reproduced here, together with their more recent clarifications for the conference. The position paper is followed by a short excerpt of exchanges preceding the discussion between Brindley and the participants in Chicago. Last minute hopes of implanting his second device prevented Brindley from traveling to Chicago. Indirect attendance was arranged via an amplified telephone hookup that permitted an exchange between Brindley and all participants. To insure optimum benefit from this exchange, a series of questions were formulated during the first day of the conference and called in to London early in the morning. Brindley's prepared answers and the exchange that ensued created the kind of exciting dialog that scientists often aim for but seldom achieve.

The work of Adams and his associates provides significant experience with phosphenes induced by implanted subcortical electrodes. This summary paper and excerpts from the subsequent discussion thus comprise a logical unit when combined with the report of the British work. Accordingly, they are included here.

THE SENSATIONS PRODUCED BY ELECTRICAL STIMULATION OF THE VISUAL CORTEX

G. S. Brindley and W. S. Lewin

REPRINTED FROM *J. Physiol.*, **196**, 1968.

SUMMARY

1. An array of radio receivers, connected to electrodes in contact with the occipital pole of the right cerebral hemisphere, has been implanted into a 52-year-old blind patient. By giving appropriate radio signals, the patient can be caused to experience sensations of light ('phosphenes') in the left half of the visual field.

2. The sensation caused by stimulation through a single electrode is commonly a single very small spot of white light at a constant position in the visual field; but for some electrodes it is two or several such spots, or a small cloud.

3. For weak stimuli the map of the visual field on the cortex agrees roughly with the classical maps of Holmes and others derived from war wounds. With stronger stimuli, additional phosphenes appear; these follow a map that is roughly the classical map inverted about the horizontal meridian.

4. The phosphenes produced by stimulation through electrodes 2·4 mm apart can be easily distinguished. By stimulation through several electrodes simultaneously, the patient can be caused to see predictable simple patterns.

5. The effects of the duration and frequency of stimulating pulses on the threshold have been explored.

6. For cortical phosphenes there is no sharp flicker fusion frequency, and probably no flicker fusion frequency at all.

7. During voluntary eye movements, the phosphenes move with the eyes. During vestibular reflex eye movements they remain fixed in space.

8. Phosphenes ordinarily cease immediately when stimulation ceases, but after strong stimulation they sometimes persist for up to 2 min.

9. Our findings strongly suggest that it will be possible, by improving our prototype, to make a useful prosthesis.

INTRODUCTION

Foerster (1929) and Krause & Schum (1931) were the first to expose the occipital pole of one cerebral hemisphere and investigate the effect of stimulating it electrically. Foerster found that when a point at the extreme occipital pole was stimulated, his patient saw a small spot of light directly in front and motionless. When a point on the medial surface of the left hemisphere just above the calcarine fissure was stimulated, the patient saw a spot of light that moved a little, but was always in the lower right part of the field. Similar stimulation just below the calcarine fissure gave a similar sensation in the upper right part of the field.

Krause & Schum (1931) found that similar localized and well-defined sensations of light could be produced by electrical stimulation of the left occipital pole in a patient who had for over eight years been completely hemianopic from a gunshot wound of the left optic radiation. This showed that the adult visual cortex does not wholly lose its functional capacity after years of deprivation of visual input, as was confirmed by Button & Putnam (1962).

The extensive observations of Penfield on visual sensations produced by electrical stimulation of the cerebral cortex (see Penfield & Rasmussen, 1952; Penfield & Jasper, 1954) relate mainly to regions of cortex outside the striate area. Where they do probably relate to striate cortex they add little to those of Foerster and of Krause & Schum, and even seem somewhat to conflict with them. However, the old German observations are so clear that they encouraged us to investigate whether electrical stimulation of the striate cortex might provide a means of giving useful visual sensations to patients who had lost the use of their eyes.

Preliminary experiments were performed to examine further whether a prosthetic device designed to do this would be likely to be useful, and to test its safety. A prototype prosthesis was then implanted into a patient. The present paper is mainly concerned with the scientific information obtained by studying the performance of this prosthesis.

PRELIMINARY EXPERIMENTS

Transmission of signals across intact skin. Since a prosthesis that is to continue to be useful and safe for years must not involve any permanent breach of the skin, it was first necessary to design improvements on existing methods of transmitting electrical signals across intact skin by means of radio waves. The improvements needed and achieved (Brindley, 1964 *a*) were to allow the transmission of a large number of independent signals through a small area of skin, and to make the receivers so efficient that nearly all the power absorbed is delivered to the stimulating electrodes.

Number of channels likely to be needed. The next preliminary requirement was to obtain by simple experiments on normal subjects a rough estimate of the number of channels likely to be needed to give useful function. The estimate obtained (Brindley, 1964 *b*) was that fifty channels should, if the corresponding points were favourably placed in the visual field, permit printed or typed letters to be read one at a time, and that 600 channels should make it possible, with the aid of automatic scanning, to achieve a normal reading speed.

Fibrous reaction to an intracranial implant. It seemed probable, by analogy with the behaviour of indwelling tubes inserted for the treatment of hydrocephalus, that any intracranial implant would become walled off from the brain by a continuous sheet of fibrous tissue, and it was necessary to know what effect this would have on the functioning of the implant. Radio receivers and platinum stimulating electrodes, encapsulated in silicone rubber except for the working surfaces of the electrodes, were therefore implanted over the motor cortex of fourteen baboons, and over the occipital cortex of four baboons, and left in place for periods ranging from 3 weeks to 2 years. A fibrous membrane was found covering the inner surface of every implant that was examined 6 weeks or more after insertion. The membrane was always tightly adherent to the implant and separated from the pia and brain by a narrow space continuous with subarachnoid space. It varied in thickness from 0·5 mm (in an animal killed at 6 weeks) to 0·08 mm (in an animal killed at 18 months). The resistivity of the membrane, measured at 100 c/s and 37° C, varied between 390 and 560 Ω.cm. It would thus be expected to have little effect either on the voltage-threshold for stimulation or on the resolving power of the implant, and these were in fact found (in the implants that stimulated the motor cortex) to vary only slightly during periods as long as 2 years.

No epileptic attacks were observed in any of these baboons, although no anticonvulsant drugs were given. One was killed before the planned date because of deep ulceration of the scalp over the implant. The rest remained perfectly healthy until the intended (and actual) date for killing them.

Confirmation of the observations of Krause & Schum (1931). In a 47-year-old patient with a meningo-sarcoma that originated in the posterior part of the falx and had invaded both occipital lobes, we stimulated, during an operation for partial removal of the tumour, forty points on the calcarine and neighbouring cortex of each hemisphere. The patient had before and immediately after the operation no visual function beyond the ability to distinguish sudden illumination of a dark room from sudden darkening of a brightly lit one. From the appearance of his occipital lobes we feared that there might be no striate cortex capable of functioning, and indeed we found that at all forty points tested in the left hemisphere and at thirty-eight of the forty tested in the right hemisphere, electrical stimulation had no effect. But at two of the points in the right hemisphere, stimulation consistently caused the patient to report seeing a spot of light in the lower left part of his visual field. We had thus confirmed that stimulation of the calcarine cortex can cause localized visual sensations in a patient who gets no such sensations from his eyes.

THE PROTOTYPE HUMAN PROSTHETIC IMPLANT

Technical details. The extracranial part of the implant (see Pl. 1 and 2 and Pl. 3, fig. 1) consists of an array of eighty radio receivers, encapsulated in silicone rubber. The circuit of each receiver is that of fig. 1B of Brindley (1964a), with $C_1 = 75$ pF, $R = 8.2$ kΩ, $L = 3.7$ or 9.1 μH. Alternate receivers in the rectangular lattice are tuned to 6·0 and 9·5 Mc/s.

The array of radio receivers is joined by a cable to the intracranial part of the implant, which is a cap of silicone rubber, moulded to fit the calcarine and neighbouring cortex of the right hemisphere and bearing eighty platinum electrodes. The working surface of each electrode is a square of side 0·8 mm. Each of the receivers is connected to one of the intracranial electrodes and to a ring of platinum strips on the outer surface of the extracranial part of the implant that serves as the indifferent electrode.

To activate a given receiver, and so stimulate the cortex through its electrode, the transmitting coil of an oscillator tuned to the appropriate frequency is pressed against the scalp immediately over it. Thus the selection of a given receiver is achieved mainly by geometry and only secondarily by tuning. The radio signals are pulsed. A commonly used and satisfactory mode is 100 pulses/sec each of length 200 µsec, but many other patterns have been tried. Various kinds of oscillators have been used, most commonly cross-coupled Hartley oscillators using EEL 80 double pentodes. To be satisfactory, an oscillator should be capable of delivering a mean power of 90 mW and a peak power (in 200 µsec pulses) of 900 mW into a receiver at a distance of 5 mm.

The 0·8 mm platinum electrodes behave *in situ* for 400 µsec or shorter pulses roughly as ohmic resistors of about 3000 Ω. For longer pulses the capacitative behaviour of the metal–electrolyte junction has to be taken into account.

Clinical details. Our patient, aged 52 yr, who had been myopic from childhood, developed bilateral glaucoma in 1962. Vision failed progressively and then in 1967 after a right retinal detachment she was left blind, despite several corrective operations. When examined in June, 1967 the patient could only recognize a flash of light in a narrow strip of the temporal field of the right eye, and hand movements in a small part of the peripheral lower temporal field of the left eye. Neither of these surviving regions of field came closer than 15° to the fovea and neither was of practical use to the patient.

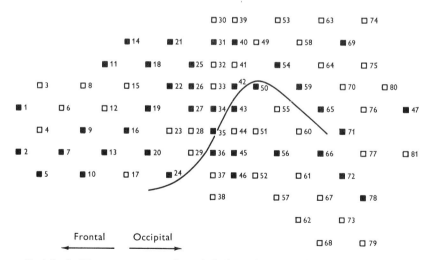

Text-fig. 1. The arrangement of cortical electrodes. Each is connected to the receiver that has the same number in Text-fig. 2. The thirty-nine electrodes that have given phosphenes are shown as filled squares. Of these thirty-nine, five ceased after some months to give phosphenes. It will be seen that the numbering of the electrodes is regular except for the displacement of 47 and the omission of 48. The heavy line shows the conjectured position of the calcarine fissure in relation to the electrodes.

Surgical technique. The extracranial part of the implant was placed beneath the pericranium and secured by tantalum screws to the skull. The intracranial part was inserted through a trephine opening. It lies mainly between the medial surface of the occipital pole of the right cerebral hemisphere and the falx cerebri, and rests in part on the tentorium. Its exact position can be well judged from Pl. 1 and 2.

General results of stimulation. These were demonstrated to the Physiological Society in November 1967, and the abstract of this demonstration has been published (Brindley & Lewin, 1968). When a train of short pulses of radio waves is delivered to one of the eighty receivers, the phosphene that the patient sees is typically a very small spot of white light, described as 'like a star in the sky', or 'the size of a grain of sago at arm's length'. This is the commonest kind of phosphene, and all phosphenes that are within 10° of the point of regard are of this kind. Phosphenes that lie further from the point of regard are sometimes elongated, the length being from $1\frac{1}{2}$ to 4 times the width. The long axis may be vertical, horizontal or oblique. The commonest description of such elongated phosphenes is 'like a grain of rice at arm's length'. One exceptionally long one, 21° from the fixation point, is 'like half a matchstick at arm's length'. The most peripheral phosphenes (1, 2, 5, 7 and 10 of Text-fig. 3) are round but not point-like. They are usually described as clouds. When pressed to assess their size, the patient likens them to peas at arm's length, but says that this is a poor description, as they differ from the more central phosphenes in lacking sharpness rather than in being definitely bigger.

Stimulation through a single cortical electrode does not necessarily produce a single phosphene. There are three electrodes (34, 36 and 50 of Text-fig. 1) for which the phosphene consists of a pair of points about a degree apart, and two (45 and 56 of Text-fig. 1) for which it is a row of three points, each about a degree from the next. Two electrodes (65 and 71 of Text-fig. 1) give clusters of ten or more dim points, distributed over regions of the visual field as much as 15° across.

When a phosphene consists of two, three or many points all in the same region, the threshold for each point is the same or nearly so; thus it is not possible to get a single point by merely weakening the stimulus. But there is another kind of double phosphene for which this is possible: for thirteen of the electrodes, weak stimulation gives a point phosphene in one part of the field, and stronger stimulation gives in addition a point phosphene in a very different part. For ten of these the low-threshold phosphene is in the lower part of the field and the high-threshold in the upper, for three the reverse.

The sensations produced by stimulation are always of light, not darkness. They do not fade during continued stimulation, and when stimulation

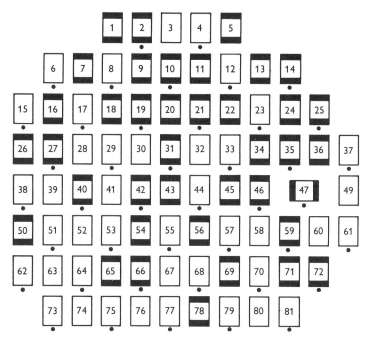

Text-fig. 2. The arrangement of receivers in the extracranial part of the implant. Those that have given phosphenes are shown with thick ends. Of those that have never given phosphenes, numbers 4, 8, 49, 61, 79 and 81 had failed electrically before the implant was inserted. A dot under a receiver indicates that it is tuned to 9·5 Mc/s. The other receivers are tuned to 6·0 Mc/s.

ceases, the sensation generally ceases abruptly. After strong stimulation, the sensation of light sometimes persists, as will be described later.

The map of the visual field on the cortex. It is well known from the observations of Holmes (1918), Teuber, Battersby & Bender (1960) and others, mainly on war wounds, that lesions of the striate cortex at the posterior pole of the hemisphere cause central or paracentral field defects, and that the more anterior a lesion of the medial surface of the occipital lobe is, the more peripheral is the field defect. High-lying lesions of the medial surface of the occipital lobe produce defects in the lower part of a lower quadrant, and low-lying lesions produce defects in the upper part of an upper quadrant of the field. Defects of the directly lateral parts of the visual field (near the 3 o'clock and 9 o'clock meridians) are not produced by any lesions of the medial surface of the occipital lobe, and the parts of the cortex concerned with these parts of the field have therefore long been believed to lie buried in the calcarine fissure.

The phosphenes produced by electrical stimulation in our patient were mapped by two techniques. The first used a hemispherical bowl ('bowl perimeter'; see Pl. 3, fig. 2) of 59 cm radius. The patient was asked to grasp a small knob projecting from a point on its inner surface with her right hand, look at the grasping fingers, and point to the phosphene with her left hand. The second technique was simply to present pairs of stimuli sequentially, and ask here to describe the spatial relations between the corresponding phosphenes. The two techniques supplement one another; the second is better for determining the fine details of the relations between phosphenes, but the first is needed to discover the scale of the map thus constructed.

The map of low-threshold phosphenes (i.e. disregarding the supplementary ones that come in with strong stimulation) is shown in Text-fig. 3. It is roughly concordant with the classical map derived from war wounds if one assumes that the position of the calcarine fissure is that shown as a heavy line. The mapping is not very regular; for example the phosphenes produced by stimulation through electrodes 18, 24 and 27 lie in this order on a straight line (great circle) in the visual field; but on the cortex 24 is very far from the line joining 18 to 27.

As would be expected from the classical map, no phosphene lies in the directly lateral part of the field. The only phosphenes between the 8 and 10 o'clock meridians are two that lie less than 2° from the point of regard.

The additional point phospenes which, for twelve of the electrodes, appear when the stimulus is strong, are greatly at variance with the classical map. It might be supposed that they are due to spread of current to a fold of buried cortex, but the fact that they are points makes this supposition unlikely. They seem rather to indicate a second map, superimposed on the classical one. When the low-threshold phosphene of any electrode is in the upper part of the field, between the 10 and 12 o'clock meridians, the high-threshold phosphene, if there is one, is always in the lower part of the field, between the 6 and 8 o'clock meridians. If the low-threshold phosphene is in the lower field the high-threshold is in the upper. The map of high-threshold phosphenes (Text-fig. 4) roughly resembles that of low-threshold phosphenes inverted about a horizontal line slightly below that through the point of regard. This resemblance is only rough, and there is no evident pattern in the discrepancies from it.

Resolving power. Adjacent electrodes are generally either 3·4 mm or (in the middle part of the implant) 2·4 mm apart. There are ten pairs of electrodes separated by 2·4 mm where both members of the pair certainly give phosphenes. For each of these pairs, the phosphene produced by stimulation through one electrode is easily distinguishable from that produced by stimulation through the other, for any strengths of stimuli. This constant easy distinguishability applies only to fairly rapid sequential presentation; for example, if the members of a pair are called x and y, the patient can always easily distinguish x followed by x from x followed by y, and either from y followed by x, if the following is at an interval of

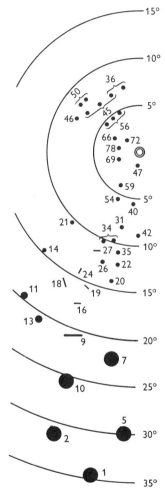

Text-fig. 3. The positions of phosphenes in the visual field, excluding high-threshold phosphenes. The symbols used indicate very roughly the size and shape of the phosphenes. Four phosphenes that are not shown in the figure are as follows. Electrode 25 gave a single point phosphene not far from that of electrode 26; it failed before it had been properly plotted. Electrode 43 gave, and still gives, a single point phosphene that coincides with the middle one of the three given by electrode 45. Electrodes 65 and 71 give large cloud-like phosphenes containing many faint points, wholly below the horizontal meridian and ranging between 3° and 15° from the point of regard.

between $\frac{1}{10}$ sec and 2 sec. When the interval much exceeds 2 sec, the distinction can be made only for a minority of pairs of adjacent electrodes, where the corresponding phosphenes differ in some quality other than position in the visual field.

When stimuli are put through two electrodes simultaneously, the phosphenes characteristic of each are seen together. If the two electrodes are remote from each other on the cortex, this is all that is seen; there is no interaction. Between some pairs even of neighbouring electrodes (2·4 mm apart), there is no detectable interaction. But for other close pairs, interactions of two kinds may be found. First, stimulation through each may cause the phosphene produced by the other to become more diffuse, so that the combined phosphene is a strip of light, though from the separate appearances of its components it would be expected to be two discrete

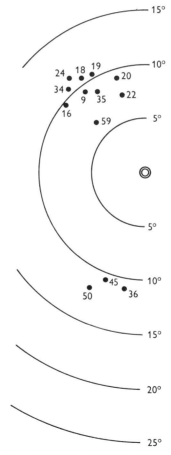

Text-fig. 4. The positions of high-threshold phosphenes in the visual field.

points. This is not a large effect, and occurs only with a minority of close pairs. When it does occur, it is little affected by whether the pulses in the two electrodes are synchronous. The second kind of interaction occurs between electrodes 26 and 34 or 31 and 34. Each of these produces a low-threshold phosphene in the lower part of the visual field, and 34 also produces a high-threshold phosphene in the upper part of the field. If stimuli a little too weak to produce the high-threshold phosphene are sent through 34, then the addition of synchronous stimuli in 26 or 31 will cause the high-threshold phosphene to appear. Asynchronous stimuli have no such effect.

By stimulating through several electrodes simultaneously, simple patterns can be built up which agree with those expected from the positions of their constituents. The number of electrodes that give good phosphenes is too small and their placing in the visual field too unfavourable to permit the patient to read, even at one letter per glance, but the pattern-discrimination achieved is compatible with the original expectation that if a prosthesis gave $50n$ good resolvable phosphenes conveniently placed in the visual field, it would permit the reading of about n letters per glance.

Effect of pulse duration. At constant frequency and strength of radio pulses, increasing the duration of each pulse makes the phosphene brighter up to about 0·6 msec. Further increase of duration has little effect, but this fact is uninformative, since the effects on the pulses of the capacities of the electrode and its 1 μF blocking capacitors certainly become significant at 1 msec, and are perhaps not quite negligible at as little as 0·2 msec. Table 1 shows an estimate, for electrode 19, of the relation between pulse

TABLE 1. The relation between pulse duration and threshold potential for electrode 19 of Text-figs. 1 and 2, measured at 30 pulses/sec

Duration (μsec)	Threshold (V)	Duration (μsec)	Threshold (V)
1000	8	60	19
600	9	40	25
400	9	30	28
300	10	20	36
200	13	10	56
100	16		

duration and threshold measured at 30 pulses/sec. The potentials given in the Table are measured on a duplicate of one of the receivers of the implant, connected to a dummy load (1·0 μF in series with 3000 Ω) estimated to match an electrode. The duplicate receiver was placed at a distance from the transmitting coil equal to the estimated distance of receiver 19 below the surface of the skin. The primary estimates of electrode properties were derived from measurements on implants in baboons, and the primary estimate of distance below the skin from X-ray photographs. All these estimates could be roughly checked by means of records of the stimulating pulses taken from electrodes on the patient's scalp. From the time constant of a pulse and the time constant of return to the base line after a pulse the resistance and capacity of the electrode can in principle be separately determined, though for various practical reasons the estimates are very rough. From the known non-linearity of the relation between the amplitude of a radio pulse and the output from a receiver activated by it (a non-linearity that depends on properties of the diode of the receiver) the absolute output voltage of a receiver in the patient can be checked with an accuracy of perhaps $\pm 30\%$, the chief uncertainty being due to the small signals picked up by many other receivers in the implant. These small signals are probably always subliminal for the cortex, but they are significant in the scalp records, since in these all of them add linearly.

The strength–duration relation for threshold at 140 pulses/sec differs little from that at 30 pulses/sec, except that all thresholds are about 25% lower.

For supraliminal stimuli, strength and duration are nearly but not exactly interchangeable. If one attempts to determine a strength–duration relation for 'constant' sensation, one obtains a relation nearly like that of Table 1 with all voltages multiplied by a constant factor, but the patient says that when the phosphenes produced by long and by short pulses are exactly matched in brightness, they differ slightly in their spatial appearance, that produced by the shorter pulse being usually a little more diffuse.

Effect of frequency. There is no sharp flicker fusion frequency for cortical phosphenes, and probably no flicker fusion frequency at all. When questioned, the patient always reports seeing flicker in every phosphene, even when the number of pulses per second is several hundred or

TABLE 2. The relation between frequency and threshold potential for electrode 19 of Text-figs. 1 and 2, measured with pulses of duration 30 μsec

Frequency (pulses/sec)	Threshold (V)	Frequency (pulses/sec)	Threshold (V)
25	29	400	35
50	27	630	37
100	21	1000	39
160	21	1600	35
250	25	4000	29

several thousand. This can hardly be due to low-frequency modulation of the signal in the transmitter, for none was detectable in the output of a duplicate receiver rigidly connected to the transmitting coil. The patient is sure that the frequency of flicker is neither that of the pulse nor twice that of the pulse; it is substantially faster. This probably excludes a vascular origin. It is very unlikely that mechanical vibration of the transmitting coil can have been concerned, as the coil was pressed against the scalp by springs attached to a heavy (430 g) hat, and no tremor of the head, hat or coil was visible. The flicker is similar for electrodes whose phosphenes are points, clusters of points, rice grains at arm's length, or small clouds. One may perhaps doubt whether a blind person's use of the word 'flicker' corresponds to a sighted person's, but her description of it as 'a rapid flashing on and off, a little too quick for the flashes to be counted', seems convincing. Even clearer is her statement that there is no difference of kind between the phosphenes seen at 20, 200 and 2000 pulses/sec. The phosphenes produced by 20 pulses/sec is described as flickering slightly, but only slightly, more strongly than those produced by the other two frequencies.

Table 2 shows for electrode 19 the relation between frequency and strength for threshold, the pulses being 30 μsec in length. The potentials were measured as in Table 1.

For supraliminal stimuli, strength and frequency, like strength and duration, are nearly but not exactly interchangeable. The changes of strength needed to compensate for the effects of frequency on apparent brightness are rather small in the range 25–4000 pulses/sec. When brightness has been equalized, small differences of spatial distribution or degree of flicker sometimes remain.

Non-visual sensations. Two kinds of non-visual sensation are sometimes produced by bringing transmitting coils up to the implant: tingling in the scalp and deep pain in the head. The tingling in the scalp is evidently due to the current that flows through the extracranial indifferent electrodes. It occurs when any five or more receivers are strongly activated if the pulses in all of them are synchronous. It is a minor nuisance which can be easily avoided by inserting delays between the pulses transmitted to different receivers.

Deep pain is produced only when strong signals are delivered to any one of four receivers: 14, 19, 31 and 40. For receiver 31 the pain is felt in the right side of the head, for the others in the mid line. All these receivers also give visual sensations. For receiver 14 the thresholds for phosphene and pain are about equal. For the other three receivers the threshold for pain is about twice that for producing a phosphene. The deep pain in the head comes on immediately at the beginning of stimulation, and ceases immediately when stimulation ceases. But if by accident it is provoked several times in succession it sometimes leaves behind it a less severe pain in and around the right eye, which fades away during the following 10 min.

It is very probable that the deep pain in the head is due to stimulation of meningeal pain fibres.

Effects of voluntary and reflex eye movements. If while stimuli are being delivered through a cortical electrode the patient moves her eyes to one side or up or down, the phosphene appears to move in the direction of the eye movement. It is difficult to be sure that the magnitude of its apparent movement corresponds to that of the eyes, but it seems likely that it does. Certainly the relation of phosphenes to the point of regard as plotted in the bowl perimeter is the same when the head as well as the eyes face the hand that grasps the fixation knob as it is when the head is turned 30° to the left or right, so that the patient, in order to look towards the fixation knob, has to turn her eyes by 30° in relation to her head.

If while stimuli are being delivered through a cortical electrode the patient's head is rotated passively, she says that the phosphene remains fixed in space, and does not move with the head.

In these two tests, cortical phosphenes behave at least nearly like after-images of retinal origin. We were unsuccessful in our attempts to produce durable and well-resolved after-images in the still functioning parts of our patient's visual field, and therefore could not check directly that cortical phosphenes and retinal after-images behaved alike.

After-effects of stimulation. For stimuli of not more than 1·5 times threshold, the phosphene always ceases instantly when the stimulus ceases. For stronger stimuli it sometimes ceases instantly, but sometimes persists for a time that is usually between half a minute and a minute, and never exceeds 2 min. When a phosphene persists, its final disappearance is preceded by a decrease in the frequency and an increase in the conspicuousness of its flickering.

Persisting phosphenes never expand or change their position in the visual field.

CONCLUSIONS

Two of our findings are wholly unexpected: the high-threshold phosphenes, with their inverted map, and the absence of any flicker fusion frequency. Our other observations agree roughly with what we hoped to find, but had no grounds for expecting with confidence. They suggest that it will be possible to make a useful prosthesis by improving our prototype, and we are working on means of improving it.

The resolving power of the cortex for electrical stimuli is especially satisfactory; it seems likely that the number of electrodes could be increased to at least 200 per hemisphere and all the phosphenes remain resolvable.

Our findings strongly suggest that it will be possible, by improving our prototype, to make a prosthesis that will permit blind patients not only to avoid obstacles when walking, but to read print or handwriting, perhaps at speeds comparable with those habitual among sighted people.

We thank the Medical Research Council for financial support, Professor P. M. Daniel for examining the brains of baboons used in preliminary experiments, and especially our patient for her careful and accurate observations during over 100 hr of testing.

REFERENCES

BRINDLEY, G. S. (1964a). Transmission of electrical stimuli along many independent channels through a fairly small area of intact skin. *J. Physiol.* **177**, 44–46P.

BRINDLEY, G. S. (1964b). The number of information channels needed for efficient reading. *J. Physiol.* **177**, 46P.

BRINDLEY, G. S. & LEWIN, W. S. (1968). The visual sensations produced by electrical stimulation of the medial occipital cortex. *J. Physiol.* **194**, 54–55P.

BUTTON, J. & PUTNAM, T. (1962). Visual responses to cortical stimulation in the blind. *J. Iowa St. med. Soc.* **52**, 17–21.

FOERSTER, O. (1929). Beiträge zur Pathophysiologie der Sehbahn und der Sehsphäre. *J. Psychol. Neurol., Lpz.* **39**, 463–485.

HOLMES, G. (1918). Disturbances of vision by cerebral lesions. *Br. J. Ophthal.* **2**, 353–384.

KRAUSE, F. & SCHUM, H. (1931). *Neue deutsche Chirurgie*, ed. KÜTTNER, H., vol. 49a, pp. 482–486. Stuttgart: Enke.

PENFIELD, W. & JASPER, H. (1954). *Epilepsy and the Functional Anatomy of the Human Brain*. London: Churchill.

PENFIELD, W. & RASMUSSEN, T. (1952). *The Cerebral Cortex of Man*. New York: Macmillan.

TEUBER, H. L., BATTERSBY, W. S. & BENDER, M. B. (1960). *Visual Field Defects After Penetrating Missile Wounds of the Brain*. Cambridge, Mass.: Harvard University Press.

PLATES 1–3 ARE ON PP. 38–40.

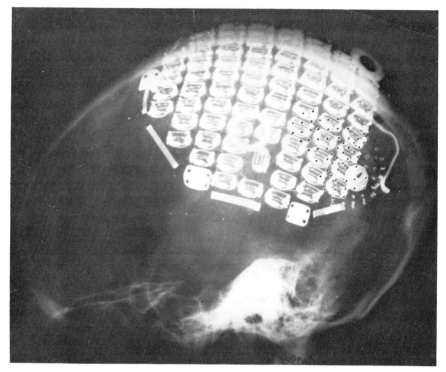

Plate 1

EXPLANATION OF PLATES

PLATE 1

Lateral X-ray photograph of the implant after insertion. The shadows of most of the electrodes are re-touched, and appear in the plate as black dots.

PLATE 2

Antero-posterior X-ray photograph of the implant after insertion.

PLATE 3

Fig. 1. The implant before insertion. Fig. 2. The bowl perimeter.

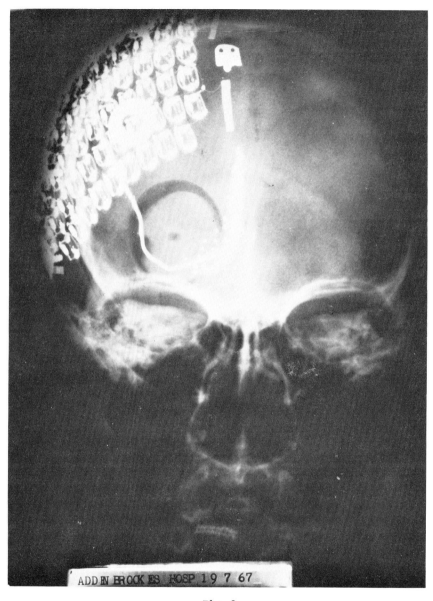

Plate 2

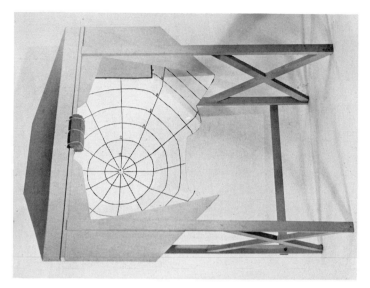

Fig. 2

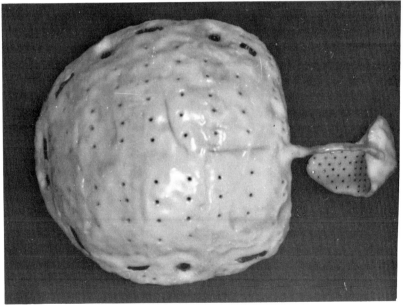

Fig. 1

Plate 3

REPORT TO THE CONFERENCE
ON VISUAL PROSTHESIS

G. S. Brindley

On rereading the paper in *J. Physiol.* 196, 479 (1968) and the preliminary reports in *J. Physiol.* 177, 44P and 46P (1964) and 194 54P (1967), I notice no important errors or substantial omissions, but there is a misprint on line 24 of p. 481 of the main paper, where "0.5 mm" should be "0.05 mm."

Several readers have remarked that the voltage thresholds given in Tables 1 and 2 are surprisingly high. That they should be slightly higher than for electrodes in direct contact with the pia is to be expected, since there is some voltage drop across the secondary dura and subarachnoid space. My methods for estimating the voltages were indeed rather unsatisfactory, and the next implant has been designed so as to allow much more accurate estimates to be made. I think that the figures in the tables are not very likely to be out by more than ±30%, but larger errors are possible if, for example, tissue fluid has tracked along minute fissures in the implant and caused short circuits. The *relative* values of thresholds given in the tables can certainly be trusted.

The patient with the first implant is in excellent health, and is in no way inconvenienced by her implant, but it is not useful to her. In February 1968, 12 of her electrodes, mostly giving single point-like phosphenes, were selected for regular testing, and these have been reexamined at intervals of from 5 to 10 weeks ever since, the latest testing being on April 21, 1969. Of the 12 selected electrodes, one failed in July, 1968 and another in December, 1968. It is very probable that the failures are disconnections within the implant, since the corresponding radio receivers, besides giving no phosphenes, contribute nothing to the scalp sensations that we attribute to current from the indifferent electrodes. The remaining 10 of the 12 selected cortical electrodes continue to give phosphenes with the same distribution in the visual field that they have always had. The thresholds (in terms of radio power at the skin, the pattern of stimulation being always a train of 12 O.8-msec pulses once per second, with 20-msec gaps between adjacent pulses of each train) have remained constant for three of the receivers, risen slightly for five, and fallen slightly for two.[1]

The second implant is completed, and will probably be inserted early in June 1969.[2] In external appearance it is very similar to the first, except that it has two intracranial electrode arrays, one for each hemisphere. The circuit is a row-and-column matrix of radio receivers, with a transistor-and-gate for each intersection. The column receivers supply stimulating current, the row receivers only base current for switching the transistors. Whereas the first implant was primarily designed for investigation, and could only have been made useful to the patient if its performance had fulfilled all of our most optimistic hopes, the second implant is primarily intended to be of direct use to the patient, and it is expected that it is much more likely to succeed than to fail in this. Our first aim is to enable the patient to read ordinary print, our second to help him to see his way about. Contrary to the immediate expectation of most of those familiar with visually handicapped patients, we think that the first task is the easier, chiefly for engineering reasons; but we shall pursue both aims energetically.

The third implant, which is designed but not yet made, will very likely be inserted into the first patient, replacing the functioning but useless implant that she has. A firm decision about the third implant must, however, wait until the performance of the second is known.

---

[1] 50% of the tested electrodes still produced phosphenes as of August 1970 (*Ed.*).

[2] Ths implant failed, on testing, to satisfy all our requirements; in particular, when soaked for some weeks in saline some liquid penetrated into important parts of the circuit. An improved second implant is being made, and will probably be inserted about June, 1970. In the first implant, there have been no further failures among the 12 electrodes selected for regular testing. (Note added in March, 1970.)

I.1.1 Telephone Conversation with Dr. Brindley

HARMON: Dr. Brindley's call is here now.

BRINDLEY: Hello.

DOTY: Who is this? Is this Dr. Brindley?

BRINDLEY: Brindley, from London. This is Dr. Brindley speaking from London.

DOTY: Splendid! This is Bob Doty, from Rochester, although I am in Chicago at the moment. Can you hear me alright?

BRINDLEY: Yes.

DOTY: Splendid! We have an audience of about 50 people here, who are very much involved with and interested in your visual prosthetic exploration. This space-age communication between us seems quite appropriate since you are the only astronaut (or "neuronaut") in the world who has gotten into the actual land of the visual prosthesis. Have you received our questions alright?

BRINDLEY: You wanted my answers to them now?

DOTY: Yes. Let's just go down the list, if you have the answers ready at hand.

BRINDLEY: I will repeat the questions quickly, because many of them fall into three or four parts.

DOTY: True.

BRINDLEY: Question 1 (a)—Did the simultaneous stimulation of adjacent electrodes alter threshold parameters toward perception of phosphenes at either or both points?

The answer to that is sometimes it lowered them a bit, and sometimes it does not alter them. I think that the lowering never exceeds 20%. If 100 is the threshold for one electrode and the other electrode has the same threshold, then when you put the two together they work simultaneously and the threshold will not be less than 80.

DOTY: Is there a mutual facilitation but quite slight?

BRINDLEY: Yes. Now question 1 (b)—If there was sequential stimulation, what is the maximum temporal separation for summation effect to be maintained?

This I never tried, but since even with simultanteous stimulation the facilitation is slight, I would expect it to be even slighter with sequential stimulation.

DOTY: Good!

BRINDLEY: Now, question 1 (c)—What is the maximum temporal separation for a summation effect to be maintained?

Well now, if that is related to (a) and (b), and really means spatio-temporal summation, where the stimuli are separated in both space and time, I do not know the answer; I have to try.

If the question means purely temporal summation between pairs of pulses put into a single electrode, usually the threshold for a pair of pulses is about two-thirds of the threshold for either pulse alone, if the interval is between 2 and 20 msec; between 2 and 20 the interval does not make much difference.

If you lengthen the interval 100 msec, there is still some summation detectable, and, at 1 sec, there is none. Precisely where between 100 msec and 1 sec it fades out, I do not know.

DOTY: This is for pulses applied to a single locus: is that correct?

BRINDLEY: Yes. Whether it is so at different places I do not know, because I have never tried.

Now going on to question 2—Could brightness be modulated by increasing the train length, with amplitude and frequency maintained constant?

Well, what I have done is to set the frequency at 40 a second; that is, 25 msec between pulses; set the duration at 30 μsec; set the amplitude at a little above threshold for a single pulse, and then put in one pulse or two, three, or four, or five, and so on.

The answer is that a pair of pulses gives a much brighter phosphene than a single one does; and three pulses gives substantially brighter than two. When you get above three pulses, however, it does not make much difference. There is only a very slight further brightening.

DOTY: That is a very important observation. I think we now know a lot more. Thank you.

BRINDLEY: All right. Now, question 3, I could not decipher. It was bad on the tape and I am not sure I have it right. But here is my conjectured translation: Did the spatial relation between any two phosphenes ever vary with the strength or frequency of the stimulation? If that is what the question meant, then the answer is no. But perhaps I may have the question wrong.

DOTY: No, I think that is correct. We were interested as to whether the phosphenes moved at all in relation to each other.

BRINDLEY: The maps made on different days did not always agree perfectly, and I am not sure whether this represents a genuine instability from day to day, or is merely because the positions were not very accurately reported. My inclination is to believe that all these apparent variations are from inaccurate reporting, and that really the things are absolutely stable: but I cannot be quite sure of that. All I can be sure of is that they are nearly stable and any variations have nothing to do with the stimulus parameters.

DOTY: Right. That answers 3, I think.

BRINDLEY: Now, question 4 (a)—What was the ratio of threshold current to maximum current producing useful increments in brightness?

A rough answer is about two; but the upper limits of the current I used were set by other effects that they produced: persistance or pain. If the currents are too strong, then the phosphenes persist, and that is the limit of safety. The brightness goes on increasing with increasing current strength, at least until that limit. Now that factor of two in current corresponds to a very large difference in brightness. It is difficult, of course, to get from the patient any quantitative statement of what it is.

I get the impression that it would be quite easy for her to discriminate 10 steps between maximum and threshold; in favorable circumstances I think she might be able to discriminate a good many more intermediate steps. I cannot say that very firmly. The question that I have just answered was 4(a): the ratio of threshold to maximal current. As question 4(b) I have "ditto on the pulse frequencies." I cannot understand this.

DOTY: In a sense, you have answered a bit of it with the pair and the pulses. In other words, if one changed the pulse frequency from 10 to 20/sec, did you get somewhat of a change in subjective brightness?

BRINDLEY: Yes. But these changes are not very large, and anyway the range of frequency that you can use is enormous, as Table 2 of the paper points out. I could go to 4000 pulses/sec, and still get an effect.

Now, question 4(c) is: What was the perceptual effect of the frequencies of less than 20? And the answer is, very strong flicker.

DOTY: Strong flicker, then, and there is no change as one lowers the frequency as at around 15/sec, the quality of the phosphene does not appear to change?

BRINDLEY: The patient did not report anything of that kind, but I was not questioning her very carefully. She said that the flicker was very strong, and I did not think it was important to ask more at the time.

DOTY: Well, that is very interesting. My reason for asking that was with the monkey experiment most of the monkeys find that as the frequency is lowered, at around 15/sec, they find it much different than at 50/sec. That is what that question is for.

BRINDLEY: I thank you for your suggestions. And when the patient next comes for testing, I will test that.

DOTY: Fine; thanks.

BRINDLEY: Now, question 5(a)—What was the maximum number of points stimulated simultaneously?

Eight is the greatest number that I have done.

Question 5(b)—What multiple stimulus patterns were tried and what were the perceptual effects observed?

Well, I tried many kinds of patterns, whatever the phosphenes happened to allow and it happens that the distribution of phosphenes did not allow me to make good letters of the alphabet. I could make a good question mark; a fairly good capital "L," and a fairly good capital "V." None of the letters were very perfect, but still they were recognizable. The question mark, though, was a very good question mark. Spatial interactions on the whole affected the pattern very little.

DOTY: That is what we inferred, but we wanted to be absolutely sure this was the case. Can she actually count them, for instance?

BRINDLEY: I am coming to that. That is question 5(c). I am still on question 5(b). I wanted to go on to say there is a tendency for them to join up. If the points are near, then what she sees when they are both stimulated together, is often not simply the sum of the result of stimulating them separately; the space in between them gets to be filled up with light. This is true only if they are near each other, and not always even then. This brings me to question 5(c)—What was the maximum number of phosphenes which could be identified with simultaneous stimulation?

The greatest number I have ever asked the patient to count was five, and she counted them quite easily. I stimulated five electrodes simultaneously, that gave discrete phosphenes, and she said at once "I see five points" and was able to describe the spatial relation of the five points.

DOTY: Splendid!

BRINDLEY: And question 5(d)—Was this result obtained for all points getting single phosphenes?

I only once tried five nonneighboring points; but I tried three nonneighboring points on many occasions, and I think this would be true for absolutely any electrodes except ones which were very close to each other.

DOTY: I see; so that the focus of attention, as it were, or the ability to process this is not dependent upon the location within the limits you have explored.

BRINDLEY: No. Now, question 6—at any time would stimulation elicit a spreading photic sensation which might be analogous to the phenomenon of scintillating scotoma.

Something analogous happened four times, in October and November of 1967. After a series of long tests, she was driven home and the next time she came she told me that for about half an hour on her way home, as she sat in the car, she saw in the left half of her visual field, stretching out to about 25° from the fixation point a checkerboard pattern. Now I did not directly ask her whether this was accompanied by headache or nausea, but I think she would have told me if there had been. There is nothing in my notes about headache or nausea, and I think she would have told me, and I assume she did not have it.

On each of these four occasions, it was continuous for the half hour, and the checkerboard pattern flickered all the time, but as you have seen from my paper, all the phosphenes always flicker all the time.

DOTY: But apparently you have no experience where the direct electrical stimulation triggered this phosphene or this spreading phenomenon directly.

BRINDLEY: Well, I think the stimulation was responsible for it, because she saw this pattern only four times in her life, and each of these four times immediately followed a test session.

DOTY: Yes, but not at any particular stimulus. In other words, if one assumes for the moment that this may be spreading depression, apparently the stimulation did not very frequently trigger the phenomenon of spreading depression.

BRINDLEY: No. I think it is more like migraines than spreading depression despite the lack of nausea and headache.

DOTY: Right.

BRINDLEY: And I think it is not a very conspicuous thing.

DOTY: Well, that is the end of our questions. I wonder if there are any quick ones from the audience. Dr. Bering.

BERING: Does simultaneous stimulation at different frequencies or current strength give the effects of shading; that is, are some points brighter than others?

DOTY: Yes. Could you get a contrasting brightness at various points by manipulating the stimulus frequency or intensities? In other words, could she get a subjective difference in the brightness among several points stimulated?

BRINDLEY: Yes. I have often tried that between two points. If I make her see two points, and then make either the one on the left brighter or the one on the right brighter, she always correctly identifies the one for which I have increased the intensity of stimulation.

DOTY: Very good! Are there any other questions? That certainly was an excellent one. Do you have any questions to put to us, or suggestions?

BRINDLEY: I do not think I have; no. I think that there is one thing I should let you know. My little report at the Conference said that we hoped to put the second implant in early in June (1969). Well, there is a little bit of delay, and it may not be until early July.[1] But on the whole, things are going as they should, and I think it will not be very long before we put it in.

DOTY: Well, we are certainly all looking forward to it. Are there any questions?

INGHAM: Dr. Doty, is that simultaneous shading that he got? In other words, were the two intensities different without them being varied?

DOTY: You are asking if he puts in identical stimulus parameters at two points, did he always get identical brightness?

INGHAM: I am saying, with the two stimuli applied simultaneously with different parameters, does the woman get the impression of shading?

DOTY: Yes, he did answer that. She did get it.

INGHAM: It is not the same answer; it is sequentially.

DOTY: I understand the question now. It is for stimulation at two points sequentially rather than concurrently, could she get a contrast in brightness? "Consecutively"—I am sorry.

BRINDLEY: I know the answer for simultaneous stimulation. She could. For

---

[1] The second implant is still not inserted, but it is unlikely to be delayed much longer (as of March, 1970).

sequential stimulation, I never directly tried it, but I am almost sure she would be able to.

DOTY: Yes, I expect that would be quite similar to a psychophysical constancy of remembering from one time to the next.

BRINDLEY: Provided the interval is not too long, I do not think there is any difficulty.

DOTY: Is there another question?

STERLING: Would you ask, did he ask the woman to compare the experience of phosphenes with her visual memory of light points? Could she equate those?

DOTY: The question of Ted Sterling's was: Could the woman equate these phosphenes with any prior visual experience which she had had? Did they seem to be real visual experiences?

BRINDLEY: Yes, certainly! She said they were like stars in the sky. This raises the question as to whether they appear to be distant or close to her, but when I tried to probe her on that, and when other people questioned her on that, she was not very consistent. I do not think she has a definite impression that they are a long way away, or that they are close.

DOTY: Well, that is certainly all fascinating. We have one quick question here.

STOCKHAM: Can Dr. Brindley estimate how many such points would fill the field that would normally be considered the visual field?

DOTY: Yes, this is an important question, as to how many of these phosphene points it would take to fill up the visual field. How many points are really available if we could get to them all?

BRINDLEY: Oh, well, this is a thing we cannot answer yet, but I can make a sort of guess at it. I think that on a sensible prophecy, the visual cortex, not including that part that is buried in fissures, the number of resolvable points is sure to be more than three hundred, and sure to be less than ten thousand; but where it is within those limits just remains to be seen.

DOTY: Right.

BRINDLEY: If you had the buried part of the cortex, then you have roughly doubled it.

STOCKHAM: Thank you.

DOTY: Well, this has been extremely useful to us, and we are most grateful to you.

We would also like to extend our great thanks through you to your patient. I expect that she is not there with you to hear this personally, but the group here wishes to congratulate her for her courage and perseverance and patience in making this very important contribution to our knowledge and to the ultimate development of a successful prosthesis.

BRINDLEY: I shall give her that message the next time I see her, which will be in about three weeks.

DOTY: Fine. Thank you ever so much, and best wishes for success with it.

I.1.2 Observations of Phosphenes in Epileptics

VISUAL RESPONSES TO SUBCORTICAL STIMULATION IN THE VISUAL AND LIMBIC SYSTEMS

J. E. Adams and B. B. Rutkin

Although the anatomical substrates have not been demonstrated, physiological evidence suggests that visual stimuli influence limbic activity. Brazier reported that photic stimulation evoked slow potentials in the hippocampus of awake man and of monkeys anesthetized with chloralose [1]. MacLean found that photic stimulation evoked unit responses in the posterior hippocampal gyrus, the parahippocampal portion of the lingual gyrus and the "prostriate" retrosplenial cortex [2]. In a later study, [3] these findings were repeated but units in the entorhinal area and in the hippocampus were unaffected by photic stimulation.

Penfield [4] clearly demonstrated that stimulation of the temporal neocortex produced complex visual hallucinations of objects, faces, persons, or scenes, as well as distortions and illusions of actual perception. He believed that this stimulation activated some memory storage site and allowed actual perceptual memory to be "rerun."

During the course of our studies of stimulating through depth electrodes implanted into the limbic system over the past six years, we have elicited visual phenomena by stimulating in the posterior hippocampus and optic radiations. These visual responses are the subject of this presentation.

We have information from 16 patients with severe intractable temporal lobe seizures who have been studied by depth electrode recording and stimulation. Bipolar electrode pairs on strands of stainless steel wire, 0.0032 in. in diameter were employed. These strands supported seven electrodes, the distance between each electrode of a single pair being 2 mm and between pairs being 10 mm. These were implanted through an occipital bur hole, 2.5 cm lateral to the midline into the posterior hippocampus. After preliminary visualization of the temporal horns of the lateral ventricle, initially by air, and more recently by Conray-60 (Meglumine Iothalamate Injection, Mallinckrodt Pharmaceuticals), the position of the hippocampus was determined from the x-ray film and transferred to coordinates on the Leksell stereotactic frame (Fig. 1). The stimulation parameters were trains of 20 to 100 cps biphasic rectangular pulses. Pulse duration was 0.5 msec and the current varied from 1 to 10 mA peak-to-peak. The subjects' responses to stimulation were recorded on a 14-track magnetic tape and, in some patients, a synchronized video tape. It was possible simultaneously to record electrocardiograms, electroencephalogram and vocal and behavioral responses. These taped records were subsequently reviewed in detail. Most stimulations were given without specific warning. The patient knew that stimulation might occur at any time during a 1½–2 hr. session. At times, after a given site had already been stimulated without the patient's foreknowledge, he would be told exactly when stimulation was on and off. This was done first to increase the patient's awareness of experiences and second to see if the patient's report would be different when he knew he was receiving stimulation.

Visual sensations reported by subjects during or after stimulations were categorized as "A," "B," "C," or "D." The "A" events were visual hallucinations described by the patient as being externally placed with content related to formed objects. The "B" events consisted of visual images with object-related content in which the images were not clearly projected onto the external environment. Thus, if a sensation was not described as having apparent reality or external spatial location, it was

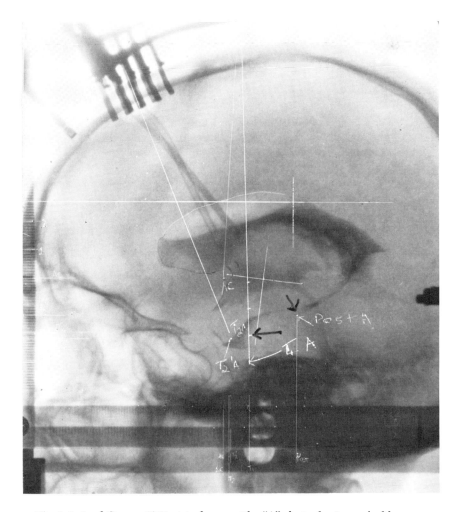

Fig. 1. Lateral Conray-60 Ventriculogram. The "A" electrode site marked by arrow.

classified as a "B" event. The "C" events consisted of elementary sensations, such as white phosphenes, colored lights, geometrical forms, etc. The fourth classification, "D" was used for visual distortions of actual perception.

The most anterior placed electrode pair in the hippocampus was called the "A" point and proceeding in a posterior direction, the subsequent pairs were called the "B" and "C" points. While the stereotactic frame was still in place roentgenographic studies were used to compare the actual position of the pairs with the intended position subsequent to implantation. In this way, the actual coordinates of the intended and actual sites could be calculated (Fig. 2).

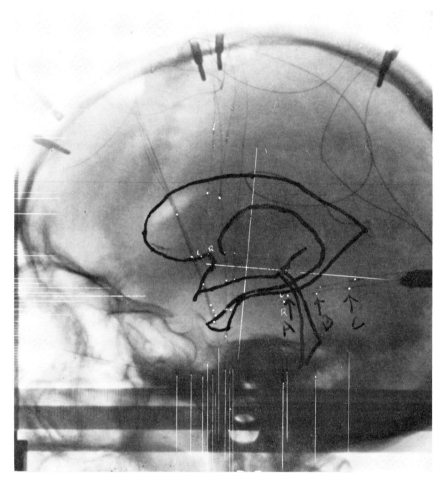

Fig. 2. Lateral roentgenogram with stereotactic frame attached in identical position As in Fig. 1. Arrows point to "A," "B," and "C" points.

In most instances the "C" point was in the optic radiation and the "A" and "B" points were in the posterior hippocampus. A primary evoked response (demonstrated by computer averaging) to photic stimulation was present at the "C" points and not at the "A" and "B" points.

RESULTS

Stimulation in optic radiation ("C" electrodes):   As might be expected, primary or "C" visual events were produced in 46 instances. Two illusory events of the "D" type (distortion of objects in the field of vision) were seen. Of the primary "C" events, the majority were white phosphenes, similar to but much larger and less constant than those recently reported by Brindley [5]. Lines or edges, usually white, were likewise seen. The phosphenes were always in the appropriate or contralateral visual field and remained constant. When the stimulus frequency was below 50 cps, the phosphenes would pulse. Above this stimulus frequency the phosphenes would appear to "flicker."

Stimulation of visual association areas: Forty-two "C" events were elicited, mostly colored, and often in the form of balls or squares, frequently in the midvisual field and not confined to either lateral field. They would frequently move from side to side and in 10 instances, in association with an after-discharge, these primary "C" events were superceded by complex "A" or "B" events.

Sixteen "A" and fourteen "B" events were elicited by stimulation in the posterior hippocampus, and eight "D" events (see Table I). Striking after-discharges were seen in association with 90% of the "A" and "B" events, and only 18% of the "C" events.

TABLE 1. VISUAL RESPONSES

Visual event:	Electrode site		
	C	B	A
"D"	2	5	3
"C"	46	20	22
"B"		6	5
"A"		8	11

The "A" and "B" events were never repeated by subsequent stimulation at the same site with the same parameters of stimulation. In other words, a new or different hallucination or visual image was elicited with subsequent stimulation. Likewise, these complex visual phenomena were usually forgotton within 3–4 min after their cessation. However, with subsequent prodding, patients could reconstruct fragments of the visual image or hallucination.

The data in regard to the "A" and "B" events show that no two stimulations of the same anatomical point produced the same hallucinations, that certain images and hallucinations were not derived from memories of real experiences, and at times, recent perceptions, ideas, or motives were present in the content of these visual events. These data do not refute the Penfield hypothesis but they suggest the need for increasing its complexity. If, as MacLean has suggested, visual impulses from the parahippocampus, they could sum with inputs of other origin and subsequently project to the hypothalamus and other parts of the brain stem to affect neurovegetative functions and emotional behavior. A neural substrate of this kind might, therefore, perhaps underlie some of the visual and emotional symptomatology of patients with irritative lesions of the temporal lobe, and explain the visual phenomena that we have described as a result of stimulating in the posterior hippocampus.

REFERENCES

[1] Brazier, M. A. B., Evoked responses recorded from the depths of the human brain. *Ann. N.Y. Acad. Sci.* **112**, 33 (1964).

[2] Cuenod, M., Casey, K. L., and MacLean, P. D., Unit analysis of visual input to posterior limbic cortex. *J. Neurophysiol.* **28**, 1101 (1965).

[3] MacLean, P. D., Yokota, T., and Kinnard, M. A., Photocally sustained on-responses of units in the posterior hippocampal gyrus of awake monkey. *J. Neurophysiol.* **31**, 870 (1968).

[4] Brindley, G. S., and Lewin, W. S., The sensations produced by electrical stimulation of the visual cortex. *J. Physiol.* **196**, 479 (1968).

[5] Penfield W., and Jasper, H., "Epilepsy and the Functional Anatomy of the Human Brain," Little, Brown, Boston, Massachusetts, 1954.

DISCUSSION

ADAMS: In regard to the feasibility of long-term implantation of depth electrodes, we have implanted radiofrequency electrodes into the thalamus and internal capsule and maintained them there for as long as six months without obvious deleterious effects. Graded radiofrequency lesions have been made and we have repeatedly stimulated them. There has been very little change in the stimulus threshold beyond a slight elevation after a period of several weeks or a month. This slight increase is undoubtedly due to changes in the electrode–tissue interface.

I would agree with Dr. Doty that, because the geometry of the visual cortex is so much more constant, a cortical implant is more logical than a subcortical implant. From a technical point of view, however, I believe that it is feasible to place an array of fine, linear electrodes in the optic radiation and a larger number could be placed in this manner. I think it probably would be as safe if not safer than placement of a surface cortical electrode.

These electrodes we have were developed for the purpose of studying epilepsy; but I think the same electrode that we have used could be modified so that each electrode bundle could have 20 stimulating points, each one 0.5 mm apart. I think one could safely implant six or seven such electrode arrays through two occipital burr holes. This would provide over 200 electrode points.

VAUGHAN: This is comparable to the number of electrodes that are being used in Dr. Brindley's initial systems. One can achieve a number perhaps 100 times as large as that on the cortical surface.

BERING: You said when you increased the stimulation there was a subjective increase in brightness. Did the phosphene also increase in size?

It seems to me that this would be simply recruiting and stimulating more fibers.

ADAMS: I cannot answer this question because we really did not question the patients closely enough on this point. I am sorry.

VAUGHAN: Dr. Adams, in the responses you described as bars, about how big were the subjective sensations?

ADAMS: Unfortunately we did not draw them. The bar would always occupy a specific area in the visual field. If the stimulus was in the right optic radiation, the bar would occupy the left upper or the left lower quadrant. They were thin bars but I would have to guess as to the angle that they subtended.

I.2 SUBJECTIVE RESPONSES TO PHOSPHENES

DISCUSSION

MINSKY: We do not know how the vision works and a few experiments like Brindley's may have tremendous benefit for everyone in getting an understanding of how vision works. There is currently a dogma that the retina does a terrific amount of preprocessing. No doubt this is true. On the other hand we know, from the experiments of Julesz, that the brain can produce an image, a rather poor quality image, I must say, but without using any of the calculations that the retina is supposed to be doing on the basis of the other experiments.

In other words, these are data that show that to an extent the brain can do without the preprocessing in the retina. This suggests with a set of cortical electrodes you ought to be able, in other words, to get something like the images that Julesz gets. They are not very good, but they are "vision."

Absolutely nothing is known, as Dr. Harmon said, of how you put punctate stimuli together to get anything like visions, images. Understanding "vision," I am sure, will help to understand how the brain works. We are in the dark about how the brain works in almost every respect. These seem to be the simplest experiments to determine something.

MACNICHOL: First of all, I would like to mention in reply to Dr. Minsky, apparently in more highly developed vertebrates the preprocessing in the retina seems to be very much less. In the cat and the monkey, for example, you do not find nearly as much of the Lettvin–type of response that you get in the frog. In the monkey and perhaps in man it appears very likely that a lot of the processing that was observed by Lettvin takes place in the brain rather than in the retina.

It seems to me that Brindley's findings provide a very good argument for trying to use the eye muscles. He indicates that during voluntary eye movements the phosphenes move with the eyes, and during vestibular movements they remain fixed with space, and so you already have this body-orienting system built in.

STOCKHAM: A point of clarification: I do not know what those words mean, because I do not know whether I am inside the reference frame or outside. What does it mean for the phosphenes to move with the eyes?

MACKAY: Can I suggest that Dr. Stockham do this for himself. Just get an after image of these various lights, staring at them for five minutes; close your eyes, and they will swing the way your eyes move.

MINSKY: The way you think your eyes are moving. If you close your eyes, they still move.

MACKAY: That is right; that is the Brindley case.

STOCKHAM: Fine! But you can just as easily have the "inside-out" situation. If any of you have tried to fly an airplane on instruments, you know that the artificial horizon is an "inside-out" instrument. Not having been initiated to the device, one might easily assume it is an "outside-in" instrument. If one does one will turn the airplane upside down within a few moments.

I think these statements about phosphene movement are sufficiently ambiguous that it would be nice to have an agreement on what they mean.

BURDE: Is it at all clear from Dr. Brindley's paper that when he stimulates, in whatever particular visual field, that he is getting eye movement directed toward that phosphene as it is projected in space?

Your assumption is that the type of input feeding into the cortex and causing these phosphenes is going to give us a directed eye movement which provides a feedback. If you are talking about a prosthetic device feeding into the cortex, that is then going to have the ends of the loop closed by having the eye muscles direct your prosthesis. I am not at all sure from what has been published that it is true that the phosphene directs eye movement.

BERING: It seems to move but probably does not move. It is probably the same spot on the cortex that is being stimulated, but this is the result of experience.

As one person using your eyes, you have to remember that this person had 50 years of their use and knew that when she turned her eyes, using the muscles, programming them whether the eyes moved or not. When they moved to the left, her eyes were looking at something to the left giving meaning to the patient when she turned her eyes, even though the same spot on the cortex was being stimulated. She sees something on the left side.

BURDE: Right. My question is, when you stimulate this field, being it is the right field, do the eyes move to the right?

BERING: No. Where the person thinks his eyes are, is where this thing is. It is a subjective relationship to where this person's eyes are directed. Then their interpretation of the location of this spot that has been stimulated on the brain is dependent on that. If they are looking straight ahead, it will appear straight ahead. If they are looking to the side, it will be on one side, or the other.

BURDE: I am not debating that at all. The relevant point I am trying to get at is, if we are talking about closing the loop, that is, the directing of the prosthetic device by what is being put in—for example, if we stimulate the left cortex, and get things projected to the right, when you close the loop you want to make your prosthetic device look to the right. If we talk about a "Cadillac," that is going to respond to interest in the input you have to determine if the extraocular muscles are going to be able to complete this end of the loop by turning toward the subject of interest.

BERING: Presumably this is one of the design requirements.

BURDE: I do not know if this is happening.

MINSKY: She says where it is; I do not see any reason to doubt it, offhand.

MACNICHOL: I think one of the important considerations is that it is apparently these phosphenes that are fixed with relation to the eyes; but when vestibular controls on the eyes are allowed, then they appear to be fixed in space; and so it would seem that the vestibular stabilizing loop is working in this blind woman, which ought to be a great help when the eye muscles are used.

STERLING: To what extent is the visual phosphene of the type produced by direct stimulation of the visual cortex related to the visual phenomenon as we know it, as it is related to optical pathways? If it is not related at all, is it possible to produce phosphenes anywhere in an array which is not associated with visual pathways?

DOTY: Concerning Dr. Sterling's question about the relation of the phosphene to normal visual experience, we had a little discussion last night as to how realistic this might be, and as to whether one could deceive an individual having a Brindley device on his cortex as to whether he was being stimulated centrally or peripherally. I contend that you would be able to arrange a situation so that the individual would not be able to tell whether his phosphene was originated by electrical stimulation of his striate cortex, or by the actual application of a matched light in his visual field. I think by some careful matching you could actually do this. It is probably irrelevant, but it might get us some useful discussion.

BURDE: I would like to speak to Dr. Sterling's question. I think when you implant the electrode, it may not matter whether this has anything to do with the ordinary visual impulse. It still may be a very valuable tool. We may be able to have a number of electrodes that are causing phosphenes that with training, in spite of being unrelated to physiologic visual impulses, will be a useful prosthetic device.

I further think, as we progress, we might find the number of electrodes that go into the brain in a given area will not necessarily be a limiting factor; but that the brain itself will limit the number of electrodes, or the amount of information fed into it, again not having to do with the normal physiology of the brain. I think these problems will be worked out.

With the type of electrodes we are using, where it has been estimated you have as many as 25,000 neurons per square millimeter in the area of the visual cortex, we are most likely getting a tremendous amount of neuronal spread. I do not believe you can relate this type of stimulus to a physiologic input.

VAUGHAN: Why is it that increasing current strength does not result in a phosphene which gets bigger? Instead, the phosphene just gets brighter.

Physiological studies by Phillips and his associates in baboons have shown that when one stimulates a cortical point and increases the current, larger and larger numbers of neurons respond at increasing distances from the electrode. One might think that would be associated with an increase in phosphene size. It is not necessarily the case, but you might suppose that; but it turns out that it is not true.

So, I think that to try to "neurophysiologize," and speculate on the basis of what we know, particularly in a negative way, to say, "it could not be this way because of the physiology," is extraordinarily hazardous.

STERLING: I think you have summarized the way you did, because in these discussions, (and I think it is by force of habit) we fixate on the neurophysiology of the visual system. Now let us look at it from a practical point of view which really has nothing to do with the use of phosphenes as a visual process.

Perhaps we ought to forget about visual physiology altogether by acknowledging that we have a technique here by which a number of points of vision can be created, and what is important is to study the parameters that determine that visual illusion.

How does it respond? What does it do with varying frequency of stimulation? What does it do in response to the rhythm of stimulation?

Look at it from the point of view of building procedures. This is the rational and practical way to proceed. If you are going to try to relate the phosphenes to actual experience, we might create an interesting experience, but without relation to reality.

VAUGHAN: One very important fact which has to be established in phosphene phenomena is the size of the visual response.

Dr. Brindley's patient described these as being about the size of small grains of rice, or "sago," held at arm's length.

A calculation as to what a sago grain at arm's length would be indicates something of a very small size. According to the published diagram, the closest these phosphenes approached one another was approximately one degree of visual angle in the parafoveal region, and this corresponded to electrode spacings of 2.4 mm.

So, unless the interaction between adjacent electrodes is of a destructive nature, by summation which would reduce the usefulness of the spatial separation of the points, one would imagine that you could get at least four times closer and still achieve useful spatial resolution of the phosphene. Now this seems to me to be a very important question to explore and assess how general the observations were in the first patient.

I believe in my paper I touched very briefly, on the problem of spatial resolution in the visual prostheteic system. The statements I made there have not been discussed by any of the other physiologists present, and perhaps there is disagreement on my conclusions, and if so these should be brought out; nevertheless, it is there.

Secondly, the question about the stability—how long the phosphenes will be functional—we have only Dr. Brindley's results to go on. It is now a year of threshold stability, stability of spatial position, and brightness. Obviously this particular kind of information is not going to be obtained in any other way than by actual direct experience.

There is animal work which would suggest that implanted electrodes of various sorts can elicit similar behavioral results, and again, I think others may want to comment on this, over very long periods of time extending, I believe, to periods of a year.

NYE: I would like to add a cautionary word, a comment in reaction to Dr. Sterling's remarks, and it is this: I think the experience of the last 20 years in neurophysiology has indicated an answer to the question of whether a reorganized input can be accepted by a human observer.

I think the evidence points in the direction that the brain has a well-organized structure, and that this structure is reflected in language, for example. It is also reflected in the way in which our visual experience is organized.

We cannot really expect to be able to use inputs which are organized in a quite arbitrary way. The evidence indicates that the information must be structured in a well-defined way so as to match the particular organizational structures which exist in the brain.

It is clear that the brain is not a plastic, general-purpose computer system which can be merely programmed by repeated experience. I think we have to acknowledge that these structures exist and that we will have to adapt the input information to meet the requirements of their organization.

SIMMONS: I would like to address a comment to Dr. Nye's remark about an organized nervous system, and the neurophysiology, so-called, or the "scrambled message concept," and whether the brain can unscramble it, or not.

A lot of information exists in hearing, language learning, and in particular experiments with deaf or severely hard-of-hearing children for which a frequency transition device has been developed. These devices transpose higher frequency sound to lower pitches which can be perceived, but the massive instrumentation required so far makes it immobile. The hard-of-hearing child comes to the laboratory, puts on the device for an hour a day and then somehow, after six months of this one hour a day, five days a week experience, an assessment is made of the child's transponder-aided hearing.

On the basis of such experiences, these devices do not appear to be much help. However, a one-hour per day sensation is not the way the brain works or the organism works. A once-a-day device cannot be transcribed in the same fashion as a 24-hour-a-day environment.

It takes two years even to begin to pick up language. I think there is a reasonable amount of evidence it takes quite a while to pick up vision. Both are 24-hour-a-day phenomena.

INGHAM: Did not some of the stimulation done by Penfield result in some very unusual effects?

VAUGHAN: This is an entirely different phenomenon. If one stimulates a certain portion of the brain, one can elicit complex hallucinatory experiences. These are not elicited from the primary visual cortex, but rather from the more anterior portions in the regions of the temporal lobe, and the effect to be gained from the visual cortex is dependent on the stimulation.

OSTER: I would like to say something about a few of the qualitative features of the phosphenes. The most extensive description of phosphenes I think is due to Max Knoll, who is an electrical engineer in Munich, and has published extensively on them. He produces very sharp square waves. That is, a very sharp leading edge. The voltages are on the order of one volt to a half-volt to three volts, actually, which you apply somewhere in the neighborhood of the temples, and he found that the character of the phosphene changes with the frequency of the pulses.

The particular psychic changes happen in the area between five cycles per second and 35 cycles per second. Sometimes people report merely a flickering which, by the way, is discernible with your eyes open, so you can superimpose it on the landscape.

He described spirals, and changing spirals, concentric circles, radial forms, etc., and he has done it with a number of patients, 600 people, actually normals and abnormals. He has constructed a chart of all the different types of phosphenes

My own experience with phosphenes, just "playing around" with it, is that they do indeed, fill the field. It presumably arises from a retinal reaction, because the major effect is to have the electrodes at or near the eyes.

The increased voltages makes them brighter, but does not change their size or character at all. Some of them do have a little color (mostly pastel shades).

You can induce phosphenes in a much more beautiful way by taking LSD, and if you do not believe me, you can ask, because I am sure you have some "acid heads" in your school who will be happy to tell you. You see colored phosphenes; pastel shades; absract figures, very sharply defined.

In the case of LSD at least, it could come back in three months or half a year, and one can see them under quite normal conditions, if one is quite fatigued, just prior to falling asleep.

There has been imported into the United States a supposed "dream machine" of Japanese origin, where you can produce your own pulses by putting the apparatus around your head. I guess they are called "dream machines" because their output is reminiscent of things you see just prior to falling asleep.

VAUGHAN: You have been talking, of course, in part about what is known as retinal phosphenes.

OSTER: Presumably these are retinal phosphenes. I do not know if it is purely the convenience of getting an electrical field into your head, so to speak. I cannot see any other place where you can get the field into your head so easily.

The checkerboard phosphenes which she (Dr. Brindley's patient) reports, as she was driven home, can be reproduced very easily on yourself simply by slightly painfully pressing with your index fingers inward (on your eyelids) and waiting a few seconds. You get a highly stylized checkerboard. I guess, it might indeed be as he (Dr. Brindley) said, a migraine headache.

MACKAY: I think in sorting through these phosphenes we have to distinguish carefully between those that affect the electrical nature of the stimulus and those that affect the time parameters. Some of those described as resulting from stimulation of the orbit are pretty well identical with those that result from stroboscopic illumination of the retina.

They are presumably the response of some higher level to the rhythm with which the whole system is being hammered. That does raise a further question: When trying particular stimulus location, might it not be important to vary not only the frequency of stimulation but also the rhythm of stimulation?

I say this because there are certain color phenomena which can result from uneven rhythm of light on the retina, and you might expect to find analogous effects with uneven electrical stimulation.

In particular, when questioning a patient, it seem important to get clues as to whether what they see represents activation of specific pattern-sensitive visual fibers, or reflects the gross vibration of the whole field. It is characteristic of the stroboscopic phosphenes, for example, that the lines you see are in extremely fine detail. The subject will report them as being etched with almost the finest resolution he can see. This seems rather unlikely to reflect the activation of specific retinal fibers.

VAUGHAN: I think Dr. MacKay is making a rather important point, which I would like to expand upon a little bit, and that is that we have to be very careful when we use the term "phosphene" to give some consideration to the physiology of this phenomenon and not lump them all into the same basket.

With reference to Dr. Oster's comment, when he referred to the visual imagery that occurs on going to sleep, this is not a phosphene. These are the hypnogogic hallucinations which I think most of us have experienced, and are presumably a phenomenon of purely central origin.

The stroboscopic phenomena that Dr. MacKay spoke of are extremely interesting and fascinating. Anyone who has done this on themselves will recognize this as a very intriguing phenomenon because of the extraordinary variety of color and pattern in the geometrical organization of these percepts which would suggest that we must, in some way, be driving at some intrinsic feature of the organization of the visual system by virtue of the frequency of the stimulus.

I do not think these phenomena are really very relevant to visual prosthesis.

BRODEY: I wanted to ask a question about Dr. MacKay's comments about stimuli, as to whether there was a background of experimentation in that area, and particularly whether there had been rhythmic stimulation, other than at a particular frequency, that is, maintained over a period of time? By "rhythmic stimulation," I mean something in the form of music or drumming.

Has anybody experimented with that? Since they use laboratory apparatus it makes it easier to turn the knob around and get a particular frequency.

MACKAY: The only thing we have done is to use paired pulses where the ratios of intervals were varied, in straight perceptual experiments. There certainly you can generate illusory contours by varying the relative timing of the two.

I am not sure that this is relevant; but it does suggest that time rhythm on that rather short scale may be a functional variable at some level in the nervous system.

HARMON: I think it is important to note that Dr. Brindley's call has answered our $64 question affirmatively: Simultaneous stimulation of multiple electrodes can indeed produce a pattern perceptual response. I think that is profoundly important.

I.3 BRAIN STIMULATION

FEASIBILITY OF ELECTROCORTICAL

VISUAL PROSTHESIS

H. G. Vaughan, Jr. and H. Schimmel

The development of a functioning prosthesis presents a unique and difficult challenge, since each of these requirements must be satisfied concurrently. In the past, a number of ingenious sensory aids have failed in practice, in part because there was an emphasis on their technological development without serious consideration of the requirements of the user. In developing an extraordinarily complex visual prosthesis, it would be easy to repeat the same error. The failure to reach a successful result could arise from but a single problem, which would render useless a substantial expenditure of effort and resources. Because this is so, a rational approach to the development of a prosthetic system demands the most careful analysis of every factor that might affect its design and implementation.

Psychophysiological Aspects of Visual Prosthesis

The basis of a visual prosthesis is found in the electrical excitability of neural tissue. This excitability permits visual sensations (phosphenes) to be elicited by stimulation of the retina or those portions of the brain which receive visual input. Although the phosphene phenomenon has been known for a long time, not until the demonstration by Brindley and Lewin [1] did we have direct evidence that a stable visual display could be achieved by stimulation of multiple points of the visual cortex. This type of display could correspond to patterns of light and dark in the environment, thus fulfilling the fundamental requirement of a visual prosthesis. The lack of such evidence before Brindley and Lewin's experiment was the single greatest deterrent to acceptance of the feasibility of the approach. The enormous complexity of the visual system, and our fragmentary knowledge of its mechanisms, had convinced many physiologists that crude electrical stimulation could hardly produce a stable spatial display. Yet, there did exist a substantial body of anatomical, physiological, and behavioral evidence which encouraged a more optimistic view— even prior to Brindley and Lewin's report of success.

The spatial representation of the external world in the visual system begins in the retina, with a reversed and inverted image projected on the photoreceptors. Each of these elements, 2.5 μ or more in diameter, responds to light from an external source approximately 0.5 min in angular dimension. This is also the maximum visual acuity in the center of the retina, which is occupied solely by cones. Due to the increasing convergence of receptors on the retinal ganglion cells, visual acuity diminishes progressively from fovea to periphery. At the retinal level, neural interactions play an important role in determining the sharpness and other features of the visual image. These complexities make the perceptual effects to be obtained from an array of stimulating electrodes problematical; but at the retinal level the dimensions are so small that an electrode spacing close enough to test the limits at perceptual resolution appears to be beyond technical feasibility. Indeed, even if one were prepared to accept a distance between electrodes 10 times the diameter of the cone, the technical difficulties in the way of developing a suitable electrode for chronic implantation appear insuperable. The retina is therefore not a particularly suitable site for an artificial input to the visual system. In addition, it is true that for a substantial portion of the blind population their pathology of vision involves the neural elements of the retina and the optic nerve.

It has also been proposed that microelectrodes be implanted subcortically or intracortically. These suggestions are also unsatisfactory. Although successful experimental stimulation by microelectrodes has been achieved, there are possibly insuperable technical difficulties in implementing a high-density electrode array. No techniques are available to place a large number of closely spaced stimulating electrodes within the brain for an indefinite period without significant damage to surrounding tissue. Yet it is clear that intracortical stimulation, were it feasible, could achieve substantially more localized neural activation, with much weaker stimuli, than stimulation of the cortical surface [2, 3]. For this reason, animal experiments employing chronic depth microstimulation are of great interest.

We now turn to the possibilities for stimulation of the visual cortex itself. Despite the existence of complex mechanisms in the retina and visual cortex specialized for signaling information on contours, wavelength, and movement, the basic spatial arrangement of the retina is preserved throughout the visual pathways. This fact was precisely established in experimental animals by anatomical and physiological investigations prior to Brindley and Lewin's work. Similar evidence in man was based upon the analysis of the visual field defects resulting from localized brain lesions following penetrating missile wounds. A few observations were made on the localization of phosphenes elicited by cortical stimulation by neurosurgeons such as Foerster [4], Krause and Schum [5], and Penfield and Jasper [6]. These confirmed, in general, the topographic representation indicated by other methods. But these early studies failed to provide critical information on stimulus parameters, phosphene size, or on the perceptual resolution which might be achieved by stimulation of adjacent cortical points. Lacking direct data from man, it was necessary to seek clues about what might be achieved by patterned stimulation of cortex from animal studies.

An analysis of the neural response in cortex to punctate light stimulation of the retina by Daniel and Whittenridge [7] established that projections of the central 10 degrees of the visual field occupy ½ of the striate cortex. The rod-free foveal region, although less than 2° in angular diameter, is represented in ¼ of the cortical projection area. This is a magnification from retina to cortex greater than 1000 times the foveal representation. This fact provides an important advantage for a prosthetic system employing cortical stimulation, since the minimal spacing of electrodes for maximum theoretical perceptual resolution would be about 100μ. Electrode separations approaching this figure can be achieved by present day microcircuit technology.

The graduation in magnification of the retinal image in the striate cortex should also affect the perceived size of phosphenes, since for a constant current density the electrodes overlaying the foveal projection will activate zones corresponding to a smaller proportion of the visual field than the more peripheral ones. Phosphene size should therefore vary inversely with the magnification factor. Hence a prosthetic system employing an array of equally spaced electrodes could mimic to some extent the normally occurring gradation of visual acuity from fovea to peripheral regions.

The gross anatomical features of the visual cortex must also be taken into account in designing a cortical prosthetic. The visual projections occupy a small region of cortex, roughly 25 cm² in total area, situated at the posterior or occipital lobe of the brain, and extending anteriorly for a few centimeters along the mesial surface of each hemisphere. About half of the mesial cortex is buried within the calcarine fissure; it is thus not available to surface stimulation. Fortunately, the important foveal projections are situated in the most exposed location, at the occipital pole. The superior visual field projects onto the lower half of striate cortex, within and below the calcarine fissure, while the inferior fields occupy the superior position. The convolution of visual cortex presents a problem for a prosthetic system, for if stimulation is limited to surface cortex, some areas of discontinuity will exist in the perceived spatial matrix. These gaps would involve, primarily, the portions of the field along the horizontal meridian which correspond to the projections situated within the calcarine fissure. The extent of scotoma, and the degree of spatial disribution will undoubtedly vary widely from person to person, due to the marked individual differences in convolutional pattern of the cortex. These differences also require us to map carefully the extent of striate cortex by stimulation at the time of implantation. Only in this way can we achieve an optimal placement of the electrode.

Doty's [8] success in training monkeys to discriminate stimuli delivered to the striate cortex at distances less than a millimeter apart suggested that adjacent cortical stimuli could be perceptually differentiated. But the interpretation of these results is difficult because there is no way to establish with certainty the cues employed by the monkey to make the discrimination. The only really adequate observations would be those made by human subjects, observations which could determine precisely the subjective character of the sensations elicited by cortical stimulation. Indeed, the observations made in Brindley and Lewin's initial experiment provide the key evidence for the feasibility of a visual prosthesis through cortical stimulation. Their initial system comprised an electrode of 80 contacts inserted over the mesial striate cortex of one hemisphere; of the 80 contacts, only 39 produced phosphenes. The phosphenes were white in color, and stable in position, size, and brightness, for constant stimulus values, over many months. With some exceptions, the location of phosphenes corresponded well with what was expected from the human retinocortical relationships (see Sterling and Weinkam, Fig. 3, in these proceedings). Unfortunately, none of them fell within the fovea; most of them did, however, occupy the central 20° of the field. As expected, there was a gap extending roughly 45° on either side of the horizontal meridian, with the phosphenes occupying pie-shaped sectors superiorly and inferiorly, adjacent to the vertical meridian. Those less than 15° from fixation were small and round, while of those more peripheral, some were elongated with axes displaying various orientations; and others were "cloud-like" with ill-defined boundaries. A regular gradation of phosphene size was not reported, but the findings are not incompatible with that prediction, since the most peripheral phosphenes were larger and less well-defined than those in the parafoveal field. Indeed, the "cloud-like" phosphenes sound to us similar to the sensation elicited by a small dim light presented to the periphery of the dark-adapted eye. Further observations will be required to define the range of phosphene size, including those within the foveal field. The elongated phosphenes at 10 to 20° from fixation also seem reminiscent of the characteristic neural receptive field shapes described by Hubel and Wiese [9, 10] in striate cortex of cat and monkey. These phosphenes might represent a selective activation of neurones representing particular receptive field orientations. The absence of elongated phosphenes more centrally might arise from the representation within a given cortical area of a larger number of smaller receptive fields which, when activated together, produce a round phosphene. Since surface cortical stimulation must activate a very large number of underlying neurons all at once, the observation of anything possessing properties similar to those of single neurons is of interest.

Brindley's electrodes were no closer than 2.4 mm apart, and the minimum spatial separation of the phosphenes appeared to be about 1° of visual angle. We do not know the minimum electrode spacing which still allows spatial discrimination, but the small size of the phosphenes, and the absence of marked perceptual interaction between adjacent simultaneously delivered stimuli encourage us to believe that spacings of less than 1 mm could be used to produce a considerable improvement in spatial resolution. The closest possible spacing of electrodes is desirable, for two reasons: first, the improvement in visual detail, and second, to improve the topography of the spatial display. Cortical enfolding produces discontinuities in the array, and also other topological distortions of the retinocortical projections. These will be reflected in perceptual effects. Hence, arrays of electrodes stimulating adjacent points of a single gyrus should produce the most satisfactory spatial map. With Brindley's electrode it is not likely that more than a few contacts lie upon a single continuous gyral surface. But a thin-film electrode conforming closely to the cortical surface, with spacing of 0.5 mm or less should lie upon a single gyrus and thus be able to create a contiguous field of about 400 points. We think that success in achieving an accurate topographic spatial array would significantly reduce the requirement for perceptual adaptation, or for difficult and elaborate technological manipulations to improve the spatial array. Even so, the well-known adaptation of the visual system to inversion lenses, and to other major distortions of the visual field, suggests that relying on the learning capability of the central nervous system may be more effective than complex topological manipulations with hardware.

For accurate localization of external objects, an artificial visual array must be correctly oriented to the position of the user's body. This is accomplished normally by neural mechanisms which integrate information concerning head and eye position and the perceived visual image. The mechanism is readily experienced. The spatial image appears to move in a direction opposite to passive movements of the eyeball, corresponding to the shift of the image on the retina. When the eyes are actively moved, no movement of the retinal image is perceived. Since input to striate cortex is topographically determined by the retinal image, it seems likely that the spatial correlation associated with eye movements occurs further on within the visual system. This inference is supported by the observation of Brindley's patient that the phosphenes elicited by direct cortical stimulation appeared to shift in conformity with movements of the eyes. It will be desirable, therefore, to link the sensor of the proposed prosthesis to the oculomotor system. This might be done by incorporating the camera directly within an artificial globe surgically attached to the extraocular musculature. This procedure is already done for cosmetic purposes, and cameras smaller than the eye are already in the offing, so the suggestion seems feasible.

One of the most critical aspects of prosthetic system development is the determination of optimal stimulus parameters. Brindley's observations established that variation either in pulse frequency or in charge delivered per pulse were effective in modulating the brightness of the phosphenes. To apply this observation successfully to the generation of a visual array corresponding correctly to the continuously changing patterns of light and dark in the environment sensed by a camera requires us to master a variety of physiological and biophysical problems. Under normal circumstancese, for example, it is the temporal pattern of neural discharge which signals variations in stimulus intensity. We think it probable that modulation of stimulus frequency will also prove best in a prosthetic system. We do know that increases in signal strength are associated with an increase in the neural population subjected to supra-threshold stimulation. It would therefore seem likely that maximum spatial resolution will be obtained by the minimum effective charge per pulse. Increases in pulse intensity are associated with undesirable electro-chemical effects at the electrode–tissue interface, and there is the risk of tissue damage through heat generation. Thus, it is clear that achieving optimal temporal patterning of stimulation will not be a simple matter; it will require extensive experimental study during the initial stages of prosthesis development.

The brain does not receive a steady neural signal, so the regular trains of electrical stimuli favored in former studies of direct cortical stimula-tion are not the optimal means of evoking a perceptual response. In normal vision, the image is shifted about on the retina by saccadic eye movements occurring at the rate of 2 to 4/sec. During eye move-ments, input to the brain is suppressed, so that the perception of the moving image is prevented, as it is shifted across the retina. A burst of neural activity follows at the beginning of each fixational pause. Maxi-mum discharge persists for no more than 50 msec, with progressive falling-off in activity during the rest of the fixational pause. In experi-ments with animals it has been shown that pattern shifts at a rate of about 3/sec produce maximal neural response in the striate cortex. These results suggest to us that cortical stimulation should be delivered in brief trains of pulses lasting less than 100 msec, repeated at intervals of 300 msec or so. In this way, we can mimic the normally discontinuous pattern of input to the brain. The mimicry could be further improved by a system with a camera linked to eye movements which gated the stimu-lation at each fixational pause.

We are sure that a human observer will be required to determine the optimal stimulus characteristics of the prosthetic system. The variety and complexity of the tests to be made, as well as the need for subjective evaluation of the perceptual effects obtained, effectively remove the task from the realm of animal behavorial analysis. In spite of this, the fears of unwarranted human experimentation have led some critics of our direct approach to demand a demonstration of feasibility in experimental animals before starting studies in man. Brindley's demonstration has attenuated the force of these criticisms. And after careful consideration of all the aspects of the problem, we are convinced that aside from the required studies of the safety of specific designs, further animal experimentation is not needed for the development of a cortical visual prosthesis.

System Considerations

In considering the information which can be transmitted by spatiotemporal arrays, three different approaches can be identified. In these displays the number of points in the matrix is the critical factor in defining the type and mode of information delivery. The first approach is appropriate for a matrix of 100 points or less; the second for 400 to 1000 points; while the third needs at least 4000 points. Although all could be produced by cortical stimulation, the first and second might make effective use of a cutaneous input. The main features of each approach are outlined below:

1. *Small matrix—coded information:* Due to the small matrix size, 10×10 or less, information must be categorized and encoded to maximize information delivery. This system cannot effectively provide a direct two-dimensional representation of space, but must abstract the significant environmental features and present them in a coded format. This approach places a heavy demand upon the development of optimal coding and display, as well as upon the learning capacity of the user. These problems are already well known in the sensory aids field and have limited the acceptance of a number of techniques for information delivery to the blind, including braille. The intrinsic limitations of this approach are severe, and it is difficult to see how it could be utilized in motility to provide more than the most elementary information concerning the presence, position, and size of environmental features. Such encoded inputs would hardly be considered suitable for a cortical device, since the limited information provided can be readily transmitted through alternate sensory channels. None of the special advantages of the visual cortex for spatial display would be exploited by this approach.[1]

2. *Intermediate matrix—preprocessed input:* With a matrix size between 20×20 (400 points) and 32×32 (1024 points), an effective two-dimensional display can be achieved. On the basis of simulation

---

[1] *Ed. note:* Unless, of course, it turns out that effective presentation of complex configurations can be accomplished through preprocessing techniques.

experiments carried out in sighted persons, Brindley [11] estimated that a phosphene matrix containing 600 points would be sufficient to permit a reading speed of 120 words per minute with ordinary printed material or careful handwriting. These experiments involved a special device which presented 10 letters at a time to his subjects. It is almost certain that the use of matrices containing 1000 points or less will require devices to adapt the input either for reading or for motility. Indeed, problems similar to those encountered with the coding technique appear in contemplating the adaptation of an intermediate sized matrix to motility applications. The combination of a suitable field range for detection of peripheral hazards with adequate central resolution for useful object identification presents a severe challenge at this matrix size. It should be noted that results of comparable effectiveness might be equally achieved at this level by either cortical or cutaneous stimulation. If the matrix size were limited by technological factors to 1000 points or less, an effort to define the limits of cutaneous stimulation might be preferable to early exploration of a cortical system.

3. *Maximum density matrix—direct spatial display:* With a 4000 point display of intensity modulated points an image subtending a visual angle as large as 10° can provide a fairly good image of a face (Fig. 1). The effects of a cortical phosphene matrix may be simulated as shown by the technique of halftone photography which permits an experimental evaluation of the effects of matrix size on object resolution. As previously noted, the observations on cortical phosphene characteristics made by Brindley suggest that a simulation of this nature is a valid one. This display size is also adequate for reading of fine print with suitable optical adjustment of field size. Even expansion of the field to the extent necessary for guidance in mobility is compatible with identification of gross objects such as persons, automobiles, curbs, and fire hydrants.

The upper limit of achievable matrix size and density with cortical stimulation is determined by physiological as well as technological considerations. We have estimated that an 0.5-mm electrode spacing would both provide adequate phosphene resolution and be technically feasible. This would correspond to a density of $400/cm^2$. A further increase to $1000/cm^2$ may be possible. If an electrode with the lower density were implanted over 10 cm^2 of striate cortex, a matrix size of 4000 would be achieved. It must be recognized, however, that electrode failures and cortical discontinuities might degrade the matrix from the ideal array. It is anticipated on the basis of experiences of paients with defects in the field of vision that a reasonable adaptation to field discontinuities will occur [12, 13].

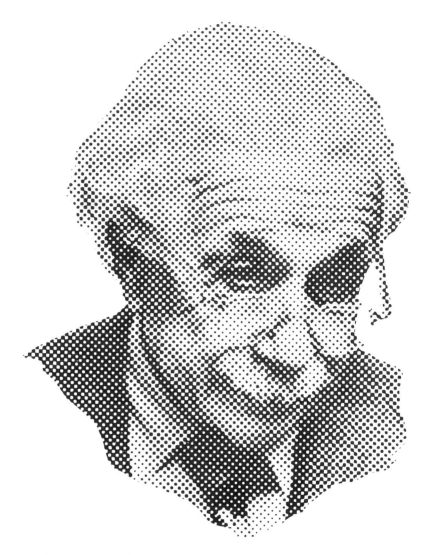

Fig. 1. Halftone photograph simulating a 4000 point phosphene matrix.

The information transmitted by a special electrode matrix of any size can be substantially increased by taking advantage of the capacity of the visual system to utilize information presented in rapid sequence as if it were simultaneous. Thus, by the technique of "microscanning" at least a fourfold increase in the effective matrix size may be achieved. The procedure would be of greatest utility for intermediate and large matrix sizes, and in the latter case would permit a 4000 point array to provide an image quality not substantially inferior to that of an acceptable television image (Figs. 2a and b). The effect of microscanning can be demonstrated by placing a perforated sheet over a photograph. While the photograph cannot be adequately resolved with the overlying grid held

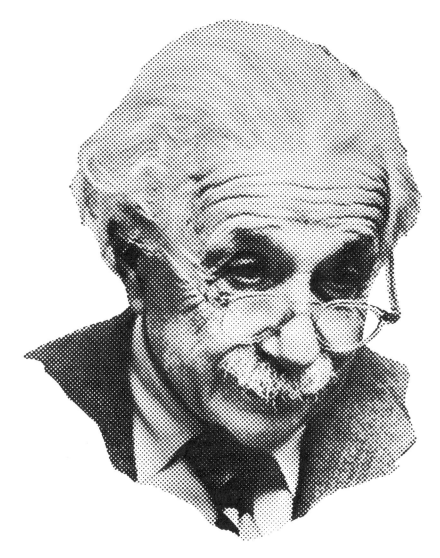

Fig. 2a. Photograph of Fig. 1 represented by a 20,000 point matrix such as might be achieved by microscanning technique.

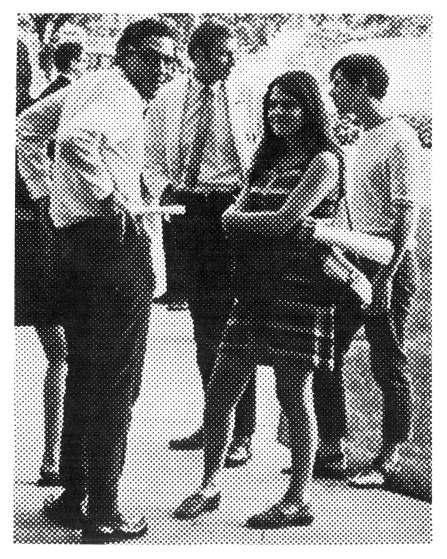

Fig. 2b. A scene occupying a field size appropriate for mobility application represented by a 20,000 point matrix. Each face contains about 200 points.

stationary, by rapidly oscillating it with an excursion slightly less than the space between holes, the picture can be made out.

In considering the technological factors in implementing a prosthetic system of this dimension, it is clear that neither feasibility nor cost now limits the maximum matrix size and density. Recent advances in integrated

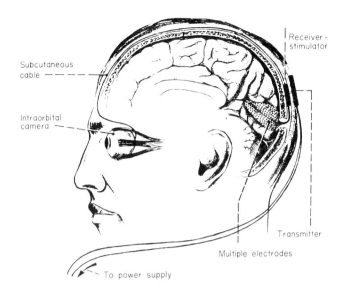

Fig. 3. Schematic representation of an ultimate prosthetic system employing an intraocular camera. All control circuitry is implanted. Only the power required for operation of the system is transmitted through the skin.

microcircuit technology permit the fabrication of a system, including camera, which could be fully incorporated within the confines of the head (Fig. 3). Although an ultimate system with camera placed within the orbit may well be a decade or more in the offing, a functioning prosthesis with head mounted camera could be produced within a three year period. The cost of system development could be surprisingly low, considering its complexity, if available components developed primarily for military, space, and computer applications could be made available and efficiently adapted for the prosthesis application. Present indications suggest that this is possible. One point is quite clear. Increase in matrix size does not entail a proportionate increase in cost. Once a modular component design is achieved, a tenfold increase in matrix size would barely double system cost, taking into account prototype development. In production, costs would be very much lower. The conclusion to be drawn from the technological situation is that, once miniaturization of system components is attempted, no significant saving either in complexity of system design or of cost is achieved by reducing the number of points in the matrix. An optimal strategy in prothesis development would be to aim for the maximum possible matrix size for electrocortical application. Since the approaches to prosthesis employing smaller matrices might still prove quite useful in patients not appropriate for a cortical prosthesis, the same technology could be applied with only minor modification to an electrocutaneous system. Since these approaches may prove to be complementary to one another in approaching the overall problem of sensory aid to the blind, we feel that a coordinated program to develop and evaluate both of these systems would be most effective and economical.

REFERENCES

[1] Brindley, G. S., and Lewin, W. S., The sensations produced by electrical stimulation of the visual cortex, *J. Physiol.* (London), **196**, 479 (1968).

[2] Asanuma, H., and Sakata, H., Functional organization of a cortical efferent system examined with focal depth stimulation in cats. *J. Neurophysiol.* **30**, 35 (1967).

[3] Stoney, S. D., Thompson, W. D., and Asanuma, H., Excitation of Pyramidal Tract Cells by Intracortical microstimulation of Effective extent of stimulus current, *J. Neurophysiol.* **31**, 659 (1968).

[4] Forester, O., Beitrage zur Pathophysiologie der Sehbah und der Sehsphare, *J. Physiol. Neurology (Leipzig)*, **39**, 463 (1929).

[5] Krause, F., and Schum, H., "Neue Deutsche Chirurgie" (H. Kutter, ed.) Vol. 49a, pp. 482–86. Enke, Stuttgart, 1931.

[6] Penfield, W., and Jasper, H., "Epilepsy and the Functional Anatomy of the Human Brain." Little, Brown, Boston, Massachusetts, 1954.

[7] Daniel, P. M., and Whittenridge, D., The representation of the visual field in the cerebral cortex in monkeys, *J. Physiol.* **159**, 203 (1961).

[8] Doty, R. W., Ability of monkeys to discriminate electrical stimulation of the brain, *Physiologist* **3**, 171 (1963).

[9] Hubel, D. H., and Wiesel, T. N., Receptive fields, binocular interaction and functional architecture in the cat's visual cortex, *J. Physiol.* **160**, 106 (1962).

[10] Hubel, D. H., and Wiesel, T. N., Receptive fields and functional architecture of monkey striate cortex, *J. Physiol.* **165**, 215 (1968).

[11] Brindley, G. S., The number of information channels needed for efficient reading, *J. Physiol.* **177**, 46 (1964).

[12] Lashley, K. S., Patterns of cerebral integration indicated by the scotomas of Migraine, *Arch. Neurology and Psychiatry (Chicago)* **46**, 331 (1941).

[13] Teuber, H. L., Battersby, W. S., and Bender, M. B., "Visual Field Defects after Penetrating Missile Wounds of the Brain." Harvard Univ. Press, Cambridge, Massachusetts, 1960.

ADDITIONAL PERTINENT REFERENCES

Button, J., and Putnam, T., Visual responses to cortical stimulation in the blind, *J. Iowa Med. Soc.* **52**, 17 (1962).

Krieg, W. J. S., "Functional Neuroanatomy." Blakiston, New York, 1953.

Shipley, T., Conceptual difficulties in the application of direct coded input signals to the brain, *in Proc. Intern. Cong. Technol. Blindness* **II**, 247 (1963).

Vaughan, H. G., Jr., and Schimmel H., "Preliminary Study of the Feasibility of Electrocortical Prosthesis" (Progress Report). VRA Grant No. RD-2064-S. Albert Einstein College of Medicine, New York, 1965.

Vaughan, H. G., Jr., and Schimmel, H., "Preliminary Study of the Feasibility of Electrocortical Prosthesis" (Progress Report). VRA Grant No. RD-2064-S. Albert Einstein College of Medicine, New York, 1966.

Vaughan, H. G., Jr., and Schimmel, H., "Preliminary Study of the Feasibility of Electrocortical Prosthesis" (Progress Report). VRA Grant No. RD-2667-S. Albert Einstein College of Medicine, New York, 1967.

Vaughan, H. G., Jr., and Schimmel, H., "Preliminary Study of the Feasibility of Electrocortical Prosthesis" (Progress Report). VRA Grant No. RD-2667-S. Albert Einstein College of Medicine, New York, 1968.

OVERVIEW OF TECHNIQUES FOR ELECTRICAL STIMULATION OF CORTICAL AND SUBCORTICAL STRUCTURES

R. W. Doty

STIMULATION OF THE SURFACE OF THE CEREBRAL CORTEX

This stimulation requires rather high intensities because of poor contact with neural elements. The poor contact arises from large pia arachnoid space in man as well as from investiture of the electrodes with connective tissue. There is some slight possibility that painful meningeal stimulation would be encountered in using such electrodes. The advantage of such placements are the significant reduction in possible damage to the brain by puncturing pial blood vessels, and the achievement of better functional localization of the stimulating current than would be the case when electrodes penetrate to the white matter. (On the other hand, if very high currents are required to produce stimulation of the neural elements, the lateral spread of the effective field might reduce the possible density of effective electrodes per unit area of cortex.)

INTRACORTICAL STIMULATION

Results on macaques indicate that thresholds are two to four times lower with electrodes which penetrate the cortex as compared with those resting on the surface, and this difference may be as much as tenfold in man. There are some difficulties in implanting such electrodes, first, in avoiding hemorrhage as the pia is punctured and second, in gauging the depth to which the electrodes penetrate, since the brain–skull relationships with the skull opened are not the same as they are with the skull closed. The maximal degree of functional localizations should be achieved, however, by properly placed intracortical electrodes.

PLACEMENT IN THE WHITE MATTER

It is possible that the threshold in the white matter might be slightly lower than that within the cortex, but this is probably not a significant difference. On the other hand, the disadvantage of placing electrodes in the white matter is that functional localization becomes confused since fibers are stimulated which pass to widespread areas of the cortex. There is, however, one very interesting possibility which deserves exploration and that is to put arrays of electrodes in the splenium of the corpus callosum. There is probably some degree of topographical organization in the callosum and small electrodes might be able to achieve some usefully localized effects.

Target of Stimulus

Certainly the elements most excitable electrically are those which are stimulated first as intensity of stimulation is increased. It has been shown for macaques that these most excitable elements are all that are required for behavioral response to be elicited from any part of the brain, and the same is probably true for man, although the situation has never been tested. Since the general structure of neurons seems designed to focus electrical effects at the axon hillock it is probable that electrical stimulation would excite cells more readily than fibers. However, since the effectiveness of stimulation falls as the square of the distance from the source and there are vastly more fibers than cell bodies in the cortex, it is quite possible that most of the stimulation might arise from stimulating axons and axon terminals as well as the cells themselves.

By appropriate manipulation of the form of the stimulating pulse, it might be possible to produce forms of stimulation which would to some degree stimulate cells preferentially to fibers or vice versa. Another interesting possibility which has received only cursory trial by Wyss in Switzerland is to stimulate the elements having a high threshold without engaging those with a low threshold. The effort here involves a gradually rising stimulus current to which the low threshold elements accommodate (theoretically) much more readily than the higher threshold elements, and thus do not fire. This has never been thoroughly tested. Thus in all currently used systems of stimulation it is the largest, most excitable elements that are stimulated with the lowest intensities; and, as intensity is increased, smaller elements undoubtedly of differing functional significance, are recruited into the stimulated pool.

Operating Parameters

Polarity

Neural elements are more readily excited at the cathode than at the anode. However, because of complex configuration of the current flow, anodal stimulation is effective, and indeed when applied to the surface of the cerebral cortex is more effective than cathodal stimulation.

Constant Current Versus Constant Voltage Stimulation

Constant current should be used wherever possible since it is the current which does the actual stimulating. If constant voltage is used, fluctuation in stimulus intensity will occur as a consequence of changes in impedance of the tissue, and such changes can be rapid and large. The current density required to stimulate is roughly the same regardless of the electrode configuration or construction; about 10^{-9} A/μ^2 from microelectrodes to metallic plates having an area of about 100 mm^2.

Intensity

As just noted, the threshold of all cells is approximately the same, so that increase in intensity of the stimulating current merely enlarges the effective radius of the stimulation, bringing a larger number of elements into play. From work on macaques, it is estimated that stimulation of only about two dozen of the most excitable cortical elements is necessary for eliciting a learned response, under the most favorable conditions. Increasing the intensity of the stimulation, which probably recruits elements of different functional significance and vastly increases the number of excited elements, does not seem to change the quality of the response to the point where abnormal convulsive activity is elicited. Fortunately, the visual cortex in primates is not very susceptible to seizure activity, and hence a very large range of stimulus intensity can be applied (in practicality, ranging from perhaps 5–5000μA). As mentioned above, however, higher stimulus currents have a rather large radius of effectiveness so that serious overlap would occur in the neural population stimulated by adjacent electrodes. The limit of discriminability here will depend upon several complex factors which it is difficult to estimate in advance.

Pulse Duration and Wave Shape

Within a certain range there is a precise relationship between stimulus intensity and stimulus duration. However, as the pulse duration extends beyond a particular time (in the practical instance approximately 1 msec), the current flow is no longer effective. The use of long pulses is thus inefficient and should be avoided to prevent unnecessary electrolysis. There are some, in fact, who feel that the electrolysis which occurs even with shorter pulses is sufficiently detrimental that efforts should be made to prevent it. This is done by using biphasic pulses (the Lilly–Hughes waveform) so that the electrolysis beginning with the first stimulating pulse is almost instantly reversed by a second pulse of opposite phase. There is a great disadvantage to this form of stimulation in that extremely high currents are required (up to 40 mA!), and it appears to be unnecessary if noble metal electrodes are used along with moderate levels of stimulus intensity. Another means of meeting the electrolysis problem (a game perhaps unnecessary, but truly adequate tests have never been performed) is to use a biphasic pulse, but one in which the second phase is very long and drawn out so as to avoid the use of an abrupt waveform which would stimulate, but have an equal and opposite current flow to that of the initial stimulating pulse and thus reverse (theoretically) its electrolysis effects. This form of stimulation is available optionally on all Grass stimulators. Stimuli approximating square waves are most commonly used because their coulomb content is readily calculated, but other pulse forms such as exponentially decaying pulses, or even sine waves (which also have some theoretical advantages for the electrolysis problem) are also effective. The difficulty with sine wave stimulation is that things become complicated if stimulus frequency is a variable, and in terms of coulomb efficiency, the sine wave is probably not as good as the rectangular current pulse. Pulse forms with gradually ascending wave front, as employed by W. R. Hess and further explored by Wyss, as mentioned above, deserve further study.

Pulse Repetition Rate

A single electrical pulse applied to the neural system is often difficult to detect without training. Thus, stimulation with trains or bursts of electrical pulses is much more common. For a great variety of systems it has been shown that the stimulus frequency is an important parameter, and that indeed many systems have optimal frequencies at which stimulation is most effective and limiting frequencies at which they no longer respond. The physiological basis of some of these frequency selective effects is vaguely understood, but much more work needs to be done. The major problem is that this frequency selectivity probably reflects several different physiological parameters of the nerve cell, including membrane time constants, refractory period, recurrent inhibition, etc. The problem is undoubtedly confused by use of monotonic stimulus frequencies which are generally abnormal for neural action which proceeds instead utilizing a pulse code in bursts having an exponentially decaying frequency. It is possible that by using more naturalistic pulse trains some improvement could be achieved in the behavorial efficacy of stimulus pulse coding which is not particularly good with monotonic frequencies. It is probable, however, that frequency modulation will never form as useful a basis for discrimination as change in location of stimulation.

Electrode Composition and Construction

Platinum or platinum–iridium is the material of choice for construction of electrodes since its rate of erosion by passage of stimulating currents is far less than that for any other metal so far examined. Silver is biologically poisonous and should be avoided, and there are, at present, a number of signs that electrolysis of such wires as nichrome or various stainless steels can produce foci of convulsive activity. There are several choices of electrode configuration. The "bipolar" configuration in which contacts are placed side by side has certain theoretical advantages in limiting the current flow precisely to the region of the two electrodes and thus achieving maximal localization of the region of the stimulating effect. However, there are indications that using a single small stimulating point with a very large diffuse and distant electrode for return (the so-called "monopolar" configuration) equal localization may be achieved. If this is actually the case, this configuration definitely has advantages over the so-called "bipolar" technique since only a single wire per stimulus point need be in contact with the brain and stimulaing polarity becomes a more meaningful parameter. (With both electrodes side by side in the "bipolar" configuration stimulus polarity is obviously somewhat confused.) Another possibility is to use "bipolar" stimulation in which the two electrodes are placed some distance apart, e.g., 1–10 mm. This situation, however, can be confusing as to localization since stimulation would probably occur at both electrode loci. It is obviously highly desirable to arrange the stimulus situation such that no leads must penetrate the skin, and microminiature techniques for accomplishing this are constantly improving. A major step forward here will probably be taken when efficient batteries are developed that can be implanted subcutaneously and draw their energy from body metabolism.

Subcortical Stimulation

Because of the greater concentration of afferent and efferent fibers (as opposed to "associative" fibers in cortex) and because such fibers are projecting into systems which can greatly amplify their effects, stimulation in many subcortical loci is effective at currents much lower than at the cerebral cortex. On the other hand, because of this concentration of usually mixed fibers of passage subcortical stimulation is likely to be much less functionally discrete, and a variety of side effects such as emotion, pain, cardiovascular disturbance, etc. may be encountered which are virtually absent for cortical stimulation. Furthermore, it is much more difficult to place an electrode accurately within a given functional area subcortically than cortically, and it is certainly much more dangerous, both because electrodes must penetrate much more extensively into the brain and because of the concentration of vital pathways in subcortical areas. Thus, unless future research uncovers some presently unsuspected advantage to subcortical stimulation, it seems that efforts should be concentrated on developing stimulating techniques to be applied to the cerebral cortex.

I.3.1 Discussion on Cortical Stimulation

DOTY: There is a possibility we have not considered: Blind patients, and blind monkeys, have very bizarre electrical activity in the striate cortex. This has been known from several studies of retroretinal fibroplasia. There is a more extensive study of this in Russia by Novikova [1] in which she examined people who had become blind in various stages of life, and in which she reported disturbances of the EEG not only in visual, but also in the precentral areas of the cortex.

In the course of experiments undertaken for entirely different reasons it became necessary for us to blind monkeys through bilateral enucleation. The electrical patterns of visual cortex were changed dramatically in these animals.[2]

The EEG at first becomes almost flat, punctuated by occasional spikes which are correlated with movements of the eyes (as measured from extraocular muscles, or by other means).

Confirming Novikova, there also appears to be a change in the activity of the motor cortex. Thus, deprivation of the visual input, achieved not by darkness but by blindness, has a very profound influence upon the electrical activity of the brain. The ramifications of this fact are at present unknown.

There is some rather tentative and still not fully explored possibility that some of this electrical abnormality is reversed by electrical stimulation. This is a very "gray" speculative kind of area we know almost nothing about, but which ultimately may have some bearing upon whether one puts a prosthetic device onto the brain, or onto the skin. Speculating for a moment, it could be possible that "exercising" neurons of the "idle" visual system might achieve some unexpected beneficial result.

[1] Novikova, M., in "Current Problems in Electrophysiology of the Central Nervous System" (V. S. Rusinov, ed.) Plenum. New York, in press.

[2] Fentress, Sakakura, and Doty, unpublished.

I would thus propose that other areas of the brain must be explored; particularly Areas 18, 19, and 20, which are related to vision and which lie upon the much more conveniently accessible lateral surface of the brain, and which we have shown in monkeys are equally capable of making all the fine two-point discriminations that one can get by stimulating the striate cortex. The monkey can respond with equal rapidity and with equal fineness as far as we have gone for electrical stimulation anyplace on his cerebral cortex.

VAUGHAN: I think it might be worthwhile to focus for a short time on the question of the temporal parameters of brain stimulation, because I suspect that these will turn out to be of very great importance in a practical sense in any functional prosthetic system. I should like to comment on the way in which the visual system is normally activated in temporal terms.

There is a good deal which has yet to be learned about this, but just to try to summarize this rather briefly, and to some extent on the basis of projections of what is known, the visual system does not receive information continuously from the environment. The visual cortex is not being subjected to a continuous pulse train. Rather, if one records from the optic nerve there are bursts of activity which are closely related to the pattern of eye movements and fixational pauses.

In normal vision, except when one is tracking a steadily-moving stimulus, the eye movements are ordinarily jerky in nature. These are separated by periods of fixation which usually last a quarter of a second, or so. These eye movements usually last in the order of 30 to 50 msec depending upon their extent.

In ordinary reading, one can record the eye movements electrically, and see that the eye is fixating and advancing across the page at the rate of about 3/sec. On the basis of both physiological and perceptual evidence, it seems that at the beginning of each fixational pause there is a sudden increase in the input to the visual system. The exact mechanism of this increase is not entirely known. If, then, the position of the eye is maintained for several hundred milliseconds, the rate of neural discharge falls off.

It is likely that this tailing off of input is related to the perceptual phenomenon of temporal brightness summation. If flashes of light are increased in duration up to about 50 msec subjective brightness will directly increase in proportion to the duration of the light flash.

If the flash is further increased in duration, the summation diminishes. There is an actual reduction in brightness at longer pulse durations, i.e., 200 msec. This is known as the "Broca–Sulzer" effect.

We also know that if the retinal image is stabilized there is an ultimate fading of the percept, presumably associated with a fall-off of retinal response. We do not know that directly. As far as I know, there is no animal work on that particular point.

Thus, one might suggest that in order to try to simulate something like this normal temporal pattern, if it is, indeed, important to do so—and I suspect that it is—one would want to stimulate the cortex not continuously but with brief pulse trains not exceeding 50 msec. Intensity would be modulated by changing the frequency and/or amplitude of the pulses within this rather brief pulse train. Proof of this belief has to come out of an actual human experiment.

DOTY: Concerning the point about the frequency of input, I agree with everything that Dr. Vaughan said. There are animal experiments of Burns and co-workers [3] which show that one has to have the visual message come in bursts through eye movement.

Kimura and I [4] studied what we called the *oscillatory phenomena* in the visual system of cats and monkeys. It is a common observation for all visual systems, that hit with a high-intensity photic stimulus, their output is oscillatory ranging anywhere from 30 up to 200 oscillations per second. We argued that the oscillations recorded centrally arise from locked discharge of ganglion cells being driven by the bipolar cells of the retina. At the striate cortex the oscillatory frequency often reaches 200/sec. At the time of writing that paper, I thought that this was an abnormal phenomenon; that one saw such oscillations only when very bright flashes were used.

This is not true. We now have repeatedly seen with unanesthetized macaques, whose visual system up to and including striate cortex, is essentially identical to our own, that every time the eyes move even in a normally lighted room there is a burst of oscillatory potentials evoked in optic tract and striate cortex. Therefore, these oscillations are an actual part of the normal visual process. Evoked potentials, which neurophysiologists have been studying under artificial conditions for so many years, are also phenomena of the real world! That is encouraging.

As to the frequency effects for electrical stimulation applied to the cortex, I take a rather dim view of the possible utility here. I found it difficult to train monkeys to discriminate on the basis of frequency alone, i.e., independent of intensity, 30/sec versus 100/sec, put into striate cortex electrically.

Similarly they could discriminate 4/sec from 10/sec, but only after considerable training. Actually their discrimination in the latter instance was many-versus-few pulses.

Spatial discrimination on the other hand was much easier for them to learn and therefore I think that we are going to find it better to code things by spreading them into different points than by modulating the frequency input to a particular point, I agree, of course, that much more remains to be tried. Dr. Brindley is in a position to try it, and I wish he would.

VAUGHAN: If you accept Dr. Brindley's observations, then one would, perhaps, want to code brightness as frequency.

DOTY: That is possible.

VAUGHAN: I say that because he seems to obtain the results that one can use either frequency or charge to produce modulation and brightness.

DOTY: But that is all one gets. One does not get a color or a movement or anything else in exchange for it.

[3] Burns, B., Heron, W., and Pritchard, R., *J. Neurophysiol.* **25**, 165 (1962).
[4] Kimura, D., and Doty, R. W., *J. Physiol.* **168**, 205 (1963).

VAUGHAN: I think that is a very good thing.

DOTY: In a sense that is true.

VAUGHAN: It would be very awkward if you did get anything else you could think about in exchange for brightness, just to make it difficult.

SCHIMMEL: Did you try to train your monkeys on the brightness level by taking two different current levels and seeing whether they could discriminate?

DOTY: Very easily. This is the way they normally solve the problem.

SCHIMMEL: You have the same point, and you are delivering at a fixed frequency. What is the discrimination in the terms of the ratios of voltage or current you have to use?

DOTY: About double.

SCHIMMEL: Apparently in Dr. Brindley's work you are not going to really double the brightness so easily by just changing frequency. I think we are involved here in frequency and number of pulses.

EZYGUIRRE: You were saying, Dr. Doty, that when you presented a visual stimulus to the monkey you had a variety of impulses, a barrage of impulses from the visual cortex. Do you find any difference in different areas of the same cortex in terms of frequency of discharge, length of discharge, etc?

DOTY: It is extraordinary. If you have, say, four electrodes on striate cortex as the monkey sits looking around a room such as we are in, each of these electrodes gives an independent picture of what is going on, and its excitability can be fluctuating independently from the others. This is revealed by the changes seen at each point in response to electrical pulses applied to the optic tract. The evoked response at each cortical point varies greatly and often without relation to changes at the other points. This probably arises from modulation of the input to each small cortical subarea by the centrencephalic system. Therefore, to get a description of what is going on at these four electrodes with reference to the environmental situation is extremely complicated.

ROBERTS: I would like to ask Dr. Adams a question with regard to cortical surface-versus-depth electrode stimulation.

In the latter instance, do you pick up spurious or aberrant electrical activity by getting into an area where extensive association tracts exist?

Further, are you not tending to get away somewhat from the discrete phosphene? You may have eliminated your opportunity to select and pinpoint the cortical phosphene less than or equal to depth stimuli.

ADAMS: I am really not in a position to answer this satisfactorily. The result of stimulation would depend entirely upon the anatomy and upon the position of the electrode. I merely think that it might be possible to develop an electrode grid in the optic radiation which, I am sure, would not be as precise as one you could get on the cortex, although we do not yet know how precise such a grid has to be. I do not think that other sensory responses would be elicited from the optic radiation.

ROBERTS: Does the efferent discharge from your stimulated areas evoke more gross visual experiences?

ADAMS: The visual responses resulting from stimulation in the limbic system did produce more gross visual experiences. However, in the optic radiation itself more than 90% of the time we elicited nothing but white phosphenes. They were much larger than Dr. Brindley's, I am sure, but at times they were quite discrete and small. Rarely we obtained colors, and usually, as I said, the phosphenes moved when the frequency was above 50 cps.

DOTY: Dr. Vaughan, I would like to add a comment on one difficulty, and that is that it might be relatively easy to get to the striate cortex in those individuals in which it is favorably located, but that is not going to be the case for individuals in whom the striate cortex does not come onto the posterior surface. In some it may be buried in the midline, and this will pose a much more difficult surgical approach.

BERING: I think it will be true for the more refined devices that if one wants to get down into the calcarine fissure with any device to stimulate it, it will involve surgery of a considerably greater degree, but it is surgery on normal structures where, again, the major risk is infection. Also with modern microsurgical techniques, the calcarine fissure can probably be entered and used for stimulation. The other problem which might come up would be an abnormal blood supply which would make the surgery more difficult. It certainly should not carry any risk of significant nature to the patient. Dr. Adams, would you agree with that?

ADAMS: Yes. I would like to add one other possibility.

If we are going to rely on a cortical prosthesis we must consider the possibility of gliosis, even though one is using inert substances or substances which are relatively inert. I think we still have to face the possibility of the problem in a long-term implant of epithelial pigmentolysis, because even Owens' work shows where there is just a very minimal dealing with membranes we do have the essential body lying unaffected. I think that has to be faced realistically.

BERING: I think this is quite true of the biological reaction to anything that is put in.

ADAMS: The visual cortex is relatively nonepileptogenic compared to other cortical areas.

STERLING: Do we have a very large body of evidence of experience telling us what happens when electrodes are implanted into the visual cortex?

BERING: Not a lot of experience with the visual cortex but about the brain in general, yes. Foester [5] in 1929 first reported punctate phosphenes from stimulation of the visual cortex. Since then, others have repeated it. In-dwelling eletcrodes and catheters have been implanted in the brain in various areas. Probably the visual cortex is the least. Wouldn't you say that, Dr. Adams?

ADAMS: Yes, depth electrodes are being implanted in patients with greater and greater frequency. They are being used to study and to treat problems of pain,

[5] Forester, O., Beitrage zur Pathophysiologie der Sehbahs & Sehsphere, *J. Psych. Neurol.* (*Leipzig*), **39**, 463 (1929).

seizures, etc. With the development of smaller electrodes, this technique is becoming much safer. Therefore, from the standpoint of safety, subcortical implants, I am sure, would be feasible. The crucial question, really, is whether stimulation of subcortical electrodes would be as useful as cortical stimulation.

VAUGHAN: One important question in subcortical systems is whether one could increase the number of electrodes with an appropriate density considering the packing of the fibers or the cells to really give you the quality of resolution that one could expect in the cortex.

ADAMS: I am sure it is a critical question. I really cannot answer it, particularly the question as to the maximum number of electrodes that could be implanted safely.

PINNEO: There is a point of diminishing return on electrodes. So, if you get them small enough so they have to be a great number, they must be more flexible and more difficult to implant. You have to use a guide of some sort, which will be stiff enough to take it down. It has to be larger in order to drive them down and this, of course, causes greater mechanical damage.

BERING: On the matter of the biological response to material implanted in or on the brain there is a great deal of experience in neurosurgery using various kinds of plastic to cover the brain as durol or bone substitutes. These do not adhere to the brain and are covered with a layer of fibrous tissue 1–2 cells thick. They can easily be removed without damage to the brain.

The physiological problems had to be solved, and this experiment is not over. A year ago Dr. Brindley wrote me that all the points were still functioning that that they had not moved in the visual field.

DOTY: I would like to point out, however, in that connection, that there is a great deal of individual variability, at least among monkeys, and among cats as well, with these long-term implants. Many of them have very slight tissue reaction, and apparently as in Dr. Brindley's case, and in those of most of our animals, there is no untoward effect.

On occasion, however, an individual animal will get a very large fibroma forming around the electrode, and this keeps growing as a tumor mass, in some cases very severely.

Thus, I think some test will have to be developed to predict the possible degree of connective tissue reaction to a foreign body in contact with the brain.

INGHAM: You have been talking about the physiological aspect of the implant on the brain, without mentioninig yet the possible long-term, or perhaps subtle effects that might accrue or might affect the thinking processes, creative activities, and so forth, that go on there. I should think there would be some material on that.

BERING: I think from experience—and Dr. Adams, I would appreciate your comments on this—but from the experience of durol repairs with plastics, filling in defects of the skull with plastics and metals, and shunting CSF with plastic tubes in and about the brain, there is a fair amount of experience now covering many, many years, and many, many people. There is nothing that has ever come up that has shown that these materials, in and of themselves, interfere with brain function. When serious tissue reactions have occurred it has usually been a technical error of not having the material to be implanted really clean.

INGHAM: But these do not displace or actually touch the cortex, do they?

BERING: They touch the cortex in the sense that the durol substitutes are in the same position vis-à-vis the brain as the electrode Dr. Brindley used. CSF shunt tubes run through the brain.

MACFARLAND: Dr. Bering, how does what you are saying stack up with Dr. Penfield's experiments?

BERING: I am including his experience in this when I speak of the general neurosurgical experience.

MACFARLAND: Didn't Penfield deliberately go in to destroy certain small areas of the brain to remove or reduce abnormal reactions?

BERING: For the treatment of epilepsy, yes.

SIMMONS: What is going to happen to the tip of a metal electrode when one passes current through it over a long period of time?

ADAMS: I can answer the question about what happens to the tip of the electrode; at least I think I can. The electrodes we use to operate on patients with Parkinson's disease do not have too much ionization, but we do lose some metal.

SCHIMMEL: If it is metal, did you use stainless steel?

ADAMS: Yes, they were stainless steel.

PINNEO: We have used stainless steel. I do not know what they look like, but the effects remain the same.

ADAMS: I think if you will examine the tip, you will probably find some iron deposit.

PINNEO: Those we have looked at we did find some, but it is not a large amount.

VAUGHAN: The answers are not all in, but it is rather clear that one is not going to use stainless steel electrodes in the prosthesis, so the data from this type of electrode is not relevant.

ADAMS: One more point that might be pertinent. It has been shown that one can safely stimulate fiber tracts for long periods. Daily stimulation of the dorsal column of the spinal cord for as long as 8–10 hours has been shown to be effective in relief of pain and has not been harmful.

REED: I listened all morning to various comments and discussion, some of the information of which was presented in the papers. There is, however, one point that is not clear to me right now. We seem to be talking about a visual prosthesis. Is there only one possible solution to this whole problem? And if so, is this the brain implant you are talking about?

Or, are there other alternate visual prostheses that we should be thinking about at some particular stage of development?

If it is this one visual prosthesis we are talking about, there are several things that really have not been clarified by the experimenters themselves.

First of all, you have not worked out all of the details about the brain implant; how long it can stay in; how long it will be effective; how long these

phosphenes will function. In addition, what is the range of effective stimulation and interpretation that you get from these phosphenes or implants, or
whatever they are? You have not even discussed, in great detail, what the
limits of perception are in relation to all of this.

I would like to ask Dr. Schimmel to "carry the ball" at this point because
there are a lot of important biophysical considerations of brain stimulation
which really have not yet been broached, and I think he might want to do
that

SCHIMMEL: Thank you for using the word "biophysical," because that is most
appropriate to the general points I would like to make.

I think people have been alluding to the "definition of vision." *Vision* is the
detection and sensation in a generalized but detailed form of remote objects
in space. In this respect I would think that there is no difference necessarily—
and I think that is the word—between trying to go through the skin or go
through the cortex, because we are dealing with a two-dimensional representation of a three-dimensional world.

I think what we are trying to get across to the brain of a living learning individual is this differentiated two-dimensional pattern. This is the most important
part: A living learning individual is dealing with a two-dimensional representation of external spatial organization.

I would like to illustrate by again taking advantage of the word "physics."
For example, if the prosthesis were working nicely on one side, and you had
something that was really functional, then if you put the left side through a
green filter, and the right side through a red filter, you should be able to
respond to color phenomena in much the same way as a normal person in the
sense that if you could distinguish between what the right side was getting, and
what the left side was getting, the light would be green or red, or a mixture
of green or red proportional to the stimulation of each side. In other words, that
would be sufficient information to tell you what the color is of the outside
stimulation, at least in kinds of a color model based on mixtures of two funda-
mentals, rather than three. From working on the prosthesis for four years I
have derived a whole series of questions. One of the important ones is, can the
field covered by a multiple electrode on the cortex become so generalized, that
it is not stationary in space, and it is changed to a much broader space?

In principle, I should think that would be possible. Just as you can use inverted lenses on a person and he can go ahead and rearrange his world, I
should think that one can take a Brindley subject and give him a visual environment to which he is slowly responding. Then he could adapt so that a narrow
area, based on his previous naive history, would be expanded into a whole
field. This would be accomplished according to the relation of the electrocortical input signals.

STERLING: I do not quite understand how you are going to expand the field.
I wonder if you would elaborate?

SCHIMMEL: What I am saying is that I would like to know the following:
Are those points in Dr. Brindley's study—and I do not think he has the hardware at the moment to answer—really in a fixed location? I think his subject's

response is based upon her previous history and knowledge as to where that point should be. Is the visual system that we are dealing with sufficiently plastic so that if the point actually were on the right but corresponding to a midpoint in a Brindley subject, would the subject gradually learn it was really on the right? As a result of feeling and learning would the subject transfer the point to its appropriate location in the real world?

VAUGHAN: Could you go back to the more concrete stimulus?

SCHIMMEL: Yes. I think that any amount of information that is available in a stable manner for which there is feedback is going to be very useful. If we had a prosthesis with only 100 points it should be extremely valuable, although it might be very difficult to get reading out of it without some very fancy computer preprocessing. It should, however, be extremely valuable because it would give blind people a much better sense of the space around them than they could get without those 100 points.

It would be the kind of benefit that you are not going to get by sitting in a chair; you are going to get it by moving around and finding out what the source is for the experience on those 100 points. So, I think from the point of view as to what is a minimum useful prosthesis, I should think 100 points would be very valuable in terms of mobility.

The question of how much further you can go is something that one cannot give a quick answer to, as to whether you can build a system with 1000 points, or 4000, or 10,000. It is something we have studied for a long time. I do not think you are going to find the answer without putting in an appropriately dense multiple electrode. If you are going to implant a system with 100 points that work, you will not know whether a system with 1000 points will work.

I think the only way you will find that out is to put in a system with at least 1000 points. Of course you can learn something by making a portion of the 1000 into a dense array and a part into a much more scattered array.

I think that is a very fair statement of the case as to why one should try to produce a maximum density system (if one can do it with reasonable effort and with reasonable cost).

In my prepared notes I have given some very simple calculations as part of the background. For example, a very early calculation was made of electric field penetration. The question being asked was, how deep into the cortex would a surface system show a different array below it? We did the calculation in the simplest way, assuming a homogeneous medium with discreet electrodes on the surface and simultaneous simulation of all electrodes.

For a homogeneous medium it is fair to say that at one interelectrode distance away, and almost irrespective of the size of the electrode, you see none of the array. It is as though there were a flat plate covering the entire surafce and acting in place of all the electrodes. For sharp points the difference between the maximum and minimum field is only 1%. That is how little information presumably would be available at a depth of one interelectrode distance.

Of course, we do not know which neuronal processes are going to be detecting the stimuli.

If the neuronal processes involved are the cell bodies, then these usually are at least 3/10 of a millimeter from the surface. If you try to use smaller inter-electrode spacing this calculation would show that you really are not gaining anything.

Of course, the calculation is very simple, and it does not take into account the inhomogeneities. The local inhomogeneities may be crucial. It is not at all clear that this calculation actually sets a limit on the practical density.

However, it is quite clear from Dr. Brindley's work, and the comments about the large number of cells which must have been stimulated, that the brain is doing something very special there. It is taking the central point right under the electrode and saying, "It is all here," and not that it is all around. Perhaps the lady knew in advance that is what she was supposed to see, but also that is what she saw. If you look at Landgren, Phillips, and Porter's [6] work I would judge Dr. Brindley was exciting cell bodies in an area of perhaps a square centimeter; yet the subject localized them as being right at the electrode, and as small as the electrode.

Therefore, it is not clear from these calculations what the limit really is as to the electrode densities that we can talk about. It may actually be less, maybe more. So, the question as to what maximum electrode density will really work is unanswered.

Let us now turn to the question of stimulus parameters. Some information on these is available in the literature. Dr. Brindley's results indicated the currents as being higher than what one would expect. He, himself, was very much surprised that he needed such large currents.

There is a comparable study by Libet et al.[7] for the cortical surface of the somatosensory area. In my report I have reproduced Dr. Brindley's data right on top of Libet's data. Libet had many subjects and none of them required as much current as did Dr. Brindley's one subject.

That is a little difficult to explain, and it may be due to the fact that a fatty membrane grew onto the electrode surrounding the Brindley subject after a couple of weeks. It may be due to an error in measurement. Brindley is not certain of his measurements. Finally the visual cortex may require higher intensity stimuli.

In any event, if you are designing a system, this kind of information is critical because you have to design for current levels three or four times higher. You have to increase your power by a factor of approximately 10–15.

This creates many more technical difficulties. So, we have this result of Dr. Brindley, which was surprising, I would say, to anybody who has been thinking about it, and according to personal conversation very surprising to him.

You may be able to achieve the same stimulus effect in many different ways,

[6] Landgren, S., Phillips, C. G., and Porter, R., Cortical fields of the monosynaptic pyramidal pathways to some alpha motoneurones of the baboon's hand and forearm, J. Physiol. 161, 112 (1962).

[7] Libet, B. W., Alberts, W. W., Wright, Jr., E. W., DeLattre, L. D., Levin, G., and Feinstein, B., Production of threshold levels of conscious sensation by electrical stimulation of human somato-sensory cortex, J. Neurophysiol. 27, 546 (1964).

but if you start out designing a system it becomes very critical as to which is the most efficient way to do it. Libet's paper has some information on effect of train length. He did experiments only on two subjects, and one gave glaringly different results from the other. My own guess is that a short train of perhaps four or five pulses would permit a stimulus with minimum expenditure of power.

Now I come to a point that I would particularly like to raise. In my report there is one other question I tried to treat, namely the possibility that the temperatures resulting from intensive simultaneous stimulation would be too high. Previously I dismissed this problem rather quickly after some calculations because I considered lower stimulus currents; but when we look at Dr. Brindley's current levels they begin to press on the border of what might be expected to be temperature rises of a couple of degrees under certain conditions of maximum stimulation.

Thus far, we have treated this problem theoretically. Now Dr. Vaughan and I have somebody preparing suitable electrodes to see, experimentally, in animals what the temperature rises really are.

As regards power requirements and temperature rise, one finds an interesting anomaly in Libet's paper. When he increases the area of his electrode by a factor of 100, he increases his current by a factor of only four and the power required for stimulation goes up by 60%.

It would be very nice if this were true for stimulation of the visual cortex, but we have no basis for knowing precisely what happened in the Libet case. The study was not carried out in a real spatial sense. I suppose you would have to go to superthreshold stimuli to identify stimuli spatially and then the somatosensory results might be different from those for visual cortex.

If we could use Libet's result on spatial interaction it would make systems design a much more simple thing, because you could increase the number of electrodes by a factor of 1000, and increase your power requirements, perhaps, by only a factor of 20. But, since we are not certain of this result, we are running into some heavy power needs, particularly for transduction through the skin. So, this is one more factor that we have been looking at, and I do not think we will know the answer except through human prosthesis experiments.

When you go to design a system you are confronted with the problem of introducing wide design flexibility, particularly in the first subject, because of lack of knowledge of the most effective stimulus parameters. You are also confronted with producing this over as wide an area as possible, and with as many electrodes as possible, to discover what the prosthesis limits are.

Now if you are going to try to include all the necessary circuitry in the first implanted system then you have to "beef up" the electronics to extravagant levels to maintain this option of diversity of stimulation to all electrodes.

On the other hand, if you could bring out a cable through the skull, you would be able to maintain these options. You would not be working with a specially designed microcircuit system. You would actually set it up so that if things did not work out the way you expected them to, and having previously determined the limits of safety, you could start to work out an entirely different program of stimulation based on the experimental results.

If we decide we have to package the whole system inside the skull to avoid an open break through the skin, we are going to have to lower the density we would otherwise use. As a matter of fact, we have had Dr. Wenke of Case Western Reserve University working with us lately and he thinks the only thing we can develop at this point, is what we call a "parallel–serial system." We have to forego the ability to stimulate a large number of electrodes simultaneously. If we do this we may lose the valuable spatial interaction effect which Libet found. If this effect exists then when you stimulate simultaneously you will need very small currents and voltages reduced perhaps by an order of magnitude.

We, therefore, have a practical question as to whether it is reasonable for a subject with a prototype system to have a cable coming through the skin.

The size of the cable, I would judge, would be about a ¼-in square, or ½ × ⅛ in for 4000 wires. It may be that we would just be bringing out 1000 wires. I have been assuming wires about 3 mm in diameter; but if we bring out 4000 one-millimeter wires then the cable will be substantially smaller (less than ⅛ × ⅛ in).

ADAMS: I think your first requirement would be difficult to meet due to the technical difficulty of the implantation and also the mechanics of maintaining such a system for a long period of time. However, I feel that we could quite safely maintain wire of 1 to 1.5 mm in diameter over a long period of time.

SCHIMMEL: One bundle of 1000 such wires?

ADAMS: Yes. We and a number of other people have maintained individuals for one reason or another with wires of this general magnitude for months, and even several years.

SCHIMMEL: If we had 1000 wires coming together in a bundle, that would be 1/10 in—10,000 wires would be 1/16 × 1/16 in size.

ADAMS: Yes, I think this would be feasible.

SCHIMMEL: And you would favor that option as opposed to compromising on density and diversity, I expect.

MACNICHOL: Is it necessary to bring out individual wires? Can't you use something like Dr. Brindley's row and column system, which means putting a transistor at each intersection? This would permit having N^2 stimulating electrodes with only $2N$ lead wires. For example: 4096 electrodes and 128 wires. That is still going to simplify things a great deal over having a completely enclosed system with radiofrequency coupling.

SCHIMMEL: I think when you do the system design and you want to maintain amplitude and frequency options, you come out with a system for, let us say, up to 4000 separate electrodes, each individually stimulated according to a pattern; but you will probably be forced very early in the game to make a parallel–serial compromise, which means that you have to divide the electrodes into groups of 10, and then go in, let us say, and stimulate 10 "families" sequentially rather than simultaneously.

MACNICHOL: I do not understand your parallel series.

SCHIMMEL: The serial system is going on in television all the time. The question is whether you are stimulating all the electrodes at one time or, whether you are going to do as they do in television. In the parallel system you stimulate the whole picture at one time. In serial (e.g., television) you go from one point to another.

VAUGHAN: It is clear that if the scanning has to take something in the order of at least 50 msec I would think that the serial address might not be satisfactory; but if it is taking, let us say, in the order of 5 msec, physiology would suggest that these points would be "seen" as simultaneous, and the temporal summation would take care of it.

One has to look at the range of pulse frequencies that one wants to use to decide whether or not one is going to depend on temporal summation of equal amplitude pulse, or whether one is going to modulate the amplitude of pulse, and so on, until one can understand what is involved in this issue.

BEDDOES: I would just like to reply to your (Dr. Schimmel) first point, which was that the thresholds were very high in this case. I do not think Dr. Brindley himself was very satisfied about it. I would like to read what he said in this report:

Just as there is some voltage dropping, my method for estimating the voltages was, indeed, unsatisfactory, and the next implant has been designed so as to allow much more accurate estimates to be made.

SCHIMMEL: He thought, however, he was accurate within 25%, originally.

VAUGHAN: Brindley is of the opinion that these measurements were accurate; but I think this remains to be seen.

LOEB: I would just like to get a few considerations without the "nuts and bolts" of this system before the group. In the first place, anyone who has ever worked with even 10 one-mm wires will think twice about working with 4000 of them. In the second place, a cable like that, to go into the brain, would have to be a couple of feet long. If the electrodes themselves had any conceivable impedance there would be a considerable problem with the stray capacitance between the wires in such a cable, aside from simply handling the 4000.

Next, with regard to using a surface-electrode, or a deep subcortical, there is the selection of power and amplitude of the signal.

One of the problems this brings up is that these electrode surfaces tend to ionize; and if we use currents necessary for stimulation at the surface of the cortex, I think it is doubtful that you can really build long-term electrodes which will stand up.

I want to bring up the point that an intracortical electrode, while perhaps a little technologically frightening, does solve a number of problems which we do not seem to be getting around in any other way.

It might require at least an order of magnitude less power, and it is important to make a dense electrode array which uses a very low amount of power, and which gives an even field. This matter of a dispersed field that is very large is going to be very serious.

If you work with a thin film electrode you cannot get very much metal into the thicknesses you have available. If you work with very large areas, the field densities require large amounts of current, although Dr. Schimmel's calculation showed that electrode surface area did not matter while you are at the surface of the cortex. With an intracortical electrode that would puncture down to at least the first or second layer of the cortex, it would be possible to use very low currents, which is desirable at this point, and to get a very dense array, which would relieve this problem of spread.

Dr. Schimmel's limits in the paper were 500μ. That is still a lot of room. I am not sure that we can afford to have the electrodes that far apart.

BURDE: I do not understand why we are coming back again to the basic assumption that we must have a dense array of electrodes. We have no idea that the nervous system, the way we are feeding information, could have any method at all of processing it. We are making a basic assumption about hardware on the basis of no knowledge.

LOEB: The nervous system at the cortex is receiving essentially a quite dense input of information.

BURDE: A different type of information—information that is physiologically arriving there by a mechanism of its own. You are talking about an external input.

You have to divorce yourself from saying that because physiologically you are receiving a million optic nerve cells feeding into the radiation, that this is necessarily the way we are going to be processing information in a visual prosthesis. I do not think you have any basis to say this at this time.

DOTY: I certainly agree with that last statement. I can hypothesize on the basis of our monkey experiments that throughout the cortex it is the most excitable neural elements that are involved in converting the electrical stimulus into a usable input. For instance, in the striate cortex, this role is possibly served by the giant cells of Meynert. There are about 1300 in the entire area striata [8] scattered roughly 1 mm apart. If this speculation should be correct it would therefore be pointless to have electrodes closer together than are the cells of Meynert.

As the intensity of the stimulation is increased, additional elements should be recruited; but the monkey gives no indication that this alters the quality of the basic effect. In man increasing the intensity of the cortical stimulation merely produces a brighter phosphene (Brindley and Lewin).

There are two other problems relevant here concerning excitability: (1) the excitability of the visual system as compared with other systems, and (2) differences in cortical excitability between different individuals.

It is a common finding in the electrophysiology of monkeys that very high currents are required to evoke potentials by electrical stimulation of the optic tract or optic radiation. Other systems, particularly the somatosensory or motor systems, are much more sensitive in this regard. Such considerations probably explain Dr. Marg's observation that currents which readily elicited somesthetic

[8] Clark, W. E. LeGros, *J. Anat.* **76**, 369 (1941).

parathesias seldom evoked any sensation of vision when the lateral geniculate nucleus was stimulated.

The other point is one which Rutledge and I [9] discovered on cats, that there is a definite individual variation in the receptivity of the cerebral cortex to electrical stimulation for one individual as compared with another. The threshold differences ranged from two or threefold, from one individual cat to the other, and this was independent of the cortical area utilized. For a particular individual if the threshold was high for one point, it was high for all. We do not understand this. Such differences might be "electrophysiological," e.g., from differences in glial barriers, electrolyte concentrations, etc.; or they might be "functional," arising from different organization of the brain.

Thus, here is another possible complication which might be encountered, and which might explain Libet's findings on the two patients.

SCHIMMEL: Libet shows that all the time, about one to three variability in the threshold.

DOTY: There may be nothing which can be done about this technically. It may be the way the nervous system is built.

VAUGHAN: [10] I disagree with the statement that we have no basis on which to decide on an appropriate electrode density. We have Dr. Brindley's data which indicate that a spacing of 2.5 mm permits effective spatial resolution; and that the phosphenes are either completely separate or maintain their relationship in space but appear to become connected with one another.

SIMMONS: The biologist approaches questions about what is going to happen in terms of predictability by asking about the action of one stimulus spot versus another, and will these integrate and form a whole?

I would propose a plea to keep it simple until those kinds of basic questions about two spots and how they interact, or three, or a dozen, or perhaps 50 or 100, how do they interact over time, among themselves, are answered before playing a very large game.

VAUGHAN: Yes. This is well taken; but there is one modification which I think is important, and that is that the density of electrodes is very critical here.

What may be true for a low density may well not hold for a higher density.

SIMMONS: Then implant a small area with a high density. The engineering problems are entirely different for 4000 versus 100; and the amount of information you can get out of that in a short period of time is not available.

SCHIMMEL: I think your point is very valuable in relation to the whole question of what might work, because in the Brindley approach, and in the approach we have been using, you have that spatial organization. I think that is the thing that is basic to creating the kind of screen. When you are in the lateral geniculate I assume that first of all, you would be exciting a massive number of neurons, although Dr. Doty told us perhaps it is just one key neuron that will give us the information.

[9] Rutledge, L., and Doty, R. W., *J. Neurophysiol.* **22**, 428 (1959).
[10] *Ed. note:* referring to the earlier discussion of electrode density.

STERLING: I think we ought to note that electrode density is not such a crucial consideration as some think. We can look at the nervous system and speculate as to how many electrodes we can get in there. But we can also study a simulated punctate phosphene and know that with proper techniques and proper learning we can use relatively few points and present a relatively complex picture on them.

Perhaps the major consideration for the induction system and for the type of brain stimulation we should aim for is not how many electrodes you get into a square centimeter, but what is it we want the thing to do?

If we want to read, then a minimal screen like that produced by Brindley is probably adequate. There is a trade-off here between optimum solution of an engineering problem on the one hand, and possible damage to brain tissue on the other. The solution may be to produce optimum information with minimal input. I do not mean "minimal" in the sense that you do, but something which is perfectly adequate—it may well be that we should look at producing a screen consisting of relatively few points; easy to construct; easy to manage; of limited danger to the patient; needing relatively low currents and potentials, and rely upon learning and preprocessing to get an optimum amount of information. Thinking this way might change the generic problem involved in electrodes versus the nervous system.

VAUGHAN: I think this point is well taken. I would like to elaborate on Dr. Simmon's point because I agree with him about the "numbers game." There is no question that what Dr. Sterling says is right, but we do have to have some reasonable estimate of what number of electrodes will give a sufficient amount of information to make a picture.

SIMMONS: That is the whole point; you have to know a reasonable number.

HARMON: The question of how many discrete points one needs in a field in order to extract information usefully and efficiently is by no means peculiar to visual prosthesis. It relates to every kind of visual display that humans use. This is a problem which has been studied over and over again, and I do not think we need to debate here how many points one needs. There is considerable literature available on what one needs to convey visual information via graphic and instrument displays, for example.

VAUGHAN: I think what we would like to have for the record is some specific information. There is a certain difference of opinion. On the one hand, I hear we do not have the information. On the other hand, I hear that the literature is full of information. What is the story?

BURDE: We do not know, with the method that we are using to feed into this cortex, (a) how much information we can present to the organism in this manner, and (b) how much input is necessary per unit area.

We do not know the basis for estimating what density of electrodes will be optimal; but to think of working with 4000 seems to me to be going way off the deep end when we currently do not even have simultaneously two spots that are 2.25 mm apart.

SIMMONS: Almost everyone agrees, at least physiologically and anatomically, that the basis for perception is an excitatory center of the activity, and the inhibitor area which surrounds it. It is probably this edge (the boundary between excitation and inhibition of neurons) that makes the difference in what is perceived.

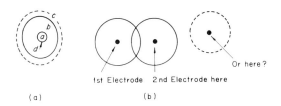

1st Electrode   2nd Electrode here

(a)   (b)

FIG. INSERT. (a) Normal incoming sensory code, where a is excitatory response, b is inhibitory surround, c is no change (spontaneous activity only), and d is excit–inhib boundary or area of major contrast in neuron activity. (b) Artificial incoming code, via electrical stimuli. (*Ed. Note*: Simmons' Figure reproduced from blackboard)

Now, if your exciting (stimulating) electrode also causes first an area of excitation (similar to a) with its inhibitory surround (generated via the local anatomical pathways of the underlying nerve nets), how much separation between electrodes will be required to make maximum use of this built in feature of the brain? Do you want inhibitory areas to overlap or be separate? What are the consequences for perception of complete vs partial separation of stimulation fields?

So, I am talking the "numbers game" in terms of what the distance is between these points. You are probably going to find, among other things that when there are electrodes positioned as shown, that these two are producing a mutually inhibitory surround, an area in which, no matter what you do, the fields are going to interact, perhaps distorting this field, or require much higher current density to activate one of them.

I have not yet heard anyone mention these problems. I say, keep the engineering simple. Answering this kind of question first and then worry about creating the entire eyeball on the top of the brain.

STOCKHAM: I would like to hear what the data are concerning inhibitory response at the cortical level.

It is understood, of course, that this inhibition is involved in a substantial part of the system, but from my meager knowledge there may not be any inhibitor at this level.

MARG: Dr. Adams and I have recorded receptive fields in single cortical units in humans; and we have recorded nine receptive fields in nine separate units, and in none of them have we been able to find any inhibitory surrounds, so I guess we are back to the "numbers game" again.

STOCKHAM: I asked because, from what little I know, it seems that in humans the inhibitory action is concentrated in peripheral, primarily retinal, elements. It would seem logical to me that at some point along the line a pattern of intensities is established as this is presented to a higher level; the inhibitory action does not necessarily need to be carried further and further.

I do not say that this necessarily proves anything. However, if the cortex is the point where inhibitory processing is complete, then it is even more attractive to implant there for the reasons that have been implied by this last 20 min or ½ hr of conversation.

VAUGHAN: Very little is known about the problem of lateral inhibition in the primate striate cortex. But I would disagree with Dr. Simmons' formulation here at a cortical level.

This may not operate at all in the same way physiologically when someone imposes a surface cortical stimulus. Again we are back to the problem of trying to equate the artificial electrical stimulus with a psychological stimulus, and I do not think this can be done.

The information we need is perceptual information. You stimulate two points. How close can you move them together and still have them discriminated? What is the interaction? What are the effects on threshold, and so on? This is an empirical question. It is not one which can be answered, to my mind, by physiological speculation.

I think one can interpolate Dr. Brindley's data, to some extent; and it looks to me as if you can have 400 electrodes in a square centimeter and still retain discriminability at individual points.

LOEB: There is a bit of data that comes mainly from the fact that the percepts which he (Brindley) reports are very small points, whereas his large electrodes must have been stimulating very large areas. So there is evidently at some point the impression of a surrounding inhibition.

VAUGHAN: This is my interpretation, but it could be considered otherwise.

SCHIMMEL: There is a very big difference between stimulating neurons and stimulating a person. There is an enormous difference. If you read Libet's work, long before the subject could consciously report that he was sensing something, there already were jerks taking place through the association paths which showed that the neurons had been activated, but not the ones that were giving him a feeling of tickling, or whatever feeling he was getting from the stimulation.

He was not getting any conscious sensation. He was being stimulated and had no percept, and yet there were neurons responding sufficiently to send signals to associated areas and make limbs move.

NYE: There may be a very close analogy here between the localization of visual phosphenes and the location of sound in space. One can do this reasonably accurately for single point sources, but if you now combine sources, either with different frequencies or the same frequency, there are complicating interactions which take place. The positional resolution of individual sources changes quite dramatically for the worse. If you were simply to predict on the basis of the response to a single source, this effect cannot be foreseen.

STOCKHAM: Has anybody counted the total number of independent phosphene locations in the Brindley map?

VAUGHAN: Yes; there are 39.

STOCKHAM: No. I mean if you extrapolated the fact that around the circumference they are large and in the center they are small, filling the entire space just once, how many points would there be?

The second question I wanted to ask is whether or not people here feel well "calibrated" to the quality of images containing between 10,000 and a million picture elements, say this big (indicating), at arm's length?

SCHIMMEL: I made the statement previously, and I think it is correct, that a very small number of electrodes would be needed if the system were developed so that a person could learn from it. Dr. Brindley's system of 40 electrodes should be extremely useful in learning about the environment because the blind now have to depend largely on sound for that; and 40 points would be a lot more information than they are getting from sound.

STOCKHAM: Imagine somewhere in the brain are stored all of the images you can possibly perceive in a library in a lifetime. When you see something you do not actually see it; it is looked up in the library and you pull it out.

It would only take 40 bits to access that library each time. This is based on the idea that you perceive a new picture every hundredth of a second and want to cover all the pictures that you could perceive in a hundred years.

VAUGHAN: I think there are some topics which have not as yet been touched upon, and a particular one which was called to my attention.

We have talked about surface cortical stimulation, and we have talked, to a certain extent, about subcortical stimulation, but we have not at all alluded to the possibility of an intracortical stimulating electrode. This may be something that one should think about seriously, since an intracortical array would retain many of the spatial advantages which accrue to the cortical side of stimulation, while permitting much more localized activation of neurons at much lower stimulus strength.

PINNEO: We know from a comparison of the animal data from surface stimulation, and from intracortical microstimulation, in other words, stimulation with microelectrodes, that the thresholds for response—and these are physiological responses—are at least an order of magnitude lower than for surface stimulation, and possibly even more than that.

VAUGHAN: Would you expand on your own experience in this area, Dr. Pinneo?

PINNEO: Most of ours have been in the motor system, where we use 2-mm spacing, which would be much greater than you would desire. I think for finer resolution I would want closer spacing; but then you get the problem of packing, how many electrodes per shaft. We have been using up to six per vertical chain, which are much smaller in terms of number, but the size is about the same. The greater number that you have in the chain, of course the greater the size of the bundle you initially put down. We have been trying to put down as many as 60.

FRANK: Perhaps I should not speak without more experience, but there is a possibility of increasing the number of electrodes in a specific area of the brain by using the "straw-in-a-gale" principle. We have a few preliminary experiments in which we have been shooting one mil, Teflon coated, platinum wires into gelatin blocks of the consistency of the brain, using a high-speed air jet.

There has not been much progress so far in control of position, but some of the electrodes have made a 10-mm penetration into a good stiff block by this technique. It looks now as though instead of trying to blow the electrode in through a small gun, we should let them be carried by a missile which is stopped just before it reaches the surface of the brain, while the electrode carries on under its own momentum. This still leaves the problem of making connections to the electrodes and insulating them, but the method looks interesting enough to be worth pursuing.

STERLING: One point made by Dr. Adams refers to the fact that if we have 200 points of phosphenes and if we can order these 200 points in a regular pattern, we can convey an awful lot of pictorial and graphic information through them. We can see from Dr. Knowlton's experiments just how much information we can get through 200 points if they are regularly placed. Thus, it may not be as crucial to produce an awful lot of phosphenes but to produce a regular array.

VAUGHAN: One of the problems with cortical stimulation, unless one visualized the possibility of taking the electrode into the fissures of the visual cortex, which is fraught with hazard from vascular damage, is that the visual field which can be generated by direct cortical stimulation will have discontinuities.

If we think about a contiguous field, this can be achieved only by putting electrodes on the surface of a single gyrus. The question, then, might come up, how many such electrodes could one place on a single gyrus to give us the kind of ordered field that Dr. Sterling is speaking about now?

Dr. Brindley, with his density of packing, probably has no more—it is difficult to be sure, but certainly not more than four or five or six electrodes on a single gyrus. So, as one would expect there were certain topological distortions in his phosphene.

If, however, you were putting your electrodes at a spacing of ½ mm, you could probably get 400 electrodes on the surface of a single gyrus.

So, this would be a 20 × 20 matrix of contiguous points, probably amassing very nicely in conformity with the visual field.

Depending on where these were in the striate cortex, they would correspond either to an area in the periphery or in the fovea; and the characteristics of the phosphenes would be expected to differ considerably.

It would be rather easy, however, to place 400 points on the surface of visual cortex and it would be considerably more "tricky" to get 400 points with similar properties in the visual radiation, or certainly the lateral geniculate body.

1.3.2 Discussion on Stimulation of Geniculate Bodies, Primary Visual Pathways

SUTRO: We have been hearing a lot about the cortex, but there are several structures that we think are very important, and a growing number of researchers in vision consider human vision to be basically binocular.

If we accept that, then the structures that interpret the two retinas become very important. I refer to the lateral geniculate nucleus, and the superior geniculate nucleus.

We are undertaking now the model of the lateral geniculate nucleus, according to the theory of Richards on how it works. There are other theories. We think this is fruitful. We hope to attempt it on the superior geniculate nucleus a little later.

The importance of all of this we think to this conference is that it is possible to automatically compute the range in the scene, and in both of the two ways that human vision is reported to do.

A number of you probably know of Trevarthan's work at Harvard, and that of others, to back these up; but there are two mechanisms of vision, the foveal which is concerned with extracting range from the central area, and then the motion or ambivalent vision, which extracts range when you are in motion.

By stimulating these and reducing the stimulation to a small compact hardware, we offer another form of prosthesis which might later be fitted in between a stimulated retina and the tie to the cortex; but it can also be used by itself with an audible output to indicate rays.

VISUAL PROSTHESIS BY ELECTRICAL STIMULATION OF PRIMARY VISUAL PATHWAYS

L. R. Pinneo

Introduction

Our approach to visual prosthesis is based on our research for the past six years on the neurophysiology of brightness vision in primates. That work was supported by grants from the former National Institute of Neurological Diseases and Blindness. The actual prosthetic work, sponsored by the Office of Naval Research,[1] is still quite rudimentary so that much of our concept of a working system is still speculative. Nevertheless, we have made some little progress and, if nothing else, we may provoke discussion and ideas in others.

The ideal human visual prosthesis will mimic normal vision, and if possible will use intact tissue of the retina and brain that mediate vision. The system should at least provide differential brightness, acuity, clear images of form and pattern, differential color, accommodation for distance, and detection of movement in terms of velocity and acceleration. To be responsive to the environment, its sensitivity to light must have a wide dynamic range with a relatively short time constant. The state-of-the-art in electronic technology, such as in video cameras, suggests that

[1] Supported by Office of Naval Research Contract No. N0014-68c-0184 and NINDB Grants NB-04951 and NB-07916.

electrical signals may be used to supply all of this information. The problem then, is to transfer the electrical video signals into meaningful stimulations of intact visual tissue of the brain.

I imagine all of us have had to begin with the same premise: In order to "see" there must be "brightness"; all other forms of vision are modifications of this sensory response to light intensity. If a prosthetic system depends upon using intact nervous tissue of the visual system in a more-or-less "normal" fashion, as ours does, then the first job is to identify what nervous activity represents "brightness," and then determine how this can be replicated in order to simulate light stimulation of the retina. Therefore, before I can describe our proposed prosthesis, I must first describe what we have found out about the neurology of brightness vision.

In our studies, we have recorded the electrical activity of the primary visual pathway, from the retina to the visual cortex, associated with light and dark adaptation, brighness discrimination, flicker and fusion discrimination, brightness enhancement of low frequency flicker, and the Talbot brightness of high frequency flicker. Most of the experiments were carried out with chronically implanted cats, rhesus monkeys, and squirrel monkeys, though we also have had an opportunity to work with humans in which verbal report was available as well as electrical activity. Also, macroelectrodes were used in most of our experiments, and the multiple units thus obtained were integrated to reflect the average amount of activity in the visual pathway. Nevertheless, our basic results were confirmed by microelectrode controls, and by others [1, 2] using microelectrode recording exclusively.

Neurology of Brightness Discrimination

During darkness or steady illumination of the retina, neurons of the primary visual pathway fire in a random fashion. The only difference between dark and light adaptation is the amount of random firing. Most of the time activity is greater in darkness than in light, though on occasion the reverse is true even in the same animal. Figure 1 is an example of multiple-unit recording from the lateral geniculate nucleus of a cat. Qualitively identical recordings can be obtained from the optic nerve, chiasm, and tract, and the optic radiations. The initial activity observed in A is that following 15–30 min of dark adaptation. At the arrow in A, a light is turned on into fixated eyes and the retina illuminated. Note the initial "on" discharge, followed by a dramatic depression of activity. Part B shows the same activity 15 min later, with the retina still constantly

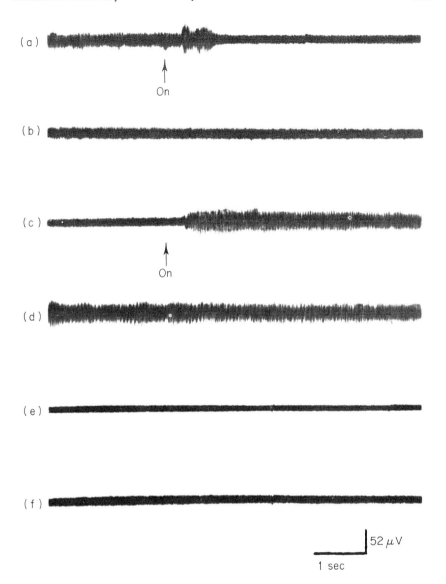

Fig. 1. Effects of illumination and of retinal ischemia on lateral geniculate nucleus activity. Set text for details (after [5]).

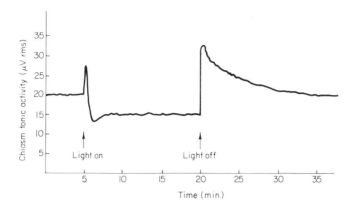

Fig. 2. Diagram of the average amount of activity of the chiasm as a function of time and the effects produced by a steady light's onset and offset (after [4]).

illuminated. In C the light is turned off at the arrow, producing a large "off" discharge. Note that after 10 min, in D, the level of discharge is still quite high. Parts E and F are control records; E shows the level of activity when the intraocular pressure has been increased over that of the blood supply, thus preventing retinal cells from discharging, while F is a recording from the same cat five minutes after death. Note the resemblance between tracings B, E, and F. Details of these experiments are given in references [3], [4], and [5].

A simple way to quantify the multiple unit activity of the last figure into a meaningful parameter is to measure the RMS value [6]. Figure 2 shows the same changes from an electrode in the chiasm, illustrating relatively high dark discharge, an on-response with the light on, depression of activity with maintained illumination of the retina, and a prolonged off-discharge after the light is turned off. (When light onsets and offsets are closely spaced, as in a flash, then the on and off discharges would merge into one transient, evoked response). If a more intense light had been turned on, the on-discharge would have been higher, the depression during maintained illumination would have been lower, and the off-discharge would have been greater.

Transient illumination of the retina, as with a flash or a rapidly moving target, has just the opposite effect. The activity of neurons of the primary visual pathway fire in a more-or-less synchronous burst, rather than randomly, and the size of the burst increases as a power function of the intensity of the transient light. A superimposed steady (background) illumination has the same effect on the synchronous phasic responses to

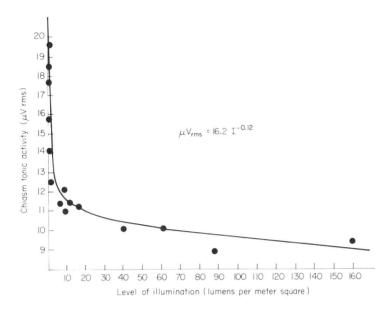

Fig. 3. Change of absolute level of activity of the chiasm as a function of the level of steady illumination (after [4]).

transient illumination as it does on the random dark discharge; that is, it depresses it. The amount of drepression is a function of the level of steady illumination, so that if the background light is sufficiently intense there is no phasic response to a flash of light. By altering the background illumination and the intensity of a transient test flash just enough to produce a detectable phasic response, one may work out a functional relationship between the two. When this relationship (as shown in Fig. 3) is compared to a Weber–Fechner brightness discrimination function (as shown in Fig. 4), and is determined from the same animal using psychophysical methods, it is found that the two curves correspond directly. Therefore, we can predict the brightness perception function of an animal based *only* upon the electrophysiological responses of his primary visual pathway [7]. With the two humans referred to above, we were able to further confirm this by verbal report [8].

Evidence for Two "Brightnesses"

The size of a phasic discharge to a light flash is not a function of the intensity of the flash alone; instead, it is dependent upon the rate of change of light entering the eye [9, 10]. Thus, a very rapidly changing

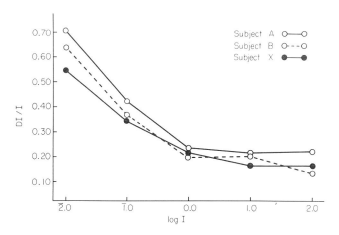

Fig. 4. Weber function of three squirrel monkeys, whose visual system activity had the same form as that shown in Fig. 3 for the same background illumination used here (after [7]).

flash of relatively low intensity produces the same size phasic response as a more slowly changing flash of higher intensity. In fact, if the increase of light intensity is slow enough, no matter what the intensity change, then no synchronous burst occurs at all and there is no increase in the visual pathway activity in response to the higher light intensity.

This is shown in Fig. 5, which is a recording of the RMS activity from the lateral geniculate nucleus of an awake, chronically implanted rhesus monkey. On the left are shown three onsets of illumination, and on the right three offsets. In each case, the level of illumination change is exactly the same, but the *time* it takes to increase or decrease the light is not. As the onset becomes slower, the size of the on-response decreases and just about disappears. Similarly with decreasing illumination the off-response also decreases in size. Notice, too, that the off-response occurs later and later in time with slower rates, suggesting that the off-discharge is inhibited until the level of illumination is decreased to a certain amount. This is illustrated more clearly in Figure 6 where in trial 1 the light is turned all the way off and the off-response begins when the light has decreased to this certain level. If, however, the light is never decreased to that amount, as in trial 2, the off-response does not appear.

Obviously both the amount of light change entering the retina and the rate at which the light is changed effect the size of the on–off response. In Fig. 7 the light is increased over a four-log intensity change at different rates of almost 2 log-units. Notice that for the very slowest two rates,

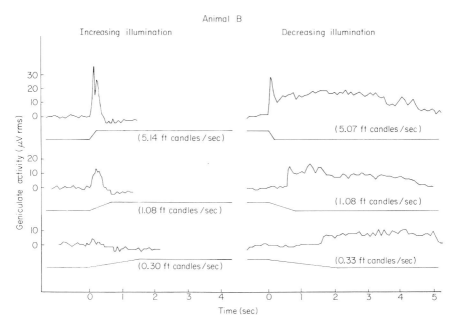

Fig. 5. Plot of lateral geniculate averaged activity as a function of rate-of-change of light illumination increasing and decreasing in intensity. The absolute *amount* of change is constant; just the rate of onset and offset is varied (after [9, 10]).

intensity of light change does not have an effect, only rate of change. Then, for some reason yet unknown, at the third rate and all higher rates, both rate and intensity change are effective in evoking the on-response. How this affects brightness is shown in Fig. 8, where human observers estimated the brightness of a light *onset*, of constant illumination change, but at different rates. Again, this is a power function as shown by the linear log–log plot.

It is apparent from these data that steady illumination and transient illumination have quite different effects upon the activity of the primary visual pathway, each producing in its own way a change in "brightness." Since both the effects and apparent mechanisms differ between the two types of light stimulation, it is reasonable to propose the existence of two "brightnesses," both of whose properties are quite different.

Flicker and Brightness

Activity of the primary visual pathway in response to a flickering light has the properties of both transient and steady illumination, depending

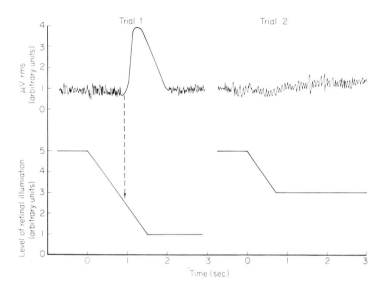

Fig. 6. Plot of geniculate activity and off-response as light is decreased. In trial 2, decreasing illumination is stopped at a level of illumination higher than that in trial 1 where the off-response occurs, thus illustrating that retinal neurons are inhibited until some critical level of darkness is reached (after [9, 10]).

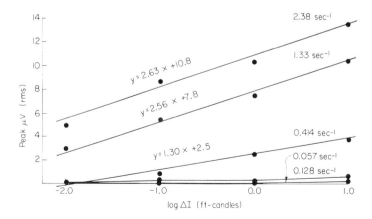

Fig. 7. Evoked on-responses as a function of change of illumination (ΔI) at five rates of change. For two slowest rates, light intensity alone has no effect, but thereafter the on-response increases as the log of the intensity change (after [9, 10]).

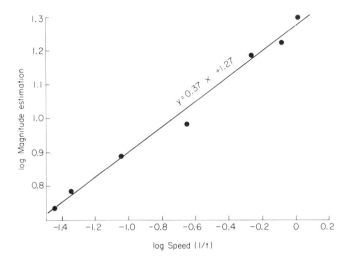

Fig. 8. Human brightness estimation of a changing light intensity as a function of the rate of change (actual illumination change is constant) (after [9, 10]).

upon the frequency of stimulation [8, 11]. For frequencies below the critical fusion level, the responses are synchronized bursts of activity which increase with intensity but are depressed by a steady background illumination. Furthermore, the sizes of the bursts increase with higher rates of light change (that is, from lower to higher frequencies) up to a maximum of about 12–16 flashes per second. At this frequency individual units begin to fuse, and the sizes of the phasic responses now decrease with frequency (Fig. 9). At the critical fusion frequency, and for all higher frequencies, the activity of the visual pathway is no longer synchronous, and in fact neurons discharge at the same random rate as they would if the retina were illuminated with a steady light of the same average intensity as the flickering light. Finally, as shown in Fig. 10, behaviorial brightness and flicker discriminations to these various light conditions, in both animals and man, follow exactly the changes in the average amount of activity in the visual pathways. Again, it was possible to predict the perception of "flicker" or "steady" light, CFF, and the brightness level of either of these two conditions on the basis of the electrophysiological activity alone [8].

Neurology of Brightness Vision

From these results and others obtained over the last few years, we have formulated a theory of how "brightness" is perceived in terms of the

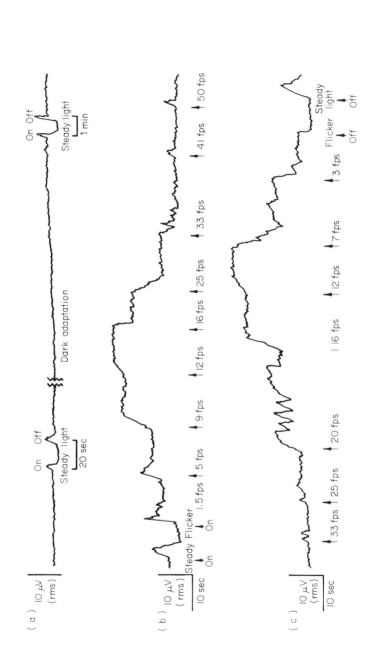

Fig. 9. Direct recording of electrical activity of human optic tract during dark adaptation (a), increased frequencies of flicker (b), and decreased frequencies of flicker (c) with intermittent light stimulation (after [8]).

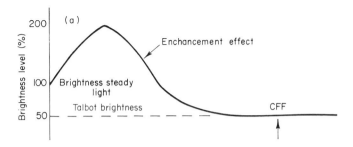

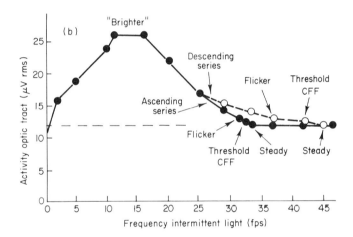

Fig. 10. Comparison of activity of human "brightness" function (a) and average amount of human optic tract activity (b), as a function of frequency with intermittent light stimulation (after [8]).

activity of the primary visual pathway. Needless to say, our particular interpretation has met with criticism from other investigators who interpret the data differently. However, their criticisms are not cogent as far as the visual prosthesis is concerned, so they will not be discussed here. The facts still remain, and it was upon these that we have devised our visual prosthesis experiments:

(1) A relatively prolonged depression of the overall activity of the primary visual pathway represents an increase in perceived brightness of a background illumination. Therefore, if we can depress the random dark discharge of a blind animal, or an intact one in the dark, then he

should "perceive" a steady background light whose intensity is related to the amount of depression by a power function.

(2) A brief synchronous burst of activity in the primary visual pathway represents a transient illumination, or flash. Repetitive synchronous discharges represent flicker. Therefore, if the primary visual pathway could be made to fire in synchronous bursts, then flashes and/or flickering lights would be "perceived" by a blind animal, or a sighted one in the dark. Furthermore, by combining the bursts with depression of activity as described in (1), then the combination of "flashes" upon a "steady" background illumination should be perceived.

To date we have been able to accomplish these changes in the activity of the primary visual pathway, but are just now testing the "perceptual" validity of these changes. First, we found that direct current polarization across the laminar layers of the lateral geniculate nucleus will produce a significant decrease in the random dark discharge as measured in the radiation fibers. By appropriate adjustment of the amount of polarization, the activity level in the radiation fibers could be made to span the range produced by four logarithms of light illumination (maximum equivalent to about 150 f-L). Polarization across the optic tract or chiasm was effective in some instances but not nearly as effective as in the geniculate. Second, by placing other electrodes in either the chiasm (or tract) or the geniculate, and stimulating with brief volleys, we were also able to produce synchronous bursts in radiation fibers comparable in *size* to the phasic response to light flashes; these were also equal to a four-log unit change of intensity.

Presently, we are training implanted rhesus monkeys in the dark to make "brightness discriminations" to these two forms of visual pathway electrical stimulation. When they reach a suitable criterion of correct responses, we will retest them in an actual brightness discrimination situation using light. If their ability to make correct discriminations is significantly better than the controls, we may assume we have replicated some form of "brightness vision" at least comparable to the retest situation.

Design of a Visual Prosthetic

If such a visual replication is possible, how might it then be used for a fairly complete visual prosthetic device? First we must in some way be able to control the activity of discrete parts of the "visual field" separately and in concert. This might conceivably be done by implantation of many vertical chain electrodes throughout the geniculate, such as we use in the motor system in our brain prosthesis for stroke. We are currently using very small electrodes of less than 70 μ diameter for production of motor behavior by programmed stimulation in the brain stem. Our experience with these electrodes suggests that an interelectrode spacing of 2 to 3 mm in all planes would provide sufficiently precise control of a discrete area in the geniculate without undue mechanical damage. If each electrode is then connected to a separate stimulator in an expanded version of our Programmed Brain Stimulator [12], so that individual electrical parameters may be selected as needed for each discrete area, then we should be able to present a three-dimensional mosaic of stimulated points representing the entire visual field

With so many electrodes, and with so many combinations of simultaneous and sequential stimulations, a computer would be required to control the individual stimulators. The input to the computer itself might be outputs from a bank of integrated circuit operational amplifiers, each in turn driven by a coordinate point or area in the sweep of a video tube. For the present we will only consider black and white representation; however, since specific areas in the geniculate related to color receptors in the retina may be identified, it is possible that a more complex signal derived from a color tube could be used to specify stimulation parameters at these geniculate sites.

In any case, analog outputs of each operational amplifier would specify the intensity of light as a function of time falling on the point or area of the tube concerned. This in turn would be sampled by the computer, which would pulse-modulate the current output of the stimulator supplying the corresponding geniculate electrode. In this way, the synchronous activity of each and every part of the geniculate being stimulated would be controlled by the brief flashes of light falling on the tube, thus providing intensity differences as a function of geometry and time in the visual field and thereby simulating pattern vision.

The level of background illumination would be determined through the computer by averaging the outputs of all operational amplifiers using a time constant somewhat longer than that of the individual amplifiers. This averaged signal would in turn modulate the direct current output of a single stimulator, which in turn would drive polarizing electrodes situated across the geniculate. The level of polarizing current, proportional to the average background illumination striking the video tube, would depress the average activity of geniculate neurons *including* the phasic discharges due to individual points of transient light stimulation. Thus, "perception" of the patterns of flashes would be related to the level of the background illumination. By proper setting of electrical parameters, this relationship could be made to follow the Weber–Fechner function and even improve upon it.

At first reading such a system as outlined here appears quite large and complicated. However, with the rate of progress in electronic circuit miniaturization, video tubes, and computer technology, it is not beyond the bounds of definite possibilities; and, while such a system alone might not replicate vision as well as desired, in combination with other techniques described at this conference a fairly adequate visual prosthesis may well be achieved.

REFERENCES

[1] Straschill, M., Kennlinien und Zeitgang der Aktivitat von Neuronen des Intensitat und Dauer, *Arch. Ges. Physiol.* **281**, 84 (1964).

[2] Straschill, M., Aktivitat von Neuronen im Tractus opticut und Corpus geniculatom laterale bei langdauernden Lichtreizen verschiedener Intensitat, *Kybernetik*, **3**, 1 (1966).

[3] Arduini, A., and Pinneo, L. R., Attivita nel nervo ottico e nel genicolato laterale nel'oscurita e durante l'illuminazione continua, *Boll. Soc. Ital. Biol. Sper.* **37**, 430 (1961).

[4] Arduini, A., and Pinneo, L. R., Properties of the retina in response to steady illuminaiton, *Arch. Ital. Biol.* **100**, 125 (1962).

[5] Arduini, A., and Pinneo, L. R., The tonic activity of the lateral geniculate nucleus in dark and light adaptation, *Arch. Ital. Biol.* **101**, 493 (1963).

[6] Arduini, A. and Pinneo, L. R., A method for the quantification of tonic activity in the nervous system, *Arch. Ital. Biol.* **100**, 415 (1962).

[7] Brooks, B. A., Neurophysiological correlates of brightness discrimination in the lateral geniculate nucleus of the squirrel monkey, *Exp. Brain Res.* **2**, 1 (1966).

[8] Pinneo, L. R., and Heath, R. G., Human visual system activity and perception of intermittent light stimuli, *J. Neurol. Sci.* **5**, 303 (1967).

[9] Pinneo, L. R., McEwen, B., and Hansteen, R. Effects of changing light intensities on retinal excitability and on- and off-responses, *Fed. Proc.*, **26**, 655 (1967).

[10] Hansteen, R., McEwen, B., and Pinneo, L. R., Changing light stimuli and retinogeniculate excitability, Submitted to *J. Neurophysiol.* (1970).

[11] Arduini, A. and Pinneo, L. R., The effects of flicker and steady illumination on the activity of the cat visual system, *Arch. Ital. Biol.* **101**, 508 (1963).

[12] Pinneo, L. R., Kaplan, J. N., Elpel, E., Reynolds, P., and Glick, J., Experimental brain prosthesis: Methods and possibilities. Submitted to *Nature*. (1970).

DISCUSSION

HARMON: Are the results for the ramp function that you get relatable to those with similar stimuli that Enroth measured in responses to ganglion cells?

PINNEO: Yes, except that we were using arithmetic or linear ramps, while they were using logarithms; therefore, we think ours are a little more accurate.

DOTY: Electrical stimulation of the optic nerve gives not just the diffuse flash of light that one would expect, but also patterns, lines, and colors.[1] I think Dr. Marg will also tell us what he has done with this. The great difficulty of using the retina or optic tract is that to get a thousand points of informational input requires an extreme finesse of manufacture of the electrodes to get at the functional units which are so much more densely concentrated; in contrast to the cortex, where a large expanse of tissue is available for the informational input. In addition, space is conveniently represented in a topographical manner at the cortex, but such consistent topographical relations would be essentially impossible to achieve with subcortical electrodes.

MARG: Earlier Dr. Sutro mentioned the possibility of stimulating the visual pathway. For reasons other than prosthetic, I did some work a few years ago with Dr. Guillermo Dierssen who is a neurosurgeon in Madrid. He was doing the usual type of procedure on the basal ganglia of the brain for the treatment of Parkinson's disease. In this operation, the neurosurgeon has to stimulate electrically with his brain probe before he makes his lesion. The probe target is relatively near the internal capsule, but if a lesion is accidentally made there the results, including a hemiparalysis, are disastrous. By stimulating, however, he can determine if he is off course and in this potentially dangerous area of the brain. As a part of this work, we stimulated with microelectrodes which were developed for neurosurgical application instead of macroelectrodes, and we recorded the reported sensations that were produced thereby. The microelectrodes were made from $1/4$–mm tungsten wire, with a $1-\mu$ tip, which was inserted in a simplified stereotaxic apparatus which led into the brain (Fig. Insert 1).

At times our electrode (Fig. Insert 2) was in the lateral geniculate area as well as in the general thalamic area. The electrode tip must have occasionally stimulated the lateral geniculate body but initially we obtained no reports of any sensations whatsoever. It was very difficult because Dr. Dierssen felt there was an error. Nevertheless, we rarely had any visual responses, any phosphenes of any sort, that would indicate the visual system of the patient was being stimulated.

[1] Nakagawa, J., *Brit. J. Opthal.* **46**, 592 (1962).

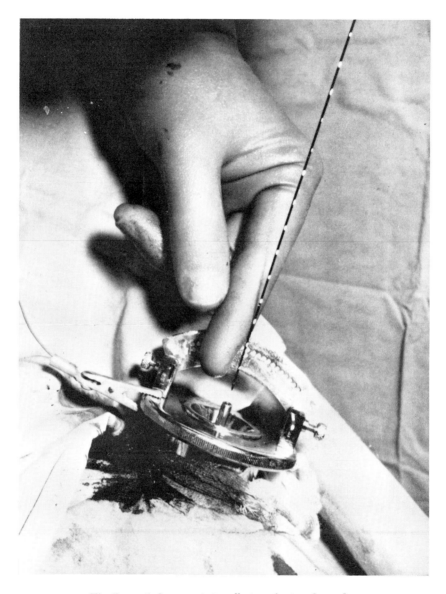

Fig. Insert 1. Stereotaxic installation of microelectrodes.

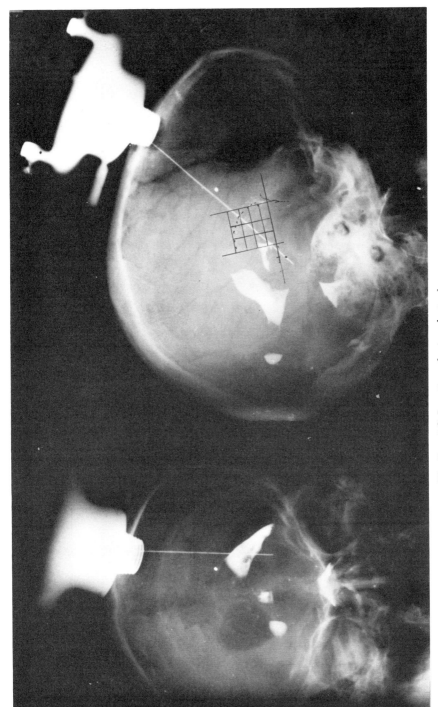

Fig. Insert 2. Location of microelectrodes.

In a series of 20 patients, in only three or four instances did we get any visual sensation reported about which we could feel confident. Even in those few people in whom we did get a reported visual sensation we could not repeat it, not even in the same patient, at the same brain site!

One patient said he saw reddish-yellow parallel lines on a white disk. As vivid as it was, and as clearly as he could describe and draw it afterwards, we never did get the phosphene again at that site. In fact, there were no other visual responses from any other stimulations in the brain of this particular patient. These results force us to conclude that it would be very unlikely that one could use microelectrodes in the visual pathways, especially in the lateral geniculate body to provide the basis of some sort of visual prosthesis.

It can be asked, "How do you know that the electrode was working, that the tissue was being stimulated?"

The same electrodes in the same patient went through the VPL of the thalamus and there, paresthesias were regularly reported from electrical stimulation through the microelectrodes.

Various types of paresthesias were reported with the same stimulus parameters and the same electrodes. Some of the paresthesias were quite small, appearing at the fingertips of the palmar or of the dorsal side of the hand. It would be more conceivable from the point of view of effective stimulation to build a prosthesis that would be in the somatosensory pathway rather than the geniculate visual pathway.

Even so, there is reported a great deal of shifting of the paresthesias from one locus to another without moving the electrode; there is also a decrement of response which is sometimes called *habituation*. This calls attention to an important point brought out by Dr. Brindley's work, that there is no habituation from his macroelectrode electrical stimulation of the visual cortex.

SCHIMMEL: I just wanted to ask both Dr. Marg and Dr. Adams a question. You described the size of your electrode surface, actually, but what kind of current and voltages were involved?

ADAMS: We used a bi-directional pulse, square wave. Usually we would get in the posterior pair a response at somewhere between 1 and 2 mA of current.

SCHIMMEL: And what voltage?

ADAMS: This would require 2½ or 3 V to produce 1 mA volt. These are stainless steel electrodes.

MARG: We used a 1–μ tip, but the insulation was pushed back somewhat further. The impedance of these electrodes was about 10 MΩ. The minimum threshold went up to about 10 V or more.

SCHIMMEL: What about in the visual system?

MARG: This is more difficult to tell. The sample of successful stimulations was very small but it left the impression that the threshold was higher.

In relation to our work in the region of the geniculate body, stereotaxic marksmanship yielding less than ideal accuracy, we were not always in the lateral geniculate body, but as frequently in the optic tract fibers or optic radiations and we still got extremely few reported phosphenes relative to the number of stimulations with microelectrodes. We have not had the opportunity to stimulate the visual cortex under these conditions.

SCHIMMEL: I think your point is very valuable in relation to the whole question of what might work, because in the Brindley approach, and in the approach we have been using, you have that spatial organization. That is the thing that is basic to creating the kind of screen. When you are in the lateral geniculus you, first of all, I assume, would be exciting a massive number of neurons, although Dr. Doty told us perhaps it is just one key neuron that will give us the information; but in either event you are not bringing up the microelectrode intensity sufficiently well, or else you are stimulating a lot of them, and there is no interpretation given to them because they have not been topologically arranged.

I.3.3 Retinal Stimulation

ICONOPHORESIS—A NEW TECHNIQUE FOR OBTAINING MACULAR VISION IN SOME TYPES OF BLINDNESS

A. del Campo

The technique to be considered here takes an image to the posterior pole of the eye and projects it by transparency and through the sclera, over the macula lutea. The image comes from the exterior and is taken through what is called an "image conduit," hence the name *icono-phoresis* [1]

The image conduit consists of 72,000 extremely fiine optical glass fibers, each one coated with glass of a different refractive index, so that an image entering at one extreme emerges from the other with remark-

[1] Greek *ikonos*: image; *phoros*: to take.

able fidelity, regardless of the fact that the conduit might be bent, curved, or tied in a knot. Fabrication principles for such conduits are identical to those used for fiberscopes. The 72,000 fibers have a cross section of 3 mm (⅛ of an inch) with a resolution of 45 tear/lines/mm, resulting in an image of extraordinary clarity. In the conduit, as in the fiberscope, the fibers are correctly oriented optically and the image entering one extreme exits with a loss in brilliancy of about 5% every 7 m.

This "optical tube" bends very easily upon heating, without harming its good qualities. Bends do not affect the image, thus permitting much more comfortable endoscopies, since a fiberscope can adapt to the patient's curvature (Fig. 1).

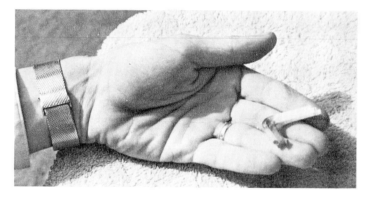

Fig. 1. The object held in the hand is made of four image conduits, as described in the text, held together. The ends are uneven because they have still to be cut and polished and also because in the process of bending, the curvatures are of different sizes.

The projection of light upon the retina, with said light coming from an opening other than the cornea or the crystal body, also produces a subjective sensation of light. By transilluminating the eye to one side of the iris (through the sclera) one perceives a very strong sensation of light. In addition, if one projects the light at a 45° angle, there is a clear sensation of seeing the retinal vessels as if they were projected on the wall. The subject integrates or perceives the illuminated field or the retina as luminous areas while the shadow projected by the vessels under the tangential light is perceived as black with such clarity that one can even see the capillaries. The important part of this phenomenon is that when some illuminated areas contrast with dark ones upon the subject's retina, he is capable of integrating figures that correspond to reality. It does not seem adventurous at this point to suppose that an image projected on the retina could give authentic visual information, even if its source is extracorneal.

There are some blind subjects with macula lutea in good condition who, for one reason or another, cannot be surgically treated to correct defects of the anterior chamber or vitreous body. It is for such cases that this extraocular technique has been developed. The image, after being received from the outside, is taken by the conveniently curved conduit through the posterior pole of the eye at the point where the macula lutea is projected. Without touching the eye, the internal extreme is fixed to Tenon's capsule in order to allow the eye free movement. The ocular end of the conduit, conveniently ground, projects the image over the posterior pole of the eye where the retina receives it through the squarer and the coroid. At first glance, this unorthodox procedure might provoke doubts as to the capacity of an image to go through the translucid coats of the eye. In the first place, experiments were conducted with enucleated human eyes where a vertical section was made and the posterior or retinal half was placed at the opening of a dark box. Images were then projected by means of lenses. The image, when correctly focused, were found to go through very well, with a loss of light equivalent to that experienced through parchment. Under these circumstances, even the image of candles in a dark room is perceived very clearly. On the other hand, conduits were permanently placed in cats (as shown in the x-ray plates of Figs. 2 and 3) and light projected on one side of the conduit was clearly seen in the fundus oculi (Figs. 4 and 5; pp. 134 and 135, resp.).

In these experiments the external extreme of the conduit was illuminated with a small flashlight or an ophthalmoscope. Not only did the pupil respond to light, but one could clearly see the eye lighting up inside. When colored filters were placed across the light source, the same colors shone inside the eye. In experiments with humans, the conduit was not installed permanently. Instead, it was pointed toward the posterior pole after experience was accumulated with an incision in the conjunctive. There was very clear visual perception when images of squares or lines were projected. These were carried to the macula and reported correctly by the blind subject. Colors were correctly identified although there is a certain tendency to perceive a constant red tint due to the transillumination of vessels and colors. Thus, yellow and blue were perceived as orange and violet, respectively.

One very important point concerns the tolerance of retro-orbital tissue (in direct contact with the conduit) to foreign materials. Experiments

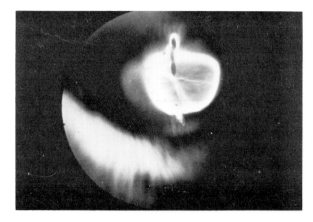

Fig. 2

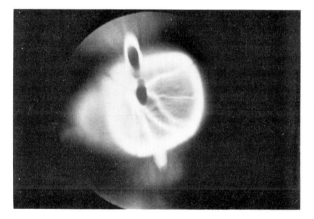

Fig. 3

Fig. 2. Photograph of fundus oculi of cat receiving light from behind the sclera. The source is an ophthalmoscope's bulb, placed against the external end of the conduit.

Fig. 3. Same as Fig. 2. The retinal vessels are clearly seen in the transillumination.

with cats showed that common glass, crystal, Teflon, polyethylene, and acrylic were accepted with no reaction. Even pupillary paralysis was absent, in spite of the proximity of important nerve bundles.

Based on this experience, we proceeded to prepare a visual prosthesis consisting of four image conduits bent in a "vee," with dental acrylic as the bonding and coating agent. The acidity of the acrylic was neutralized by immersion in a solution of 5% NaOH for 48 hrs. (This step is essential.) The resulting surface has an effective diameter of 6 mm, with 288,000 points of information being provided. At present, this represents a type of "tunnel" vision, but it is expected that improvements can be made. Although visual perception will be correct with regard to vertical orientation, the bend in the fiber produced an inevitable mirror-like inversion from right to left. This will require retraining. Optically correct images will be projected on the external extreme of the conduit by means of a lens mounted in a pair of spectacles. The ocular extreme of the conduit was carefully ground with a spherical mold whose diameter approximated that of the eye, so that the concavity is parallel to the external aspect of the posterior pole. Similarly, distortion is minimized by grinding the conduit's external extreme flat and perpendicular to the logitudinal plane.

Work is continuing on the placement of electrodes in cats on the optic nerve, chiasm, optical tracts, geniculate body, and occipital cortex in order to optimize the optical pathways.

DISCUSSION

HARMON: In the system you diagram the lens presumably forms a real image. Why not have a prism in that system to take care of the left–right reversal?

DEL CAMPO: You mean a prism to convert from right to left?

HARMON: Yes, so we get a normal projection.

DEL CAMPO: I think that would be one of the solutions.

LOEB: Have you given any thought to making the image that the person sees

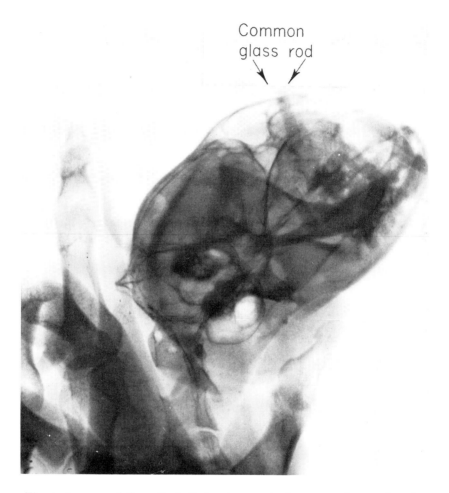

Common
glass rod

Fig. 4. An x-ray of the cat's skull showing a rod of common glass implanted in the orbit in order to find out the tolerance of retrorbitary tissue to foreign bodies. This was excellent.

steerable using the extraocular muscles? At the moment he sees only exactly what his head is pointing at. Is that correct?

DEL CAMPO: This is the conductor that gives you a sort of tunnel-like vision, straight ahead; but if you make it larger I think that even the thing could be made to mushroom out, and that this is a problem of manufacturing.

LOEB: If the subject wants to track a moving object, he has to move his head.

DEL CAMPO: He has to move his head, yes.

COGAN: Dr. del Campo's technique depends on stimulating some intact photo-

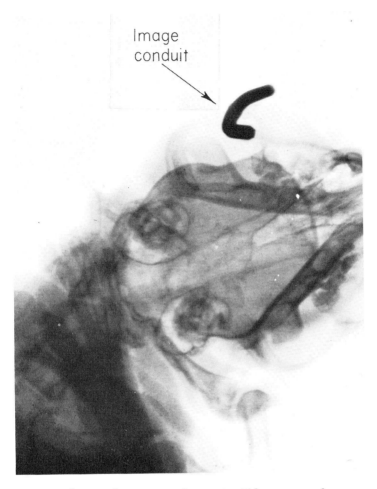

Fig. 5. An x-ray showing the image conduit in situ. Tolerance was also very good.

receptors in the retina, and I cannot conceive of any patient in which this would be indicated. It certainly would not be indicated in retinitis pigmentosa, where the photoreceptors have disappeared.

The case of vitreous hemorrhages is not relevant since the hemorrhages either clear up or else lead to blindness from detachment of the retina which would not be suitable for the "light pipe."

The retina does not stay in place. The hemorrhage does not stay there permanently. I just cannot conceive of any patient where there is an intact photoreceptive device to which this would be indicated.

DEL CAMPO: What you say represents a long drawn out question. In retinitis pigmentosa, the thing seems to be a matter of degeneration, and apparently when this happens there is nothing to do. Retinitis pigmentosa is known to be a progressive disease. It has no treatment. It may last for years.

In the abnormal eye, however, the pigmentary layer is situated closest to the proximity of the center of the eye, while the receptors are located more closely to the choroid.

The light, the image, must go through the thick pigmentary layers in order to reach the photoreceptor element. What I am doing here, trying to do, is project the image backwards. In other words, the image will be projected more closely to the photoreceptive elements without having to cross the pigmentary layers. This is one of the ideas.

BERING: This is not unrelated, as a technical matter, with the use of fiber optics. By utilizing fiber optics, you can expand the field to be much larger, and bring it out so it would be much smaller outside. And by using different lenses, from wide-angle to telephoto, you could project pictures of various sizes or have a zoom lens. From the point of technical optics, however, there are a great many variations that could be used in this kind of situation.

DEL CAMPO: I have no experimentation on phosphenes to report; I only have experience with external stimulation by electricity. I might say, however, that phosphenes have been produced on people who have no eyeballs, and they have been demonstrated for years. The possibility of any retina elements or functioning optical nerve being present is, of course, out.

I say that you can produce phosphenes easily by placing the electrodes almost anywhere. For example, if you place one of the electrodes in the cranium and the other one on the leg, all you have to do is raise the voltage and you get the experience of light.

This experiment was done in the 17th century by Leyden, who produced a discharge with a condenser. He produced the sensation of light in a normal subject. Now for the question of whether this stimulation produces phosphenes in the retina. I did experiments on blind subjects several times. The experiment consisted of incising precisely the conjunctiva and getting on the back of the sclera and stimulating with an electrode which as you mentioned this morning, needed rather high voltage.

It produced burns and some other discomfort; but there is a sensation of light, very pinpointed, which, in the presence of retinal elements follows the inversion pattern. You stimulate the upper half; the sensation comes from below, and vice versa. Also, the degenerated optical nerve produces phosphenes, too. I do not mean it is conducting nerve impulses but just conducting electricity, because it has salt and water, and it will get to the cortex eventually; the same as if you put the stimulation on the outside, on the back, or anywhere on your forehead.

If there is any damage in the retina, the optic nerve would degenerate too and the type of signals it might conduct could be of little use. The retina can be used for sending information. If there is retina, with damage of the crystal and/or vitreous body, there are other ways to send the image back, which are not electronic.

I developed a technique tested only on cats so far, where by using an image conductor, you make sort of a "periscope," which takes the image back and projects it through the sclera, where it stimulates the retina.

In other words, you are bypassing the eye and projecting an image on the back of the eye. The important aspect in the phosphenes that we produce by extrnal stimulation, as with the one you mentioned, is that it produces sensations of light in people without eyes, and it goes through the trigeminal nerve.

This may sound a little bit unorthodox, but we were able to pick up occipital potentials in cats by stimulation of the trigeminal nerve. You get potentials from the reticular system, and everywhere else, but they are interpreted in terms of light provided they remain within a certain frequency and the subject feels this as a flickering light provided he is within that frequency. If you go on above that, then you are out of range and you feel electricity but no light. All of these facts, I think, are pertinent to what we discussed this morning.

BURDE: Would you explain in detail fully exactly where that electrode was placed? I do not understand how you can take that position. You have stated the ganglion cells will not react to any stimuli and now you claim that you are stimulating them.

DEL CAMPO: Theoretically there is damage of the retina, all the retinal layers, but not always. Let us say there is a hemorrhage behind, or a detached retina. Supposedly the elements are destroyed. This is something you cannot determine. You are working by memory from other cases.

Suppose the ganglion cells in some cases do not suffer damage. If you stimulate by using a luminous source you get no sensation of light. In other words, the ganglion cells seem to act only as an interconnector of the light-receiving elements. They have no capacity for transmitting signals themselves to interpret as light, unless the stimulation is electrical and not luminous.

BURDE: You are stimulating from outside the sclera. I do not understand how you can be sure you are getting light to the ganglion cells when you do not know the pathologic conditions which exist.

DEL CAMPO: I am talking about the damaged ones. There is no way of finding out if the ganglion cells are intact. I am talking about cases that have definite damage of the retina.

BURDE: Dr. Cogan addressed himself to this problem when he spoke this morning.

As far as we can see, anatomically, both by light and electron microscopy, the ganglion cells are intact in disease processes such as retinitis pigmentosa. You can perform animal experiments where one can destroy the photoreceptor cells selectively. Spontaneous activity in the ganglion cell is noted in these animals as well as light evoked responses in certain strains of albino mice.

From your description there is no way of being certain what elements are viable. In these conditions some receptor bipolar-ganglion cell elements in tandem may remain intact. Further discussion at this time seems fruitless.

VAUGHAN: I do not think it would be at all acceptable to state that effective stimulation of the ganglion cells could be ineffective in producing phosphenes, because these are the normal elements in the visual pathway, which discharge into the optic nerve, and into the visual cortex. So, if you are, in fact, stimulating them, it would be inconceivable to me that you would not have phosphenes.

DEL CAMPO: The point is, in the cases I have seen I had no way of knowing whether the ganglion cells were damaged or not, because no further study was made on the patient.

COGAN: Dr. Adams mentioned complex hallucinations. Were those experientially, or were they formed?

ADAMS: They were formed hallucinations, that is, ones projected into the environment, as I have mentioned. The patients would see friends or people. The other type we have described as a "visual image," and here the visual event was more inside the patient. It was not projected to the environment, yet it was still very vivid, like a dream. One might describe this response as a visual "dreamy" state, not really projected as true hallucination into the environment.

BERING: Weed and Cornell have reported experiments similar to those of del Campo, and in their work visual sensation was reported only when there was some intact retina and visual pathway present.

COGAN: Among persons that are blind a substantial number have retinitis pigmentosa (or choroideremia) in which the photoreceptor cells of the retina are destroyed but the ganglion cells remain intact indefinitely. I wonder if any consideration has been given to special prosthetic devices for this type of disease in which the ganglion cells could be stimulated directly. Is it possible to place a silicone sleeve over the back of the eye with implanted electrodes which could be stimulated analogous to the silicone prosthesis on the brain? We know from abundant experience in retinal detachment surgery that silicone is well tolerated on the surface of the eye. I confess I have not thought this through very thoroughly but I would think this group of patients offered a special case in which electric stimulation of the retina might have merit.

STOCKHAM: I wanted to ask Dr. Cogan what is generally understood about the kind of activity that would ensue if one were to excite the ganglion cells of the retina with an image directly analogous to the light image that falls on the retina?

Specifically you might assume that in passing from the receptors to the ganglion cell level there is a transformation in the image iteself. If you were not to take that into account, what might you experience?

COGAN: I think we would induce no more than phosphene. When, for instance, I stimulate my own eye electrically, I get a diffuse light sensation in the corresponding part of the field.

STOCKHAM: Bright? Very bright?

COGAN: In the dark it seems bright, similar to what one produces on rubbing one's eye.

STOCKHAM: I would not classify that as bright; by "bright" I meant glaring.

COGAN: One turns the eyes to the opposite side and massages the sclera through the lid.

STOCKHAM: What about the other, implicit, part of my question? How dramatic, or how minor, is the transformation between the light image and the neural image?

COGAN: I am not aware of any serious attempt having been made to stimulate the retina by focal points. There is, of course, the choroid and a substantial thickness of the retina between the sclera and the ganglion cells. As far as I know, no serious attempt has been made to study the responses in some people who have lost their photoreceptors.

SCHIMMEL: How about in animals?

BERING: I know of one paper concerned with two point electrical stimulation of the retina. As Dr. Cogan described, one does get phosphenes. It is difficult to say whether they are glaring, but they are very much the same kind as Dr. Brindley derives, punctate, depending on the size of the electrodes.

The electrodes used which have been used for this are about 1 mm diameter, but if you get them sufficiently far apart you get two separate spots of light.

I have not, however, heard of anyone doing the thing that you are talking about where the photoreceptors have been destroyed.

Again getting back to this general question of what other ways there are to stimulate the visual system. There are other places that one might enter the visual system. The reason for using the visual system for a prosthetic device is that this is the system which in the brain is organized to process and interpret visual information. Why not use what remains of this system which is designed to do it to help anybody who has lost his vision?

In theory one should be able to enter the visual system at any place from retina to cortex, but each place might require a unique device. The best possible place from the information processing point of view is to enter through the retina when you have the whole system.

It would seem to me ideal if one could stimulate the ganglion cells. This would also be the easiest from the preprocessing point of view.

The fact is that Dr. Brindley and Dr. Lewin have put in a device that stimulates the brain. This changes everything from a practical point of view and stimulates many to follow this approach. I am convinced it will work and will give people useful information.

It is also possible theoretically to stimulate the optic nerve, the optic pathway, the lateral geniculate bodies, and the optic radiation. All of these are possible places to enter the visual systems. Each of these places of entry would require different devices and there are different problems in doing each.

The cortical stimulation has been done and shown to work, and so this is one that everybody talks about, and reasonably so; but there has been some thought regarding other plans of stimulation.

DOTY: I just wanted to comment on Dr. Cogan's suggestion that the ganglion cells could be stimulated in those retinas in which they survive.

In a paper in *Experimental Neurology* [2] Nancy Grimm and I discussed this, and showed that one could stimulate the retina electrically and elicit rather

[2] Grimm, N., and Doty, R. W., *Exper. Neurol.* **5,** 319 (1962).

localized potentials at striate cortex. This, however, to be practical, required the placement of the electrodes directly on the retina. Efforts to stimulate the eye through the sclera, while successful, required currents which were many-fold greater than the direct retinal stimulation, and therefore they would undoubtedly be painful in the conscious human being and would also give a great deal of spread so that discrete stimulation would not be obtained.

Therefore, I feel it is impractical to think in terms of stimulating the surviving ganglion cells through an externally-provided prosthesis to the eye, and one would, instead, have to think in terms of some impossibly complex way of getting an electrode array into the eye.

BERING: This might be possible, but needs surgical research to develop the technique.

DOTY: There is an interesting possibility raised by the experiments of Karli in Strasbourg,[3] who found that mice in which the photoreceptors degenerated completely as a result of a genetic defect nevertheless could distinguish light from dark, apparently on the basis of some inherent photoexcitation of the ganglion bipolar cells. I think the use of extremely intense illumination thus might be worth exploring in some such individuals.

VAUGHAN: This phenomenon actually has been studied, in the 19th century. Probably the best experiments were done by Giles Brindley, who used himself as a subject, and performed the rather heroic procedure of inserting electrodes behind the eyeball to get these electrodes as close as possible to the sensitive retinal elements rather than doing as most of us have done, putting electrodes around the orbit. As far as I know, this is probably the best attempt to get spatial resolution from retinal stimulation.

Dr. Brindley's observations suggested that the spatial resolution that could be achieved, even by getting the electrodes in the back of the eyeball in this rather crude fashion, was rather poor. In other words, he could get patterns in one quadrant of the visual field; and there might be some color and brightness gradients. They were, as you mentioned, rather complex kinds of experiences, not at all like the punctate, stable, white phosphenes that he described from cortical stimulation.

BACH-Y-RITA: I heard you gentlemen refer to the perceptual information gathered from eye muscle movement, and I have heard it before. The eye muscles have been my major research interest for a number of years, and I have to point out that there does not seem to be any noticeable perceptual role of eye muscles, although man has extraocular muscle spindles, as do cattle and sheep. Some primates, cats, rabbits, and rats do not have any; and it seems the squirrel monkey does not have any stretch receptors at all. It would seem from behavioral, neurophysiological, and other evidence, that the eye movement is signaled not by feedback from the eye muscle, but from the motor output to the eye muscles. So, I do not see that this would be necessary as a part of any prosthetic device.

Remember, any prosthetic device mounted on the head would be in rela-

[3] Karli, P., *Prog. Ophtal.* **14**, 51 (1963).

tion to the very fine movements of the neck, and these have quite fine proprioception.

BERING: The thing that the eye muscles do is tell you where your eyes are looking because you are programming the eyes to turn in some direction through the motions of the eye muscles, you would use this as a feedback for the controlling mechanism, and you would then have internal control of the prosthetic device.

I agree that it is not proprioception from the muscles—it is the programmed direction of the muscles which is important.

MINSKY: You would lose control because you know you would not know where it is looking. He is saying there is no way to tell where your eye muscles are going to look.

BERING: You can close your eyes and move them to the right or to the left.

BACH-Y-RITA: If you close your eyes, and you are in a dark room, you think your eye is moving. That has been shown by quite a number of people. Also, if the conjunctiva is anesthetized and the eye held immobile with forceps (in the dark) when the subject attempts to move his eyes, he thinks he has completed the movement.

VAUGHAN: I think this discussion is very important. It has been a misapprehension in neurology and psychology for almost a century that some type of kinesthetic feedback is necessary for normal motor behavior.

You are undoubtedly familiar with the recent work on deafferentiation of the limb musculature, which has shown that when all kinesthetic informaiton is eliminated and visual feedback is eliminated, that monkeys are still capable of performing skilled motor acts. It is true that if the eyeball is restrained from moving when you "will" it to move, a false impression of movement will occur.

Nevertheless, in the absence of restraint the monkey can go climb about his cage and perform rather incredible feats of motor dexterity without any visual or kinesthetic feedback, utilizing only this internal motor program.

So, I do not think that the absence of sensation or afferent information from the eye muscles, does not impair the validity of this very important concept that has been emphasized by Drs. Brodey and Johnson.

This, I think, is an essential component not only of the normal visual apparatus, but of any useful prosthesis, whether it be by way of the sensory system or utilizing the remaining visual apparatus.

JOHNSON: I would like to suggest to Dr. Bach-y-Rita there are a considerable number of feedbacks from the tissues surrounding the eye which the central nervous system uses.

BRODEY: We are not talking about feedback loops in the old sense; that is, as you know it. It is very different. We are talking about the whole loop rather than some particular feedback loop, so that when the whole eye moves the input to the eye is changed.

Again we will go back to the eyes, and it is peculiar that we are out of the game of cybernetics in the old sense, in a peculiar way, because now instead of talking about a small amount of information returning to alter the direction that the system is moving, we are talking about any output really fundamentally affecting the total input.

SIMMONS: You are not talking, as I understood previously, about the kinesthetic being more favorable, or any one central, and going back to itself being more favorable than the use of two centrals, then?

BRODEY: No. Really what we are talking about is what we have found in our explorations, that one sense by itself is useless.

As one increases the number of senses, one increases the skilled power that one has. But we are interested in bringing "dialog," to use that word that some people do not like, closer, and it is difficult to get dialog between the hands and the eye, as compared to a hand and another hand, because the hand and the hand are sort of the same system, of the same style, of the same movement, of the same time nature. You can get a more delicate exchange between things that are much alike than you can between things that are very different.

SIMMONS: At least you do not notice the difference as much.

I.4 PREPROCESSING OF VISUAL INFORMATION

The visual scientist and the engineer have carefully built an interface between hardware and nervous tissue. Whatever the deficiencies of any such system might be, they can be corrected in part by introducing percepts in a way that allows the nervous system to handle them more easily. Whatever the strength of any such system might be, it can be enhanced in some way by taking full advantage of the ability of the nervous system to view a complex image. Thus, the addition of digital logic to process pictures and present them to the nervous system becomes an integral part of the prosthesis. Accordingly, the computer scientist becomes involved.

This session turned about three major topics:

(1) To what extent can a particular combination of phosphene points be exploited? To what extent can complex information be presented on a relatively sparse display surface? The position papers of Sterling and Weinkam, and of Knowlton demonstrated various methods by which pictures can be formatted and presented for blind and sighted individuals.

(2) There have been many ways to manipulate a picture. Now, the computer has introduced new dimensions and new flexibilities to this process of picture enhancement. The presentation by Stockham provided a most vivid demonstration of these possibilities.

(3) There is also a subtle area of subject and object interactions. perhaps we learn to perceive not only through visual experience with visual objects, but also through somesthetic and kinesthetic sensation resulting from repeated handling of the variegated environment. Brodey and Johnson, while not using computers, do make use of the kind of mechanisms which become an important adjunct to any simulating system.

The discussions were further enriched by two presentations, one by Carr and one by Nagy. Carr pleads for formulating theory before further development of picture processing techniques. It was a curious plea, betraying the natural science bias which is not shared by the more empirical biologists and physicians. Nagy described how terribly difficult it is just to implement the recognition of machine letters that are produced as different typesetting fonts.

There is just so much time for any discussion. The complex topic of automatic pattern recognition did not ever emerge. This was an unfortunate omission because this topic most likely will be a central focus of future discussions. An explanation for this deemphasis is well expressed by Harmon in his opening remarks to the preprocessing part of the proceedings:

HARMON: We shall be talking, in part, about information, coding and flow, and the amount of display needed in order for humans to achieve certain levels of perceptions. One can play "numbers games" with respect to data flow rates, but one must be careful, I think, not to do so. Each retina, for example, with 10^6 ganglion cells might transmit along the optic nerve as many as 500 spikes a second in each axon. If these spikes are of uniform amplitude, then we can estimate on the order of half a billion bits a second which could be transmitted along the optic nerve. Contrast that, however, with what every psychophysicist knows, that transduced rates, through the human, for typing, whistling, speaking, or reading, say, are approximately 50 bits per second.

No matter how complex the central processes are, input data overload has to be avoided. A major problem in all sensory-aid and prosthesis design is how to constrain and to encode many classes of input signals to achieve effective handling of the environmental data and to do so with minimum stress on the user's remaining sensory channels.

Preprocessing is intended to make these all-important condensations and input selections. We shall include discussions of analysis and display, in terms both of software and of hardware.

PREPROCESSING OF SENSED INFORMATION FOR ANALYSIS AND DISPLAY

T. D. Sterling and J. J. Weinkam

The idea of systematically adapting a signal to the information-processing capabilities of a perceptual system to facilitate its discrimination from other signals has not been extensively considered until now. Information gathered by a variety of sensing devices was and still is presented to physically handicapped persons more or less as raw input with the hope that the nervous system will be able to learn to respond appropriately. Effectiveness of an "aid" has always depended on the ability of the user to learn the meaning of the signal that was produced by it.

With the development of digital logic technology, it is now possible to modify a signal and present it in such a way that the nervous system can learn to understand its meaning much more easily and reliably. For instance, it is possible to translate the content of a printed page by spelling out words or pronouncing them, by representing words as a constant flow of easily understandable signals to the skin, or by using a punctate phosphene screen (such as developed by Brindley) combined with scanning techniques. There is no reason why signals could not be presented to more than one sense at the same time. A combination of tactual and auditory display might easily lead to faster and more efficient "reading" than the use of either sense by itself. Certain sounds could be made to indicate the direction of moving obstacles. Vibratory stimuli could be used to supply information about the type of obstacle encountered. Even crude pictures of obstacles in the environment could be displayed on a punctate screen or as a matrix of tactile points.

The present state of computer technology permits intermediate processing to control displays in almost any desired shape or form. However, it is necessary to marshall the present state of the art and translate it into a working structure before an investigator can effectively incorporate preprocessing concepts into prosthetic technology. Specifically, it is necessary to develop:

(1) convenient methods to study computer-directed display sequences;

(2) a suitable command structure (or "descriptive source language) by which investigators can form and manipulate images at will. Implementations of this command structure must be sufficiently versatile to allow investigators with limited computing facilities to utilize them;

(3) optimal methods for converting software solutions into properly packaged hardware components for practical prosthetic devices.

It is necessary to point out that the progress of preprocessing for display will depend on the success of constructing algorithmic languages for display manipulations. In principle, these languages are designed to relieve the problem arising from the fact that computer control of patterns and shapes requires a considerable amount of programming. Much of this burden can be removed from the human programmer by developing specialized "compilers." These are translating programs which permit the user to state his processing needs in a simplified source language consisting of relatively familiar terms. The translating program then converts the user's commands into the necessary sequence of machine-language instructions. Thus, much of the final programming is actually done automatically.

The usefulness of preprocessing can be best investigated through the powerful simulation techniques. These, in turn, depend on computer languages that give to the investigators the power to manipulate "percepts" flexibly—through whatever sense they might be presented eventually to the blind viewer. Given the possibility of manipulating visual material in the form of much more comprehensive codes, it may well be discovered that even the limitations of the skin as a communication medium are far from exhausted. Furthermore, such tools provide vehicles for exploring the possibilities of combining a number of dimensions which

support and enhance perception, especially the visual illusion of phosphenes. Such dimensions as time, spatial organizations, and different
modes of sensory input can be combined to form entirely new experiences and perceptual units by which the visual environment may be
interpreted with facility and accuracy.

This language is designed to simulate a system such as that depicted
in Fig. 1. The system consists of a camera which may be pointed at a
scene, circuitry to analyze the pattern "seen" by the camera, and a screen
on which the information is displayed as a set of discrete points. A person
using such a device would move the camera about to scan the scene and
would hopefully be able to recognize properties of the scene by observing the changing pattern on the screen.

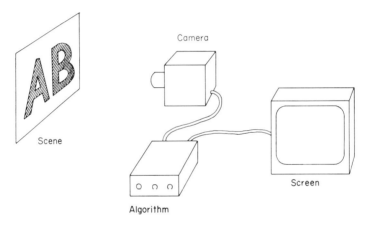

Fig. 1. Schematic of visual processing system.

PROSIS simulates a simplified version of such a system in which the
scene is restricted to be a two-dimensional black and white representation, the algorithm applied by the circuitry is assumed to have certain
simple properties, and the path of motion of the camera is assumed to
have a simple mathematical representation. Data structures in memory
are used to represent the important features of the system, and commands
are provided in the PROSIS language to manipulate the contents of these
structures and thus control the operation of the system.

The important data structures are:

(a) SCENE—which represents the scene seen by the camera. The language contains commands to enable the user to insert objects of any size
into the scene at any desired location.

(b) DICT—which is a dictionary containing the drawing instructions for various objects. Commands in the language enable the user to describe any object to the system in terms of a series of lines and arcs. This information is stored in the dictionary and may be used at any time to draw any combination of objects on the scene.

(c) MAP—which contains a list of the location, size, and shape of each phosphene or point of light which the system can use to display images.

(d) PARM—which contains the parameters which describe the path of motion of the point on the scene at which the camera is aimed. This path is described in terms of the sum of three elementary motions: a linear motion, a horizontal sinusoidal motion, and a vertical sinusoidal motion.

TABLE 1. SUMMARY OF PROSIS COMMANDS

	Command	Function
Definition of objects	DICTIONARY	Initiates entry of instructions into the dictionary. A parameter OBJECT specifies the name of the object.
	LINE ARC	Specify each line or arc of the object in terms of coordinates in a unit square.
Drawing on the scene	ERASE	Erase previous contents of the scene.
	INSERT	Insert object into scene. Parameter OBJECT specifies name of object; other parameters specify size and location. Besides the objects in the dictionary, simple objects such as LINE, ARC, CIRCLE, TRIANGLE, and RECTANGLE may be specified.
Specification of the path	PATH	Specify scanning path. Simple paths such as LINE, ZIG-ZAG, and SPIRAL may be specified by name, with additional parameters to control the speed of motion along the base line and the relative rate of the sinusoidal motions with respect to the linear motion.
	START	Begin displaying the pattern which results from scanning the current scene as specified by the current path information. The display continues until a key is depressed on the display console.

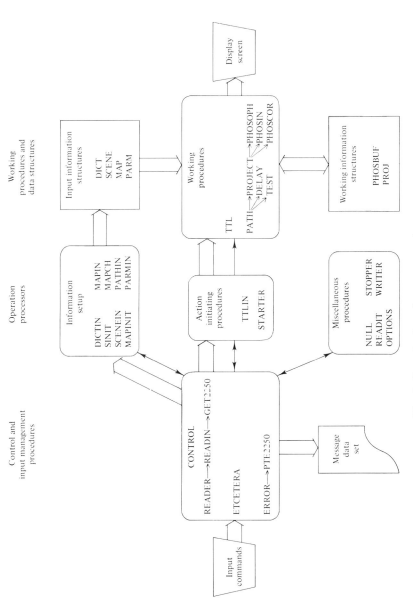

Fig. 2. Organization of PROSIS procedures.

Some of the principal commands are summarized in Table 1. In addition to the commands shown in Table 1, the language contains commands to direct the system to read in a series of commands from tape or disk which would contain dictionary entries, description of the phosphene screen, etc. There are also commands to assist in recovery from errors and to print out diagnostic or reference information about the state of the system.

Figure 2 depicts the organization of the entire system. The various programs are grouped into blocks with rounded corners and the data structures are shown in blocks with square corners. Data flow is indicated by double arrows and flow of control is indicated by single arrows.

(A film was then shown that had been produced using the PROSIS language described above. The figures described here are still taken from this film.)

Figure 3 depicts the phosphene distribution obtained by Brindley, displayed on the IBM 2250. Figure 4 shows a representation of a fire hydrant using a hypothetical phosphene screen on which the phosphenes were somewhat more regularly spaced than on the Brindley screen. (The film concludes with a number of simple geometric shapes, letters, and words being moved across the simulated Brindley display screen.)

DISCUSSION

BRODEY: Can you read these?

WEINKAM: Yes I can, but I have had a bit of practice and, of course, I have the advantage of knowing what is on the film.

BRODEY: Can you read a strange message?

WEINKAM: I can do so fairly easily as long as it consists of letters I have seen before. Every time a new letter is introduced it takes some getting used to. The point is that you have to fixate on a point on the screen, and that is somewhat difficult. You tend to scan the whole picture and cheat a little. One thing that makes it considerably easier is to increase the scanning rate. When we were

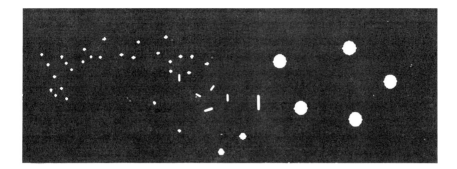

Fig. 3. Simulated Brindley screen.

editing this film we could crank the material through the editor at any desired speed. Letters were easy to recognize if you cranked rapidly enough. They seemed to pop out.

HARMON: Have you tested otherwise uninstructed observers on their ability to identify objects or letters correctly?

WEINKAM: Not by any systematic basis; we have shown the film to small groups and people have volunteered opinions on what they thought they saw. After viewing the film for the first time, most of the people had difficulty in identifying objects displayed on the Brindley screen, although a few have correctly identified them. Most people can identify A, B, C, triangles, circles, and so on after seeing them. All in all, I think it is pretty clear that with some practice one can learn to discriminate quite accurately.

CARR: Have you considered alternative transformation, such as making a one-for-one transformation so that all the information is present on the Brindley screen but topologically distorted?

WEINKAM: We have not attempted that, but our program is perfectly capable of it.

STERLING: Actually, we used the "picket fence" principle. The idea is to act as if the picture is hidden by a picket fence. Then we imitate the action of the fence moving by the screen and try to see what is behind it.

BERING: There is a fallacy in the "picket fence" principle as applied to visual stimulation. In the picket fence principle, as you move by you pick up impressions with the entire retina. When one part is not seeing something because it is blocked by a picket, the next part is stimulated. Punctate stimulation of the visual cortex provides stimulations only for a group of particular points. The entire visual field is not filled as is done when passing a picket fence. It is as if the source moved by the fence with the same part of the retina always occulted. Sterling and Weinkam's work is most fascinating but the most difficult part, as Dr. Weinkam has said, was keeping one's eye focused on a central point. When we did this on-line using an IBM 2250 screen we put a small piece of tape on it. It helped considerably.

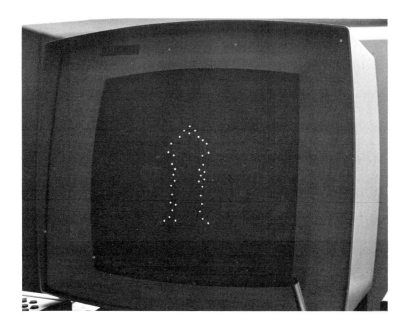

Fig. 4. Hydrant image generated by PROSIS.

Despite these problems this is an extremely useful and interesting way to see what kind of results might be coming out; and I think anybody who is developing an electrode for this kind of stimulation is well advised either to get this program or do something of a similar nature to see what the end product might look like to a blind viewer, what kind of learning he would have to be able to do and what kind of information he can really receive.

PINNEO: I have two points. The first is that we are viewing this with our eyes. Now I wonder what the difference is between this and the actual cortical experience, which may be a different thing. The second point is, that while watching the Brindley screen I noticed that I was not recognizing on the basis of the actual "A" but on the pattern or sequence of two or more things that would occur. So, I needed only a couple of pieces of information to identify the "A."

Therefore, you do not really need to represent the entire letter in each case, but simply this sequence of patterns that corresponds to "A." These were recognizable to me; in fact, earlier recognizable to me than actually seeing the letter "A" or "B" or the triangle.

WEINKAM: It would seem that for high speed reading one would probably want to develop a compressed code to represent letters, but I think one would also want to keep the ability to try to view the entire object. In the case of reading, this would give one the ability to read an unfamiliar font right away without changing any circuitry or ground prisms.

STERLING: Dr. Pinneo brought out two important points: What is the relation between viewing this with the eyes and a blind person's "perception" of the "visual illusion"? It may be fairly safe to assume that if a sighted subject cannot make sense out of a particular scanning method, a blind individual implanted with electrodes producing a Brindley-type screen will not be successful either.

I do not know whether the opposite is true, but certainly if we use a computer on a sighted subject, then we would eliminate some scanning techniques which are useless, or less effective than others, and yet obtain some clues before hooking up a subject.

The second point is that we are then able to develop new sets of codes, with each succeeding set representing an improvement over its predecessor. We are able to do so before sitting down with the blind subject.

HARMON: In that case, I would raise the question as to why go to all the trouble of having this tye of presentation? Why not do it tactually?

STERLING: Let me put it this way: We have to learn and see what we get out of an implant. We cannot do that tactually.

JOHNSON: I wanted to ask Dr. Sterling to clarify one sentence which appeared either in his talk or in some earlier discussion. I am taking it out of context. "The usefulness of preprocessing can be investigated only by use of these languages and simulation techniques."

STERLING: If we want to experiment with a subject, and it does not matter whether it is to be done in a visual, tactile, or auditory mode, and if we are going to say, "I'd like to move a particular image by at a particular rate using a particular type of movement" it would be very difficult to do this if we had to write a program each time we wanted to change the image or modify some of the scanning parameters. (It would be even more difficult if we had to build a special piece of hardware each time we wanted to make such a change based on previous experience.) The time between experiments would then be what it is today in psychophysical research where a single investigator may be able to perform no more than two or three experiments a year.

On the other hand, if we have a computer controlled display technique and a good source language which will permit us to instruct the machine in a very flexible way, we can decide what we are going to show and construct each presentation or modify right then and there.

JOHNSON: I was wondering if you would accept the alternative of a hand-held or subject-mounted analog device.

STERLING: Analog devices will do, but they are not as flexible as digital devices. Each of the pictures you saw was developed by one or two instructions. It was really a demonstration of how flexibly such a langauge could work, what you could see with it, and yet how easy it makes the manipulation of images.

NAGY: I would like to register agreement, especially, Dr. Sterling's comments about the special languages. However, it is my impression that no one who has developed a special study language, after removing all the "bugs," has enough energy left over to apply the language to any problem not related to the language itself.

STOCKHAM: I would like to make a comment on that. I developed a rather modest special-purpose language to manipulate images on the TX-2 Computer at the Lincoln Laboratory.

This language consisted of approximately 25 basic processes. For instance, adding two pictures together; creating mirror images, and so on.

I used this language extensively for a period of a year and a half without changing it very much after it was finally created, and I could not have done a thing without it, at least without also killing myself in the process.

I found that it was very desirable, however, to have an associate build the basic pieces of the language for me, to my specifications. That allowed me to concentrate on the design of the language, which is an essential ingredient, and also allowed me to have energy left over to use it.

POLLACK: To apply some more realistic perspective to those people in the group who may not be experienced with the design and use of languages, Dr. Knowlton developed a language and has been using it routinely for a period of five years. We will see a film that is a very striking demonstration. It was prepared entirely in this language.

STERLING: We have taught our procedures to Dr. Bering, and we are using them ourselves for other purposes. Dr. Bering happened to pick up the operational rudiments in approximately 15 minutes. We are using our system for various other display purposes so we are really not that naive.

VAUGHAN: It is a good idea for this type of development to take place, because it will certainly be useful in prosthesis development. I think, however, that pictorial display of the work provided by Sterling and Weinkam may differ substantially from the format required in the prosthesis itself. This will create a visual display that can be perceived by sighted individuals; but the transformation of this visual display that may be necessary for tactile or cortical input, may be quite different.

I am wondering whether the computer language will, in fact, be able to take care of that kind of transformation without an extraordinary amount of additional work.

STERLING: This is exactly what we are talking about now, and the answer is yes. If we have an array of points on which we want to move, say a line, from left to right, then what the program will do is generate a line of a given size and move it as indicataed. We would phrase the instruction according to our own scale system, as for instance, move Array 20 from right to left—and the computer would generate a line, check what angle we want, and then simulate a set of points so that a line is moved across them at the rate at which we want to move it.

VAUGHAN: There is a very important limitation in the demonstrations given here of what has been called the "Brindley screen." It has been assumed that this screen is to be at rest in a way which does not correspond to what I would think would be an optimal way to address this screen.

Now if the language is going to be able to be useful, it must be useful to someone who wants to program cortical stimulation. What one is going to have to take into consideration, at an early stage, is the physiological transformations that are going to be required; and at the present state of knowledge I submit that it is very difficult to state what these might be.

STERLING: Let me mention something I omitted before. It is our object, also, to create a compiler which will enable the investigator to write new command structures with some limitations.

SUTRO: I wanted to ask about their example of a man going across the scene. Why not use the television camera and the computer, as several of us have it set up, and actually have a man do it, and use the signal from the resulting tape as your input?

STERLING: If we wanted an experiment concerning a man walking across the scene, then we can use the television system. But, under some conditions the picture of a man could not be shown. Then we may want to present the man as a stick man, we may want to present the man as two parallel lines; or as a circle, with a cross on top.

POLLACK: One of the most common misconceptions about these artificial languages is the assumption that in order for them to be designed, the potential user has to be able to anticipate every contingency under which they would be put to use. This is not true. One of the most important, fundamental features of a well-designed language, is something that has come to be known as "open-endedness." Although an extensive set of primitives is provided, included also is the ability for combining them to synthesize more complex commands which, to the user, are no more complicated to implement than the simple commands with which he started.

MINSKY: Dr. Pollack just said what I was going to mention. It is difficult to anticipate some physiological transformation that could not be expressed in terms of a good set of primitives. It is conceivable that you might come up with one, but one would have to extend it.

I think with regard to Dr. Sutro's remarks, among the kinds of activities you want the system to handle are things like, yes, having the man walk from left to right, and I think Dr. Sterling's point that you might want the man to be represented by a stick figure, or by the edges of the television image, or something similar, is important.

Another part of the language, however, would provide that while he is moving from left to right, you would transform the image in such-and-such a way if the occulomotor system asks for this or that, and so the language has to have programmed into it the possibility or responding in reasonably fast time to other physiological signals one is going to provide to it.

This reactivity is probably an essential part of any prosthetic device that will make the subject feel he is moving the Brindley screen over the image rather than the image over the screen.

I think some of us felt we could read the images going by past the screen if by chance our eyes were drifting in the proper direction, and then one had this effect.

I guess my major plea is that a laboratory that does this is going to be fairly expensive, and fairly complex, and it will not work unless it has rather good people in it. So, it probably should be proposed on the basis of a perceptual, basically visual perceptual, laboratory.

There is not any in the country, although Dr. Sterling's laboratory, and our laboratory, are experimenting with such things, and probably even aside from the particular application of visual prosthesis there certainly is a need to have a good experimental physiological stimulation laboratory in the country, perhaps two or three, and I think that would justify developing these languages and the associated facilities with them, whether or not it leads to a cortical stimulation device or, in fact, any prosthesis for the blind.

COMPUTER SIMULATION OF PUNCTATE SCREEN DISPLAYS

K. C. Knowlton

I want to show you some slides and some movies which were very largely inspired by Dr. Sterling and Dr. Weinkam, and demonstrate, I hope, the kinds of "games" you can play and the kinds of questions you can begin to ask, assuming that what you, as sighted people, are seeing is somehow like what the blind person would see.

Let us assume that what you see is similar to what the blind person with the electrically-stimulated cortex would see. (For that matter, as soon as one can demonstrate differently, then one can presumably build the proper interactions, into the computer program and improve the validity of the display for experiments with sighted people.)

Let me show you 16 movies quickly. They are simply a sequence of films taken under 16 conditions. That is to say, I am taking four variables and questioning their relative importance: (1) a regular screen versus an irregular screen, like Dr. Brindley's; (2) the laterally restricted Brindley area versus trying to get down into what I think is the calcarine fissure, in which I believe lateral vision is mapped; (3) the Brindley density versus four times that density of points; and (4) bilateral versus unilateral prosthetic vision.

I think questions like these are very crucial at this point, because answers to them indicate which way the surgical and electronic technology should first try to go.

Figure 1 is a pseudo-Brindley screen of 26 phosphenes. The ones on the top of the screen are double, which seems to be what is happening in the Brindley case; Those in the center of the screen are individual points; The ones at the bottom are lines in four different directions. I have ignored Brindley's very large, nebulous phosphenes at the bottom.

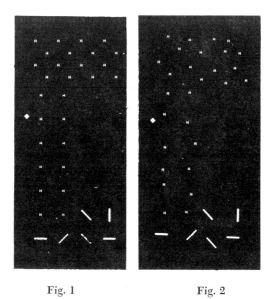

Fig. 1   Fig. 2

The next figure (Fig. 2) is simply the same thing, 26 phosphenes here randomly displaced, but still within their original squares; this approximates the kind of thing that Dr. Brindley had: half of a dumbbell shape, if you continue to ignore the large phosphenes at the bottom. Next (Fig. 3) is one with four times as many spots. This represents 104 phosphenes regularly arranged. Figure 4 shows the same thing, with the 104 phosphenes, displaced.

Figure 5 we have presumably bilateral vision, and I have left the original ones a little bit brighter so you can see, in successive slides, just where the original field is. We have now 52 phosphenes regularly spaced. Figure 6 is the same thing, but with the random displacements. Next one is the regular arrangement of four times as many, which gives 208 phosphenes (Fig. 7). The effect of displacement is shown in Fig. 8.

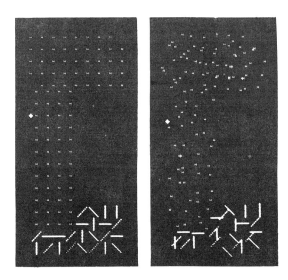

Fig. 3   Fig. 4

Figure 9 is with lateral vision, assuming that you can get in the side area there, and you see what my approximations here have been. I have arbitrarily extended the region of lines to move a little bit upward and to the side; the region of doublets has been extended down and to the side. There are 43 phosphenes here. Figure 10 goes on with random displace-

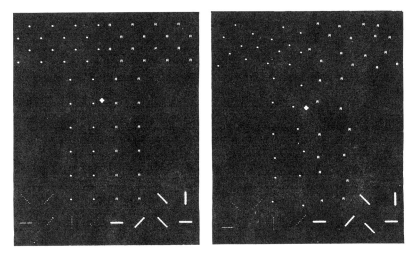

Fig. 5   Fig. 6

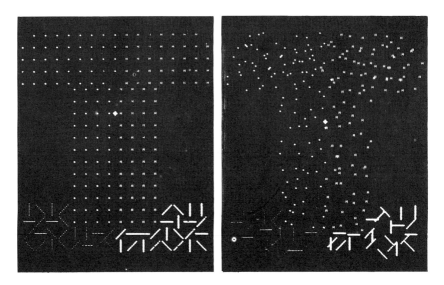

Fig. 7   Fig. 8

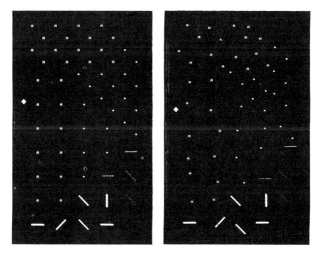

Fig. 9   Fig. 10

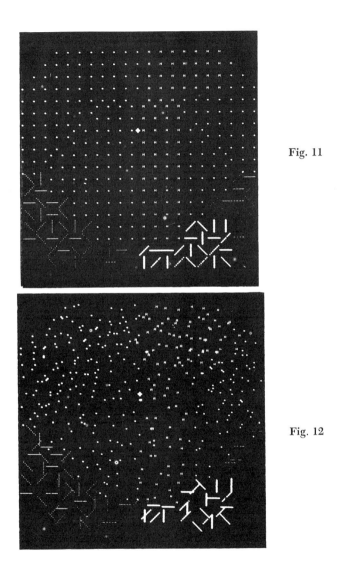

Fig. 11

Fig. 12

ment. Figure 11 shows four times as many. This gives you 172 in half of the visual field and Fig. 12 is one with random displacement, and still with 172 points.

The final series brings us to a large number of points. Figure 13 is a regular array of 86 phosphenes. The effect of irregular arrangement is seen in Fig. 14. Figure 15 is the very best of the 16 shown here. This is

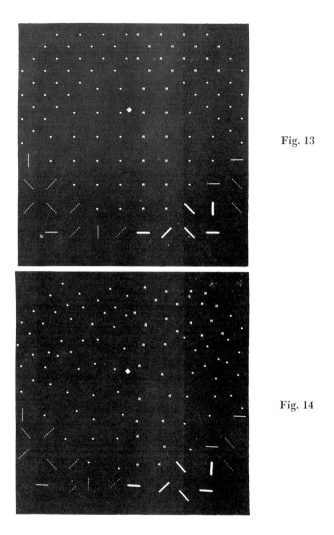

Fig. 13

Fig. 14

304 phosphenes, quite regularly arranged. The last one (Fig. 16) is still the same 304 phosphenes, but juggled around slightly.

Those are the 16 slides that define the variation in the film I have prepared. The movie consists very simply of four geometric figures, moving from right to left, and then a four-word sentence. I will present it in exactly the same order, and, I hope, you will begin to get a feeling for the importance of the various things that I talked about.

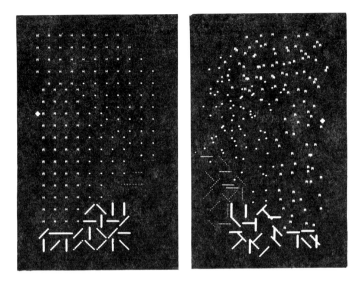

Fig. 15   Fig. 16

You cannot really start to answer questions here without putting people through training sequences and real tests, and with some real judgment as to whether or not they are fixating at the cross. (Film is shown during talk.)

DISCUSSION

KNOWLTON: How many of you could read the message? Apparently some of you could.

MANN: What was the rate?

KNOWLTON: The rate was approximately two characters a second.

DOBELLE: Would it be any easier to read it if you went slower?

KNOWLTON: Yes. It was at sound speed. I had planned to show it at silent speed. So, you can imagine it lasting 50% longer, and you could have seen it better. There is one point I want to make here: In each of these 16 presentations there was exactly the same information content. That is to say, the large letters on the fine screen were devised from the information in the coarse screens.

The letters themselves were actually devised on a 5 × 7 grid column plus a couple of extra lines down below for the tails of the *i*'s, *j*'s, etc. The information in the two presentations (unilateral versus bilateral) was exactly the same, and the fact that your response to each presentation was different demonstrates the whole reason for involving the visual cortex in a visual prosthesis. That is, the visual system is built for seeing two-dimensional patterns.

The thing that I want to go into right now is some real testing. I want to make training sequences of longer sentences and put subjects through a sort of reverse order training program, going down to fewer and fewer phosphenes, in a resrticted area, ultimately down to the actual Brindley area except that I want to go to the right half of the visual field instead of the left half. I think that for purposes of reading, Brindley has chosen the wrong side, because if we want images flowing from right to left, it is best to show the actual material on the right and hope that the subject can visualize it a tenth of a second later on the left, and thus "see" the whole picture: the immediately prior material visualized on the left plus the current material actually presented on the right. This, I think, makes much more sense than to have him see it on the left and try to "visualize" it having been on the right a tenth of a second earlier.

Then, after subjects have been trained for 5, 10 or 50 hours, I shall actually test them for many different modes, even though I have told them previously that their job was only to learn to read the Brindley screen. The test should therefore give us a feeling for the importance of the four different parameters we have been considering.

Furthermore, there may be other questions that you think are important that can be programmed in this fashion.

DOTY: When I read the last filmed example, which was the first one I could really read, I did so only by saccadic movement. There is a problem of scanning. I am not quite sure how the brain-applied prosthesis is going to do that, but perhaps the subject could scan the field by his own movements and this would accomplish the same results.

KNOWLTON: That brings up another matter; actually, we have been asking two kinds of questions. One is: What kind of prosthesis do you want? What arrangement of electrodes is best? The other kind of question is: Given a particular configuration, what kind of encoding is best, including what kind of control by the subject? Ultimately, one will undoubtedly want some sort of feedback where we monitor, say, the person's head and eye position, and if he looks to the left the movement of his head or eyes is to the left, the display slows down; and if he looks far enough, the thing stops. I think Dr. Minsky has a display something like this. Did you not have some kind of motion where you essentially held the acceleration constant or somehow controlled the velocity of the display?

MINSKY: Yes.

KNOWLTON: Obviously, you want to be able to back it up; conversely, if things are going well, and reading is satisfactory, the user can look to the right and in a sense anticipate. He is looking this way because he wants to get on with the reading.

DOTY: Certainly in the evaluation of these displays by sighted subjects one must be very careful to eliminate or control, or understand, the saccadic scanning.

KNOWLTON: It is a whole order of magnitude more difficult experimentally to try to fixate images on the retina, and it involves a lot of equipment. It seems to me at this particular point that getting 10 times as many people, or requiring them to put in 10 times as many hours, gives us perhaps more information. We should, of course, be really conscientious about monitoring the subjects' eye motions during the testing.

I am surprised that you (Dr. Doty) said you actually scanned, because these were going by pretty fast.

DOTY: Possibly I did so because we are currently doing research on eye movements.

BRODEY: I think when we consider the projection of possible tests we get a divergence developed between two points of view. In the one situation, we put the test on the screen, and we have someone looking at it passively, without any real control over what goes over the screen. We now have a great deal of data that suggest that having control over something that we are learning about facilitates the learning process.

Instead of the projected tests, let us take the situation where we have the Rand tablet and where someone is scribbling, or writing, or making letters on the tablet, and the computer is being used to go from the Rand tablet letters to letters which are displayed on the Brindley screen. The person then gets into the loop. Now let us assume that not only is he scribbling the letters himself, but he is also required, in some way, to make a statement of whether he has those letters, or not. This statement may be made by some means of which he is not necessarily aware. For instance, schizophrenic response, or some recognition which may be his personal style.

Then the computer moves into the situation of changing the speed at which his own writing is displayed to him, so that he is really in a loop which is now made responsive to his own style, his own control, even more elaborately than he might have done with his own hand,. In this way we are beginning to learn how to close the loop.

Let us say that in addition we move the Brindley screen from far outside to a cap with a master cell over his eye. We are gradually approximating the real situation with regard to a single subject. Elaborating this, we get a series of subjects, for each of whom a tailor-made situation is developed.

BLISS: I am struck by the great similarity between what has been described here and the tests that have been carried out in my own laboratory with computer generated patterns in which letters of the alphabet are presented both tactually and visually.

In our experiments we have, in the visual case, measured eye movements while subjects read from a "moving belt" of printed text. In the tactile case, we have conducted experiments with and without feedback in which the subject could have control over the speed, or how the information was being presented. I think there should be more communication between these two kinds of research because there is a lot of commonality here.

MACKAY: I feel this is a very salutary series of demonstrations. If anyone has over-sanguine hopes of what a blind person with 60 or 100 implants may be able to do, particularly the first one with the Brindley screen, this suggests to me that for many purposes it would be of advantage to us to have a much smaller selection from the total number of available points. I do not know how many other people have this impression; but if the Brindley screen had been reduced to something like 16 points in a regular array, and then registration carefully selected, perhaps a decent recognition job might have been done where this was impossible as it stood. I wonder whether anyone has used the program where the subject's eye movement could be used to control the advance of the scanner, so as to see how much easier it might be to recognize these patterns if the subject can do his own pacing in a pseudo-saccadic manner.

HARMON: That might even be possible with the line prosthetic situation.

MACKAY: Indeed, yes; but it could be done more easily with the computer, I would suppose.

MURPHY: I have a couple of questions for both Dr. Knowlton and Dr. Weinkam about the matter of scale, i.e., the size of the screen versus the size of the letters. Were large or small projections on the same screen more effective?

In the second place, the experience that we have had for some years in teaching optophones, visotactors, and, presumably Dr. Bliss's experience with tactile devices which provide a complete map, would imply that it is possible to learn the code, at least at the slow rates comparable to the view that you are showing; however, that learning does take considerable time.

There exists a systematic course for the optophone developed at Battelle Memorial Institute, so it might be interesting to use the words from that same course with direct stimulation and give the same tests. Then we may have some idea of whether the learning curves should vastly improve on the very slow rates that are possible with the single line of only nine vertical cells.

KNOWLTON: I do not know what the letters should be like. For a given screen, would you prefer a crudely drawn font where you can see the whole letter at once, or a carefully drawn letter of which you can see only part at one instant:

WEINKAM: We did try small letters, but they did not show up too satisfactorily.

MINSKY: If we take any printed materials, take a piece of paper, and cover up the bottom two-thirds of a row of lower-case characters, we can see that we can just about read it. If we cover the top of the printed characters, we have much more difficulty. So that if we knew we were looking at letters, we could cut off the lower half of them and I think we would double the rate of comprehension, perhaps with the same number of points.

STERLING: Very good!

KNOWLTON: We can go to the extreme of using only six dots, and present braille visually. This would not make very much sense, and I would expect that the reading speed would not exceed (and would probably be less than) what a good braille reader can do.

The point is that just to read the standard English alphabet cannot be the goal. This is a flexible, general system; you can use the Greek alphabet; you can invent or devise anything new that you want to make in terms of symbols —anything you can draw, in this case, on a 5×9 screen, which provides a theoretical repertoire of 3×10^{12} different characters. Perhaps you would want to use several thousand of them.

COMPUTER AIDS IN IMAGE STORAGE
AND PROCESSING

J. Carr III

It is apparent to me that visual prostheses already exist in great quantity. The television system, throughout the world, is one that is very well known, although not recognized as such. Every sighted person has his visual capabilities extended manyfold. A second device, which is just beginning to make its way felt but which will probably be tied into this first television-oriented visual prosthesis network, is the display computer. The two examples described at this conference (Weinkam and Knowlton) give an illustration of how one can compose and construct visual moving images.

I think the experience of Dr. Minsky and his group on a computer-aided visual system in using computers is one that should be studied. The work at Stanford University represents work in which the translation of visual information is being investigated very intensely for other purposes. The theories and technologies of radar systems, which are communication devices which involve visual displays, obviously are very germane to this undertaking.

It would seem to me that one is compelled to conclude that there must be a very thorough simulation of these systems before one goes very deeply into the human brain, because in a certain sense this is not a visual prosthesis alone; this is a brain prosthesis, as Dr. Minsky has said. As soon as you make entrance into the brain-pan, you will find you are proposing to do many things other than just presenting visual images.

Among the scientific theories, there is not available for solution of this problem one analogous to that which was present in preparing to go to the moon. In that case there was available a very complete theory of dynamics; a theory of gravitation, including very elaborate theories of relativity which went into very great detail.

On the other hand, as I interpret what I have heard here, there is no theory on the development of phosphenes in the brain, and no development of a theory at all on the preprocessing of this information once it gets inside the brain. Therefore any attempt at this sort of simulation must, indeed, wait on such theories being developed.

I have one comment about Dr. Knowlton's presentation, to support the contenion that we are, indeed, talking about *brain* prosthesis.

It would seem to me that Dr. Knowlton can apply a transformation to his randomized screen to "clean it up" and make it look like the regularized screen if that should turn out to be a better presentation; that such a transformation could be developed by a digital preprocessor which would be presumed to be small enough to be mounted either inside a human being, or on the outside, if you can resolve the process of penetrating the skin, which seems to be a very difficult one.

It should be possible for a human subject to have some sort of personal control of this transformation that should allow what appears to be a highly distorted structure to be brought into more regular form. If one can develop some technique by which the user can "tune" this transformation, using a digital computer, or a set of circuits, this would allow him to bring the crude image that he has originally into something that is more easily usable by him. Thus, I think the use of the ability of the human system to adapt may possibly be less effective than an alternative attempt to have an external system preprocess and adapt for the subject.

We have a DEC-338 computer, which is still a fairly expensive device (but recently a much cheaper machine at $15,000 has come out) which, when equipped with a very inexpensive digital magnetic tape, appears to be a complete system which can be connected as a satellite computer to a larger machine. Using this arrangement, we have developed two animation systems for producing moving images like those you have seen, but we have not experimented with exact presentations of the types that were shown here.

We have generated mainly line drawing and stick figure animation. One can, through the use of local definitions and push-buttons controlling such a system, develop a stenotypist-like control, or a piano-like control, or a typewriter-like control, so that by pushing buttons one can, in a certain sense, "play" images on the screen.

We have produced moving images like those that were described at this conference in periods of a half-hour to an hour. This was done by filing away within the machine previously-generated images, various transformations, which have themselves been defined in terms of previously-defined transformations, and by calling these out, either by typewriter, by light pen, or by push-buttons. This can be done on-line, at real-time speeds, using a relatively inexpensive system.

Our experimental system allows us to store and retrieve images very effectively by a process which the television engineers call "delta modulation." This takes the *difference* between succeeding images and files those on tape rather than filing the images themselves. It turns out that one can store large quantities of simple pictures on very simple magnetic tapes, and this may be very useful for the sort of experimentation that is going to be needed for developing this prosthetic system.

DISCUSSION

HARMON: I am very much in sympathy with your plea for theory to develop this prosthesis idea. Certainly space travel, if developed on a purely empirical basis, would end in disaster. Would you also argue, however, that one should not proceed empirically in the present situation?

CARR: I am not a physician. I think I personally would only proceed with the very thorough agreement of physicians in this situation.

BERING: Historically, a great deal of progress in medicine has been made by ad hoc advancement, and a lot of physiological theories come "after the fact" of the practical applications.

THE IMPORTANCE OF NONLINEAR
IMAGE ENHANCEMENT IN
VISUAL PROSTHESIS DESIGN

T. G. Stockham, Jr.

While some of us have vicarious knowledge of what goes on in the retina when natural images are processed, very few of us have studied for extensive periods to gain a quantitative feeling for what those signals are like.

Of course, the retina is a part of the visual pathway between the eye camera and visual cortex. Many people envision this pathway as a transmission device which carries a physical light energy image back to the visual cortex in some form or another. Indeed, that is a vital operation, but the visual pathway is not only a transmission pathway—it is also a transformation device. While we are all aware that the physical light image that falls on the retina is transformed, very few of us are as conscious of its character and importance as, perhaps, we should be.

Figure 1 points out what some of these transformations are like. This image is a typical gray scale. Each different rectangular area is a uniform

This research was supported by the Advanced Research Projects Agency of the Department of Defense and was monitored by David A. Luther, RADC, GAFB, N.Y. 13440 under contract AF30(603)-4277.

shade of gray, and each appears to be approximately as different from its neighbor as the neighbor is from the next one. At the bottom we have a bright white bar, and at the top we have a dark one. Each successive amount of darkening seems to be about the same as the previous darkening. In fact, however, this image progresses exponentially from white to black with each successive darkening a factor of two from the previous one. This suggests that the visual system is logarithmically sensitive; that is, it transforms an exponential staircase into what appears to be a linear one. This is in agreement with the Weber–Fechner law.

Fig. 1. Gray scale illustrating the visual system's logarithmic transformation.

Figure 2 shows a classical optical illusion called the "simultaneous contrast illusion." The two small gray rectangles are exactly the same shade of gray. There is just as much light reflected from the square on the right as the one on the left. (This, of course, can be quickly verified by a reflection densitometer.) The rectangle on the right which is surrounded

Fig. 2. Simultaneous contrast illusion.

Fig. 3. Mach band illusion.

by a light field appears darker than the one on the left which is surrounded by a dark field. This can be accounted for by a kind of spatial
filtering process in which the slow variations are attenuated, and the
rapid ones are accentuated, or at least left alone.

In Figure 3 we have still another optical illusion, the classical Mach
band illusion. The bottom of the bar is all one light shade of gray; the
upper is dark. In between there is a uniform transition from light to dark.
Yet, to you and to me, the subjective situation reveals a light band of
overshoot on the bottom and a dark band of undershoot on the top. These
bands are known as Mach bands and are also explainable by the accentu-
ation of rapid variations and attenuation of slow variations.

Now let us observe a possible model for this. Figure 4 is an image
processing model. On the left is a transformation which changes physical
energy into its logarithm, known to photographers as "density." Next
there is linear filtering which, in the visual system, can be accounted for

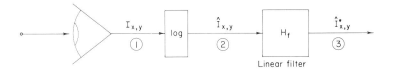

Fig. 4. Schematic of image processing system.

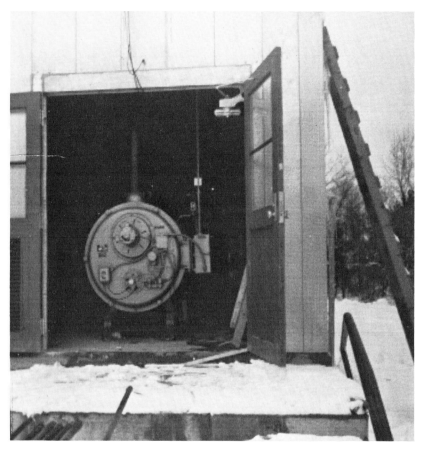

Fig. 5 Computer-processed picture composed of 340 × 340 points.

by the neural interaction in the retina. Think of this model as a kind of image-processing device that could be realized via a computer or some special hardware. The two elements in the figure might be a model for a part of the transformation that takes place in the visual pathway.

Now in Figure 5 we have the first of a series of real-world images.[1] Each of these real-world images is a computer-processed photograph consisting of 115,600 points of light, 340 × 340 points on a side, with approximately 250 shades of gray possible at each point. It represents a

[1] For an alternate description of these images see: Oppenheim, A., Shafer, R., and Stockham, T., Nonlinear filtering of multiplied and convolved signals, *Proc. IEEE* (August 1968).

resolution quality approximately one half as high as home television. However, home television will usually look much worse than this because while the technology is capable of producing better image qualities, the industry is not pushed to provide them.

This real-world image appears via a silver emulsion which is limited in its capability to handle dark and light values and thus cannot portray scenes with large dynamic range without distortion. This scene has a very large dynamic range, because there is a lot of light outside the building and very little inside. Let us pass this scene through the abovementioned model taking the logarithm and attenuating slower variations according to an appropriate frequency response.

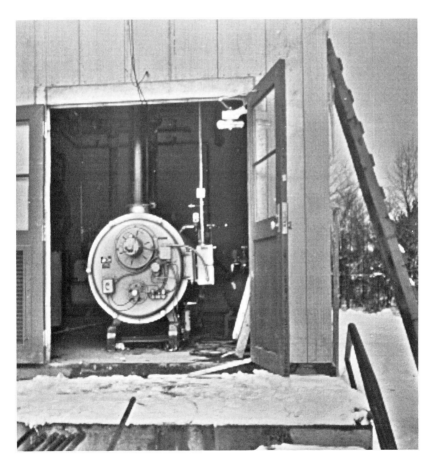

Fig. 6. A 10,000-point picture after image enhancement.

If slow variations are attenuated to half their original amplitudes and the amplitudes of fast variations are doubled, the image shown in Fig. 6 is achieved. The difficulties with dynamic range have been overcome and it is possible to see into the building, as well as outside of it. In addition, the perceptibility of objects is stronger than in the original. This image, again, is a 340 × 340 mosaic, and the "phosphenes" are capable of assuming approximately 250 shades of gray from dark to light.

For an idea of what a picture would look like with 10,000 points arranged on a regular grid, concentrate on the area of this picture which just surrounds the boiler. Imagine a square which occupies approximately

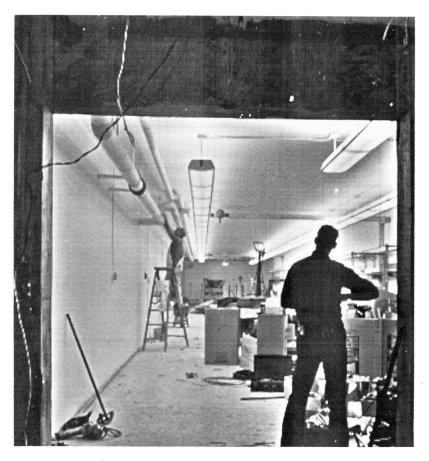

Fig. 7a. A 100,000-point display after image enhancement.

one-tenth the area of Fig. 6 thus dividing the 100,000 points for the total picture down to 10,000 points. (Perhaps a better idea can be obtained by holding a hand up before the eye, making a hole through thumb and fingers, and concentrating on that small portion of the picture.) It gives a bit of an idea of what could be obtained as an impression of the real world through a 10,000-point rectangular array, amplitude modulated appropriately.

Figure 7a also contains 100,000 points with shades of gray enhanced by the image-processing device that gives you a sort of super-retina action. Figure 7b is an outdoor scene with lots of detail. Figure 7c indicates the same object closer up.

Figure 8a is an original unprocessed 340×340 point scene, with Fig. 8b representing sort of an outline picture processed by a computer. The computer-processed image depicts three different shades of gray rather than a continuum. Concentrating on one-tenth of the area of this outline gives an idea of what can be done with a 10,000-point, three-shade or two-shade iconic attempt. Incidentally, it takes 100,000 bits to specify this outline. The other images conain about a million bits each.

If the retina is exposed to a square rooted picture as in Fig. 9a, the result is the same as the original, except that it produces a half amplitude signal inside of the logarithm. The picture fits well into the dynamic range of the medium, but the details are washed away. In contrast, Fig. 9b makes the image appear brighter by squaring the light image which is equivalent to doubling the logarithm of the image. This results in almost pure white and pure black everywhere in a semisilhouette.

Figure 10 is what one might see if someone managed to kill off all of the neural interaction in your retina. In other words, if one were to come along and eliminate the Mach band illusion and the other illusions which are associated with the low-frequency attenuation, the world would probably look as if viewed through a piece of ground glass. In addition, if the logarithm conversion is not made, one might attain a picture similar to this one combined with Fig. 9b in which we had a semisilhouette.

The next four figures depict a noise study. Figure 11a is an original picture without computer preprocessing. By superimposing a pattern of random noise whose energy is approximately half of the picture itself, the result shown in Fig. 11b is obtained. Adding the same amount of noise to the logarithm of this picture and then viewing the picture in terms of light energy produces Fig. 11c. Finally, by adding the same noise to a picture which has not only been logged but has also been enhanced as per simultaneous contrast and Mach band phenomena, the effect shown

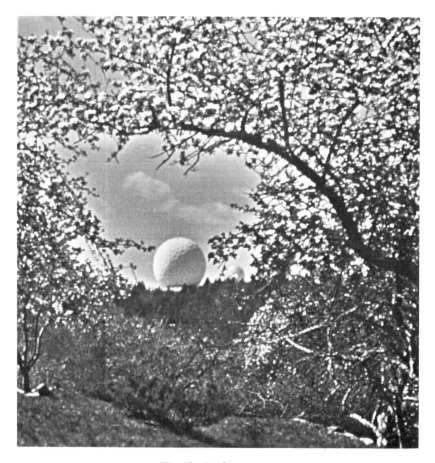

Fig. 7b. Outdoor scene.

in Figure 11d is obtained. Thus, by utilizing the logarithm and attenuating low frequencies, an image can be protected from disturbing forces (additive noises in this case).

If the visual cortex were to be presented with a very high fidelity replica of a physical light energy pattern as it might fall, let us say, on the foveal surface of the eye camera, the results encountered might be as poor as the frosted glass scene, the semisilhouette, or even worse. However, by using a preprocessing method of the type described, one could possibly avoid such disappointment while simultaneously protecting the image against any disturbing influence such as noise.

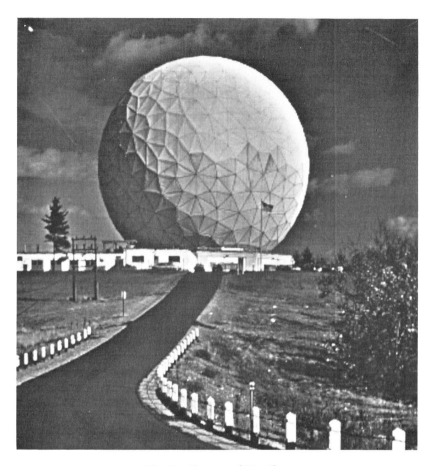

Fig. 7c. Close-up of Fig. 7b.

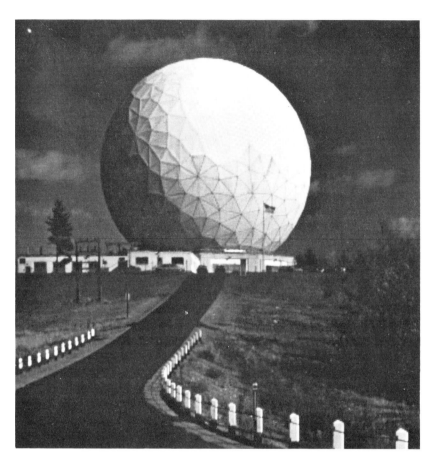

Fig. 8a. Unprocessed scene.

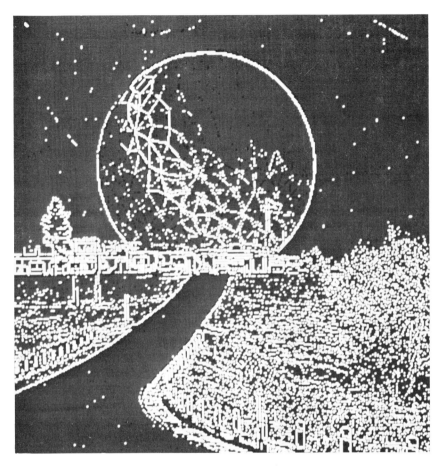

Fig. 8b. Outline display of Fig. 8a after processing.

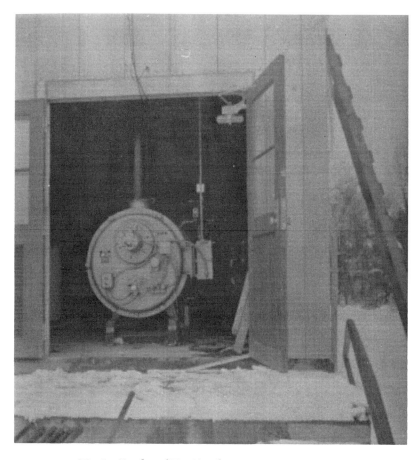

Fig. 9a. Display of Fig. 5 with square-root processing.

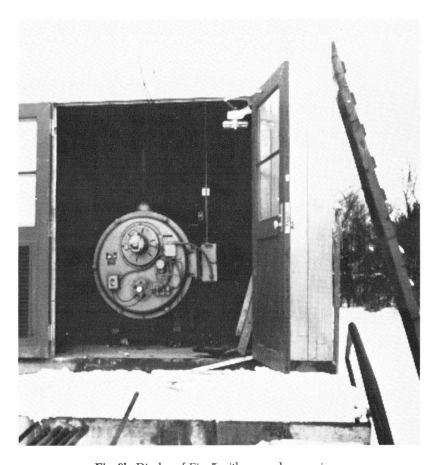

Fig. 9b. Display of Fig. 5 with squared processing.

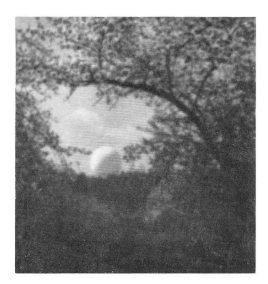

Fig. 10. Display of Fig. 7c with neural integration suppressed.

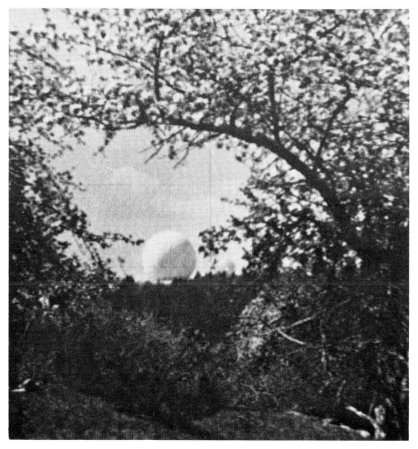

Fig. 11a

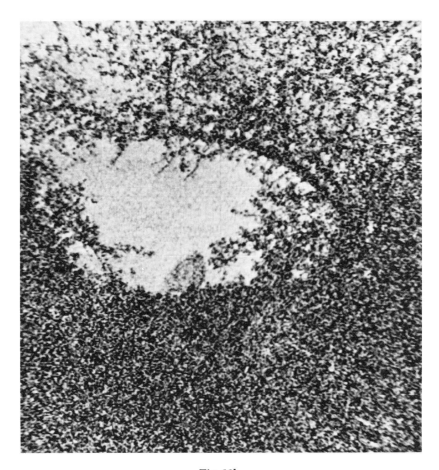

Fig. 11b

Fig. 11a. Reference display (without preprocessing).

Fig. 11b. Display of Fig. 11a with random noise superimposed.

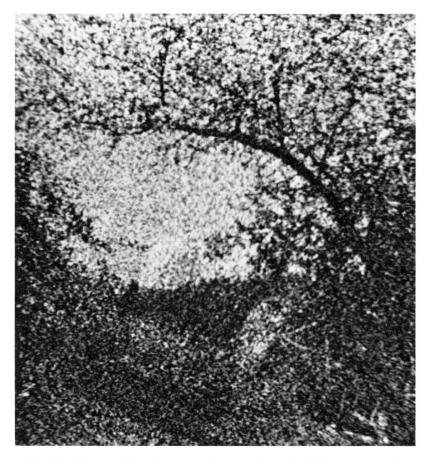

Fig. 11c. Display of Fig. 11a with random noise logarithmically superimposed.

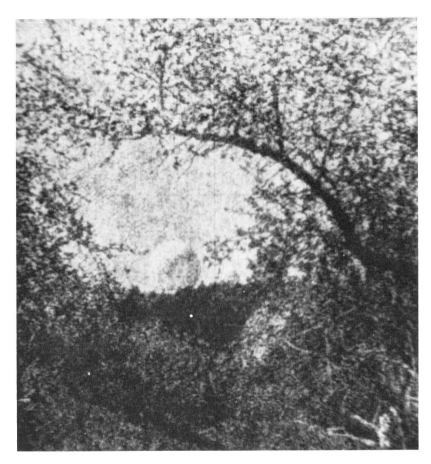

Fig. 11d. Display of Fig. 11a with superimposed random noise and preprocessing.

DISCUSSION

BERING: I think this brings up a very important point relative to cortical stimulation. When you stimulate the cortex the phosphenes you get are of constant illumination. It seems possible to get various shades of brilliance from nothing up to something terribly bright which means half tone pictures, if density is great enough, or some partially degraded image.

STOCKHAM: I would like to say two things in that vein. First, we know that gray scale information is passed along the visual pathway. How it is encoded at various different points may not be clear, but presuming there is some encoding at the cortex, how to excite is a question of breaking the code. I believe there are people who understand this problem quite well.

The second thing I wanted to point out is associated with the question you asked: What will pictures look like if they are not resolved isotropically?

If you fixate on any point in an array of 100,000 squares, there are too few squares in the foveal area, and in the periphery there are too many. The physiological map of visual space onto the cortex is like a checkerboard, with great big squares in the middle and little ones on the edge.

If you had 100,000 squares shoved around in the right way, a lot in the foveal area, a few in the periphery, you might be able to obtain the same image quality as is associated with many more points under standard circumstances. Ten or 20 years from now, or who knows when, you may be able to obtain this kind of illusion through cortical stimulation.

HARMON: Inasmuch as most of the phosphenes are modulated light, one might have to look where color is, or brightness.

STOCKHAM: That is why I say, why are these phosphenes *pure* white or *pure* black? I do not really *know*. But let me suggest if you are not very careful about how you excite them you can quickly use up all the dynamic range capability they might have in every dimension, tone, color, and whatever.

The point is that if you presented them directly with a low contrast physical picture they probably would be immediately saturated into some sort of colorless pseudo-silhouette.

I was struck most strongly by some experiments which I did concerning sound, in which I took the logarithm of sound waves. When you look on the oscilloscope at sound waves that have been carefully logged in real time, you find tremendous variances in wave shape from what you expect to see, having been trained on oscillograms of regular audio.

I suspect that most people who have seen a lot of video signals would be shocked if they spent some time in the laboratory looking at carefully logged video. The effect generally is that the log video signal does not change very much as the scene gets brighter or dimmer. One does not see a lack of activity in dimmer or in brighter situations. The major surprise is that almost all of the information concerning the scene is contained in a *very small* band of amplitude near the top of the log video signal. Most of the negative going activity in these signals is almost irrelevant.

JOHNSON: I assume that you are taking the original picture from tape, processing it either on a linear or a section at a time, and then displaying it. How long does this display take?

STOCKHAM: With my equipment, which is not designed to display quickly, these displays take 5–10 sec.

JOHNSON: Suppose you could take a degraded image, that is, take points spaced further, what percentage of this, then, could you store in memory at any one time?

STOCKHAM: The last picture which I showed was somewhat fuzzy and fit into approximately 3000 or 4000 36-bit words. The others take 32,000 36-bit words, or a little over a million bits.

JOHNSON: There would, perhaps, be made available to you an eye movement monitor so that a subject looking at this picture could have a very degraded picture in the surround, and have the density of points increase where he was looking.

STOCKHAM: Certainly! Splendid!

JOHNSON: And then, applying the various image-processing techniques to the points displayed would begin to show a considerable enhancement of what the subject can take off of the picture when he is the one doing the looking.

STOCKHAM: Right.

LOEB: I would like to point out that in addition to the number of points, and the density of the points in the field, these pictures reveal another aspect of resolution. The actual points here are immediately adjacent to each other. There are no intervening spaces of "unstimulated" black, as we might call it, as in some of the other pictures presented here.

I think that this may be a very importat thing with regard to the resolution obtainable. Many of the prostheses which we consider may, for technological and possibly physiological reasons, be incapable of obtaining phosphenes large enough and close enough to fill the interphosphene area.

COGAN: May I ask Dr. Stockham, if it is possible to put these phenomena in unsophisticated terms, such as "glare" and "halation," and opacities in the media? Specifically in your noise picture, is that what you infer a person complains of when he uses the word "glare"?

STOCKHAM: No. I suppose we are inconvenienced by the fact that my vocabulary is electrical communication vocabulary, and many of you do not have that vocabulary. We have all done photography and had some connection with it.

A very grainy picture, indeed a super-grainy picture, developed in a pot of boiling water, is very noisy; that is to say there are undulations of black and white on the film that have absolutely nothing to do with the scene to which it was exposed. That is what I mean by "noise."

In the visual pathways there is a lot of noise, too. Presumably the visual pathway carries an image from the retinal pigment back to someplace where it is abstracted. I presume the visual pathway is a relatively noisy, somewhat "statistical" device. I guess some of the cells work, and some of them do not; some of them fire when they should not, and so on. You might find if you measured one of these images as it would appear at higher neural levels that it would be a lot noisier than you might expect.

Consequently, I wanted to show how, by conditioning a picture through appropriate preprocessing, you could make that picture look less damaged by the same amount of noise at some point in the transformation.

You might ask yourself, how the visual pathway transports an image of the real world which may have a thousand or million-to-one dynamic range through a set of nerves which have frequencies that vary between fifty and a thousand pulses per second (a dynamic range of twenty-to-one)?

If we jam that thousand-to-one picture into that range, what are we going to get? We are going to get a semisilhouette. Everything will be pure white or pure black; very little between. What I am suggesting is that by taking the logarithm and throwing away smooth components, a picture will fit in this limited transmission medium and still portray the gamut of detail we are used to perceiving.

MINSKY: We have an eye tracker with computer display, and very soon shall be able to put up pictures and have the resolution increased in the foveal area so if anyone wants to peer into this they can come around.

STOCKHAM: Will these be gray-scale pictures?

MINSKY: Four gray scales, namely, eight levels. They will, however, have a foveal concentration where you look, probably a little too slow to be completely realistic.

Would you consider having quadruple rays of electrodes? This is a situation where a certain number of electrodes might be set up in groups, such as pairs or quadruples, with closer spacing, so you could have a coded representation of the edge direction or something like that and you might get quite a bit more out of a given number of retinal points than to have them in a regular array. I suppose only direct experiments will show whether these grouped electrodes are any good.

BEDDOES: Did you (Dr. Stockham) try log functions? Did you try anything else such as hyperbolic tangents? I ask that because you get some pronounced infinities in your pictures.

STOCKHAM: No. I used the logarithm for a very definite reason: It is the only convenient mathematical transformation that will map multiplication into addition. Images as you encounter them are basically products of an illumination field and a reflection field. I wanted to transform that product into a sum, so I could conveniently separate the two through linear filtering. It seems to me this is a natural signal-processing phenomenon that the retina is more or less designed to do.

BEDDOES: I think the hyperbolic tangent would avoid infinity.

STOCKHAM: The fact that there is no such thing as negative or zero light intensity avoids infinity.

MACNICHOL: I am sure this is why you mentioned the hyperbolic tangent, but it seems to have at the present time a justification in retinal physiology which the simple logarithm does not have, and a good many of the relations between the input in the retina and some of the electrical signals coming out of this retina show a very close fit to this hyperbolic tangent relationship.

STOCKHAM: I do not go along with the hyperbolic tangent except as a method to obtain saturation. For purposes of my discussion here, today, saturation is a secondary consideration. Of course without saturation my model predicts that we ought to see well in arbitrarily low light and certainly we do not, so it needs saturation but the logarithmic relation is a much more basic one. The hyperbolic tangent is an excellent saturation model, however.

MINSKY: Aren't they the same, except for very small values, $e^x + e^{-x}$, I would think?

STOCKHAM: How about $(x^2 - 1)/(x^2 + 1)$ which is a hyperbolic tangent saturating a logarithm?

INPUT SIGNALS FOR AN INTERPRETIVE READING AID

G. Nagy

This paper examines the various forms of input to a reading aid for the blind, irrespective of the output form.

In view of the widespread commercial usage of optical character recognition (OCR) devices, the first question is whether any of these machines are suitable for adaptation to the needs of the blind.

Readers are now available for reading *stylized fonts* on credit cards, cash register rolls, and invoices, *handprinted numerals* inscribed in boxes on sales checks and questionnaires, and *single font* or *few font typewritten* material in fairly restricted formats. There is no machine available to read unformatted typescript in a majority of the more than 300 typestyles marketed by U.S. manufacturers.

Machines for reading typeset text are not yet generally available, and here also there is little to be hoped from immediate commercial developments. While in a typical novel or biography there would be only about 120 symbols, with exceedingly simple formatting, there is relatively little demand for coding this type of material in computer readable form.

Most of the text required for automatic abstracting, indexing, extracting, and other information retrieval operations is much more complicated in format, involving one, two, and three columns of print, illustrations, mathematical expressions, headings, subheadings, labels, footnotes, super-scripts, and other anathema to automatic formatting schemes. Examples of such material are United States patents, legal case histories, news-papers, and technical journals of all types.

Altogether there are about 300,000 different symbols in use in the printing industry. This number encompasses not only the various styles, such as *roman, gothic, cursive, extended, condensed,* etc., but also varia-tions in the *point size,* which, unfortunately, does not correspond to simple scaling.

In a single publication of the types listed above, one may encounter 500–1000 different symbols. This includes the main body of text, passages in boldface or italic, titles, references, ligatures (fi, ffi, fl, ffl, etc.), Greek letters, and other miscellanea depending on the subject matter.

We must conclude that it is unreasonable to expect the early develop-ment of a completely autonomous reading machine capable of coping with a significant portion of the normally encountered typeset text. It is more likely that the first commercial machines will have to operate in an *interactive* mode, with an operator to guide the scanner to the areas of the page to be processed, to label selected symbols either before or after the reading operation, and to perform some manner of postediting or proofreading.

It is, of course, quite conceivable that many of these operations could be performed by a blind person. For instance the amount of information required to set up the format control for a fairly complicated page cor-responds to what one would see about 10 ft from the page, or to a resolu-tion of about 100×100 grid points. This much information could be conveyed to the blind by tactile or auditory means.

In contrast, a raster scan of about 2000×2000 lines is necessary to yield the minimum of 20×20 points per character block required to identify a printed letter by either man or machine. Note that this refers to a binary video display of the scanned page, rather than to a specially created, "character generator" display. For the latter, 7×9 grid points would be ample, but of course the character would have to be identified before such a display could be generated.

A flying spot scanner capable of operating in a stable manner at the specified resolution over long periods requires a cathode ray tube and driving circuitry an order of magnitude better than current domestic television. Lower performance tubes would require precise and there-fore expensive means of moving either the scan field or the paper to expose different regions of the page. A nonprogrammable scanner, such as a drum, moving mirror, or other mechanical device is penalized heavily by the amount of computation required to locate lines of print and to isolate characters among the millions of bits of information generated by a fixed raster scan. In either case, a fairly flexible processing unit is necessary in order to control the order in which the characters are recognized and to generate the output. That is why current commercial reading machines, performing simpler tasks than those envisioned here, cost several hundred thousand dollars.

These readers operate at the rate of 1000 to 2000 characters per second, and there are no significant savings to be obtained by operating at a much slower speed. Thus, it seems that reading aids to the blind operating in the interpretive mode will have to be centralized operations at first, serving several "clients" rather than individuals.

It is, of course, well understood that a blind reader could tolerate a much larger error rate than most computer operations. He is capable of taking advantage of contextual information in a very sophisticated manner. None of the commercial machines use context at all, and to the writer's knowledge, even experimental work has not progressed beyond the use of letter bigram or trigram frequencies and simple dictionary look-up schemes. Thus there is hope of significant savings in the proofreading and error correction phase, and in operating at a lower than customary reject rate.

There still remains the question of pictures. We do not know what to do about pictures, except that band-reduction techniques investigated for use in television transmission allow a compression ratio of about 10:1 in ordinary gray-scale photographs. Line drawings such as graphs, flow charts, and engineering drawings allow a much greater reduction.

The whole problem of automatic text reading is a transient one which will probably disappear in a few years, both with respect to commercial readers and as reading aids for the blind. Even now digital computers are used to control typesetting operations in whole or in part in several printing plants; it certainly seems unreasonable to use one computer to set up the type, and then another to read the print. Meanwhile, however, we must do the best we can with the last few hundred years' accumulation of printed matter.

DISCUSSION

MANN: If I may make a comment with respect to your last remark, with regard to type composite tape translation by computer into Braille, that was demonstrated in the fall for the first time on a major scale when a new novel, "The East Indian," was simultaneously published in print and in Braille, using a type composite and the dot system translation program of MIT. So, I agree with you.

MINSKY: But it is only a matter of time before reading machines will be easily accessible and of use. The commercial type reading machines are not even general-purpose computers yet.

NAGY: That is true; right.

MINSKY: Nevertheless, I disagree with the idea that it takes a person to format the page. That is something that is relatively easy to program. Nobody has bothered to do it yet. Also, I do not believe the availability of tape from the compositors will be an important factor. It will be much more routine to put the book in a reading machine and get it back from the machine in good form; it would be just too much trouble to get hold of tapes from publishers.

INGHAM: The other issue with the typesetter tape is to start storing the whole book and arrange for higher information retrieval on a text basis. There is no reason why you would want the whole book once the text is available.

MINSKY: But information retrieval programs that do not have access to the whole text are doomed to disappear as a very primitive stage of information retrieval. Most information retrieval systems do not have enough computation to understand what any of the words mean; whereas, modern programs are beginning to understand the sense, the intent. So, I think word systems that depend on key words are at the peak of their development.

INGHAM: I am not proposing keyword approaches. I am proposing, given the whole text there, the user can start flicking through it without having to make hard copy reproductions for use on the machine.

STOCKHAM: I want to make a point, and ask a question. I am sure we are all aware that when Dr. Nagy mentioned four million total points (to present a replica of a page of text that can be read by a human) he means much higher total resolution than we have in the visual system.

Take any page and focus on the centermost letter. You cannot read the whole page without moving your eyeball. Accordingly, the number of points that we need to stimulate cortically in order to be able to read this page, with a tracking system, would be much less than four million points.

NAGY: I suggest this is the number of addressable points you would have to have in the system.

STOCKHAM: You do not suggest I look at four million distinct points in reading this page?

NAGY: No, 2000 lines across the paper corresponds to the minimum resolution required to identify a single letter.

STOCKHAM: The other point I wanted to make was this: You said the bandwidth, reduction ratios for printed text and drawings was considerably greater than those so far attained for pictures of the real world. I would like to have you clarify that, because I was under the impression that it is not significantly greater. For instance, the picture that I showed of the apple orchard was a 10:1 bandwidth reduction from the original.

When I was at the recent Bandwidth Reduction Conference at MIT, people who talked about coding images of printed text and drawings were talking about compression ratios of perhaps 15: or 20:1, which is not, in my vocabulary, a significantly greater reduction.

MINSKY: That is without letter recognition.

STOCKHAM: That is right. Dr. Nagy, did you include letter recognition in reduction to codes?

NAGY: I did not make any statement about bandwidth reduction in textual material. I was talking about the pictures you might find. Your pictures are much higher in resolution than you would be likely to find in most publications.

STOCKHAM: I made the statement about pictures written in some language.

BEDDOES: He talked about line drawings.

STOCKHAM: You are right. Your statement about line drawings—let me ask my question in terms of that.

NAGY: The compression is greater than you can achieve on photographs.

STOCKHAM: Do you mean twice as much is much greater?

NAGY: No; 10 times. It depends on the line drawing, of course.

STOCKHAM: Okay. Let us consider a weather map. Let me just repeat what the people at the Bandwidth Reduction Conference said. There were some people there who have studied weather maps and coding in depth. For weather maps, as they are transmitted via facsimile scanners today in this country, there were some theoretical discussions which showed reduction ratios approximating 20:1. This is only twice as much reduction as the kind of pictures I showed. Weather maps are extremely cluttered binary drawings; they are not as simple as five or six triangles.

NAGY: Most engineering drawings are predominantly and primarily horizontal and vertical.

STOCKHAM: They showed those, too. The figures they gave for them seemed to hold water for me. They were considerably higher, but they did not approximate 100:1 or 1000:1.

EXPERIMENTS IN SELF-LEARNING CLOSED LOOP SIMULATION

W. M. Brodey and A. R. Johnson

Progress in direct accessing of the cortex by electrical stimulation allows us seriously to consider prosthetic systems which either bypass disrupted human–environment interfacing systems, or augment those already functioning normally. This conference bears upon the former. The study of either application benefits the other.

Direct accessing first brings the thought of blindness being undone by transducing light phenomena into electrical phenomena recognizable by brain: an exercise in finding the "right" transducers and filters. Many simple transducing systems have been fashioned in this mode but none has received more than passing interest from the blind. Though the devices have often fulfilled their designer's requirements, the blind complain that the information received is not worth the effort. The idea of an artificial eye, like an artificial heart, is intriguing. How can such a device be rendered congenial to the user? Can the task be simplified by alloying technological sophistication with dependence upon the user resources to provide the prosthesis with the "grasp" of active looking, rather than the simple "two-point threshold" of being shown?

The point is not a trivial one. Raw sensory information, passively received, has little meaning for the recipient unless he has the opportunity to explore it actively. As a passive observer, you might have an object pressed, moved, rotated, or otherwise touched to your hand and in the absence of any response on your part you would find it difficult to make an identification. However, allow but a fleeting moment of grasp of the object and its identification can be immediate: the process of grasping, as organized by the object itself, is the descriptor that is recognized. The behavior of the perceiver engaged in applying his perceptual apparatus to the environment forms the percept [1, 2].

This paper will particularly emphasize, and perhaps exaggerate, the effective use of the *effector* aspects of the perceptual system. As noted above, this aspect is often given design importance only as an after-thought; complex user participation in looking for/at what he wants to see we believe, is essential to congeniality of the system. The user twist-ing hand dials is not what we mean. We are concerned primarily with interfacing systems which organize themselves to explore the environ-ment in a somewhat autonomous way, and in whose behavior the user participates as one removed from the sense data. This is the kind of participation with which we are now beginning to become familiar.

For the purposes of argument, we will propose an embodiment which has not yet been realized in hardware but which is technically feasible. We will suggest later the steps of simulation which may be necessary for its actual design and fabrication. The focus of our interest at this confer-ence is upon the fundamental qualities of the interfacing system rather than upon its structural details. We hope that later conferences will bring more detailed entelechies to review.

Consider a prosthetic replacement for an excised eyeball which has been attached to the periocular muscles both mechanically and by way of stimulator electrodes which can cause those muscles to contract. No other means of attachment nor of signal transduction is proposed. We wish thus, to define an active search process which will elaborate an interface with the higher-resolution positional control loops conceivable via direct cortical stimulation.

Within the eyeball itself are: (1) an optical system with a single lens and variable iris, (2) a retina of a few tens of photosensitive elements covering perhaps 30° of visual angle and distributed in depth over the useful image planes, (3) a microminiature special-purpose hybrid com-puter with sufficient conditional programming logic to render it capable of self-organization, (4) output control channels for muscular stimula-tion, iris control, and perhaps a simulated retinographic potential, and (5) battery power supplies.

Consider the prosthesis to be a multiple-goal, multiple-actuator, self-organizing controller [3]. Designs and applications of these controllers are available in the literature on control systems but have not heretofore been applied to prosthetic systems. In this case the prosthesis experiments with the photosensor changes produced by muscle stimulation, adjusting the muscles so as to achieve goals defined as various spatiotemporal distributions of contrast boundaries on the simple photosensor retina. The purposive behavior of this system as a whole may be seen to be that of accessing for itself functional aspects of the visual information available from the environment. Its behavior is autonomous yet simple and recognizable. This loop of the final composite prosthesis is like a seeing eye dog (or reader), not yet aware of fine detail of what is wanted. The dog (or reader) is autonomous. The user does not have to teach either how to perform his usual routine.

The user is engaged in delivering his own signals to the periocular muscles in the "normal" way and also in manipulating the surroundings musculature: lids, cheek, brows, and in moving his head so as to redirect his attention or so as to experience the prosthesis as he modifies its normative behavior. He overrides or harnesses the prosthesis using the fact that he can change the state of his periocular muscles and thus change the effect of the prosthetic stimulation. The dialog which takes place between the user and his environment is by way of their mutual steering of the prosthesis. The extraocular means by which the subject normally constrains the movement of his eye in "attending" can serve as reinforcement to the prosthesis in learning the desired relative priority of the available goal structures. That is, he can *train* his prosthesis to *grasp* in a preferred manner.

Some objections have been raised to the effect that the periocular muscles are not controlled by a "gamma system" and have no muscle spindle afferents which can deliver kinesthetic information of eyeball position to the central nervous system. We acknowledge the objection in its specifics but find it somewhat empty in principle. A prosthetic eyeball may certainly be made sufficiently irregular in shape to provide unambiguous cues as to its orientation; and in any case the focus of our attention is to promote the use of what normally would be considered as output information instead to be useful *input* information if in fact it has arisen from a self-organizing system which is actively dealing with one or more aspects of the environment in real time.

The burden of our argument is this: that in the replacement or enhancement of perceptual apparatus, one must provide a purposive system whose behavior is indicative of the information to be perceived. The processing in the brain–visual cortex loop now has a visual context for recognition and interpretation. Information delivered by direct cortical stimulation enters into the user's experiments of looking/seeing. In the absence of an "effector mapping," however, direct access from transducer to brain is unlikely to offer means whereby the user may evolve a broad spectrum of familiar identifications. He is also unlikely to incorporate the prosthesis into his body image unless its identity for his is in terms of behavioral modes in which he participates.

If a simulation of the proposed prosthesis were to be undertaken, consideration would have to be made at the outset as to the replacement of each transactional channel that is lost due to the removal of the prosthesis from the subject's periorbitum. Initially, perhaps, a head-mounted "eyeball" would suffice. An eye movement monitor might provide positional data, and stimulating electrodes could deliver to the skin around that eye an indication of the position of the artificial device with respect to the axes of the head. In no sense, however, should such a simulation be expected to provide the kind of synergistic learning experience which a more closely integrated and cosmetically acceptable prosthesis would make possible.

Restoration of the interconnectedness of the visual system effectors with sensors may make scientific analysis by older methods more difficult, but provides for real-time study of the user's expecting, search, recognizing what was searched for or what was completely unexpected. It allows study of the user's efforts to maintain his information level within workable limits by changing his tactics for visual experimentation, if not his strategy. The user who can learn to use his prosthesis with increasing elegance of control will, we think, actually integrate it into his body image. This is not likely to occur if the prosthesis is an elegant camera to be extolled for its pictures rather than its congeniality with its user's moment-to-moment changing style of and need for picture taking.

We are going to be talking about the situation where the input and the output, and the transforms between them are now connected so that the output again becomes the input.

We want to talk about the actual person who is the user being in the loop, because when you connect the output back to the input, you are really connecting through the field of activity and behavior, and we want that field to be modifying the whole system at all times. So, we want the actual use of the device, the behavior with the device, to be modifying how the device operates.

What we are saying is, something that I think we all know, but perhaps have not said quite this way. The computer is now capable not only of operating in terms of the transform, but also helping the person to use the device. All of this is happening simultaneously. Each one of us here so far has talked about a piece of it, and our effort is to think about the whole getting together.[1]

I do not know what part of the slide is being projected on my face. You do; you can see it. I have a hand mirror here, so that perhaps I can see it, too.

How can I find out what procedures to go through to determine what is being projected on my face? I could use you as super-preprocessors just to tell me what is on my face. That does not help me in the future if I do not have you around. The next step is that you could tell me what to do. If I can find the letter, and I can, "C," you could tell me what to do in order to keep the white color in these. All I have is two sensors here (indicating eyes). All I can see is what is coming out of the bright bore of that projector, and I can see it with either eye, so I have two sensors I can carry over the field, and you can tell me what to do to move through the shape of a "C," let us say. Helping me through one letter may teach me a little bit of how I could go through letters and what letters are like.

What must I *be* in order to discover letters, shapes, and objects to which I want to pay attention in this scene?

Let us go on to the next slide. It might be interesting to someone to know that this is a one-way street, but you do not really have to scan across here and read the letters. It would be enough if you had something such as an arrow out there, something that could behave in such a way that by my feeling its behavior I would know there was an arrow.

The most interesting thing in this next scene is perhaps the red shoes. They really caught my eye. They are not quite as red as in real life. Suppose I had a device that was looking for or would respond to something interesting; a couple of fast-moving bright red objects might be interesting to it. It is the movement that counts. The prosthesis does not have to really know what is up and what is down, because if it is moving with respect to you, you can feel it aiming up or aiming down. One would want a prosthesis to give you a "feel" for distance, and what it might mean to walk up to it and walk along the surface or up to that surface. I would want a prosthetic device to give me an idea that moving my hand out to it would be appropriate, but it is not something that you look at so much as you would feel.

We want to show you the business of connecting the input and the output together, i.e., closing the loop. We are now moving a television camera over toward the monitor. There it is in the monitor, and now we

[1] *Ed. note:* A slide is shown with Dr. Johnson standing between projector and screen.

have a feedback situation where the camera is looking at the monitor, and within that loop there develop patterns that are quite unstable. The monitor seems to be "fooling around" with itself. We have some movies of this, and the small ambient changes in the elements of the monitor and the electronic circuit in the room will change what happens in that loop. Then I can put my hand in the loop, and when I do that it is very sensitive, but it does not do just what I expected.

The system is interacting with the hand only in a visible way. I cannot feel anything with my hand. It is a visual loop, as it were, and I am trying to interact with my hand, but if I were blind I could not see the effect I produce.

Our self-organizing eyeball has a camera with a retina in it of 13 cells. The connections to it are at random. I do not keep track of what is connected to where. The behavior of the eye, as it looks, up and down, and left and right, is driven by "McKibben" muscles. Each of these consists of an air balloon inside a braided tube, and when the balloon is inflated the muscle contracts and it feels very animal-like. This is all hooked up to a computer. The inputs to the computer are from the retinal cells, but again at random. I do not care where the changes of information are coming from. The program in this machine is a simulated self-organized controller. In this particular program the eyeball is simply trying to look for the maximum light. It is trying to maximize the number of photocells that see light, rather than dark.

One goal is to maximize the number of cells that change within any sample interval, thus representing a form of behavior toward contrast boundaries. If you say, "I want the number of cells that change from dark to light to be as equal as possible to the number of those that change from light to dark," then you will tend to hang onto contrast boundaries once you find them.

I have not gone any further than that, but I have some ideas. You can change the purpose depending upon what it is that seems to be useful to the person in the loop.

We are illustrating, again, a motive approach. Our technology is rather primitive. I am not steering that camera very much; it is sort of steering me at this moment with my hand on it. You can see the muscles contracting and relaxing. There will be some pictures with the device just by itself.

We are thinking of this kind of a device being in a prosthetic eyeball connected with the muscles. The muscles being, as it were, controlled by stimulation at the output from the controller. So, you have this dialog going on between *your* input and the input from the device in common at the muscles.

The scope pattern, which is very faint right now, is showing the goal structure and the goals are shown in an up-and-down direction. The goals that are being pursued are the horizontal lines moving up and down, and the output to the actuators, the vertical lines going left and right. The desire remains fixed in place. Whatever form the object happens to have at that moment will continue in form.

This would mean that the editing that takes place for the Brindley screen could take place as a function of the interaction between the person tugging on the muscles, which are activating this interocular procedure, and the interocular procedure itself trying to follow rules of behavior that it has developed for itself.

Just for the record, the control program that is simulated in the computer is a controller designed and devised by Adaptronics, in McLean, Virginia, which is what they call a "Probability State Variable Controller." In this case, it is programmed to operate on up to six actuators in the pursuit of four goals, although I am only using one goal at the moment. It is programmed so that instead of playing the usual game of going through a long list, it is essentially playing the game of hot and cold; that is, as the device moves toward the goals that have been set up for it, or it has set up for itself, it is rewarded, more or less.

The device does not make a measurement on the world and then try to do a transformation on that, deciding what to do next that will make it go better. It learns by doing. It keeps a record, not a moment-by-moment record, but sort of a history in an up–down counter of successful trends in a second derivative. It will reverse what it is doing if the trend turns bad, but will continue in the way it is going if the trend is favorable toward achieving the goal.

This system does not care if one of the actuators is defeated. It will continue to operate, not quite as well, not quite as fast, at a lower resolution. There is a "graceful" degradation, which is the current term for its kind of gradual failure. The interesting point is that you feel this—you put your hands on this object, or on the muscles, and you get the feeling of something that is so dynamic it is almost embarrassingly alive.

REFERENCES

[1] Gibson, J. J., "The Senses Considered as Perceptual Systems." Houghton Mifflin, Boston, 1966.

[2] Johnson, A. R., Organization, perception and control in living systems, *Indust. Management Rev.* (MIT) **10** (2), (1969).

[3]   Barron, R. L., Self-organizing control: the next generation of controllers, "*Control Engineering,*" Part I (Feb., 1968); Part II (March, 1968).

[4]   Brodey, W. M., and Lindgren, N., Human enhancement: beyond the machine age, *Instit. Elect. Electron, Eng. Spectrum* 5 (2), 79 (1968).

[5]   Brodey, W. M., and Lindgren, N., Human enhancement through evolutionary technology, *Instit. Elect. Electron. Eng. Spectrum* 4 (9), 87 (1967).

DISCUSSION

STOCKHAM: I would very much like to hear Dr. Brodey and Dr. Johnson say something more explicit about this. Do you think you can help us out a little bit? Can you "shift gears," so to speak, to outline a little more specifically and explicitly about how this might be an aid?

BRODEY: Let me start by saying I do not think what is required is psychological sophistication. There is a different point of view that we have been trying to build throughout the meeting, which is the view of speaking in terms of the loop rather than in terms of input–output. If you want us to do what other people have done, namely, to take the elements of the loop and describe them separately, we can.

Part of the impact of doing it this way, even though it is hard to understand, stems from the demonstration, which was set up to describe a whole loop with a person in the loop.

STOCKHAM: I understand that.

BRODEY: If you want to talk about the use of this for blind people, we will say at this point we are not in the busines of designing. We did not design this for use by blind people.

On the other hand, we are making a set of suggestions for whomever is building the "Cadillac" model; and the suggestions have to do with how you get a person into the loop where he is governing what information is available to him.

Let us consider, for a few minutes, that we are concerned about the practical problem of editing the material that is to go into our prosthesis, the intracranial prosthesis.

It is possible, I think, to find, and again to look for, patterns or features in the way that the man and this sort of thing operate and interact, so you find locations where he is tugging one way while the prosthesis is going another; and he seems to want to look in a particular way. He finally takes over the prosthesis, and surely at that point he would get material from the camera, as it were.

This is a technique of trying to decide what the man wants to look at, and as he looks at it he then gets a feeling of this being his own looking rather than the passive system which compels him to take the incoming information.

JOHNSON: Let me make a somewhat philosophical statement about the behavior of this sort of device. The central nervous system is engaged, if it is engaged in anything, in trying to discern the meaning of the object and the events around the organism.

I know that Dr. MacKay has presented outstanding topological descriptions in the past as to what the definition of meaning is in terms of the probabilities of events that can be associated with what is happening, but let me give a more behavioral one for the moment. Meaning is embodied in the appropriate response of the organism to the event or object that is being perceived.

The devices that we are interested in are ones which are, at all times, engaged in appropriate response, so that there is an interfacing loop, as it were; there is a self-organizing loop that is interfacing you with the environment, and you are sharing a part of that loop with it. You are not interested in the sense data which that loop uses. It is operating in a fast time with a lot of data, some of which may be irrelevant; but what is relevant to you is its behavior, and from that behavior you discern the meaning of what is out there. You make the identification of objects and events.

MACKAY: I should only like to try to use a simplifying analogy, and it will be oversimple, I am sure. Suppose that you had in your hands a powerful magnet in an environment which included iron objects. Then, as you waved this magnet about with your eyes shut, you would find your hand being pulled this way and that and you would sense the location of iron objects, in a different way, a more kinesthetic way than if you merely had a beep signal reflected back when an iron object was in the vicinity. And you would do this without attributing any "goal" to the magnet in your hand.

My question is, would it be sufficient to illustrate what you are saying to think of your artificial sensor not so much as being like a seeing-eye dog, which is somewhat like a person, but as something like a magnet sensitive to a variety of different things, not only iron, but objects of a particular shape, and so forth. If so, then you could say what you have developed is a series of selective skills, rather than bringing in the rather abstruse and perhaps over-personal notion of goals.

JOHNSON: We like using the word "role" these days, rather than "goal"; that is, this behaving object takes on certain roles with respect to this particular environment.

The principal point, however, that we want to get across is that the way it interacts with you is in the same modality as your movement of it. It is a physical response to a physical movement, not an auditory, or a phosphene feedback. Now we are not saying this substitutes for implanted electrodes. We are only including this as an enhancement device for forming percepts.

MACKAY: With respect to that, the magnet would do if iron was all you wanted to locate.

BRODEY: The magnet is fine, particularly the magnet, not only in the sense you have been using it, as a sensor, but also as an actor; that is, it is searching out.

LOEB: Did I understand you to say that you felt the visual prosthesis should have a certain amount of its own searching built into it, and its own goals?

BRODEY: That is right. In this situation, let us say we have an edge-detecting purpose built in. It would be looking for edges, and following edges itself. Then you would override it if you particularly did not like that edge. You wanted to get into another territory where it might follow other edges that were more interesting to you.

LOEB: Suppose you had this device inserted into the eye socket, and it was attached to the extraocular muscles. Is there any reason why you would need anything like this? Is there any reason why you could not rely on the normal tracking system which is elicited by the percepts in the cortex, presuming you have a decent image in the cortex?

JOHNSON: We have not suggested any connection from there to the cortex. We have only been talking about a self-organizing eyeball connected to the muscles with no connection to the cortex at all.

I do not think that much exploratory behavior comes back from the cortex. I think it is a much shorter loop than that, and we are trying to circumvent that loop.

LOEB: Are you saying, then, that a person who is blind does not have the tracking pathways?

JOHNSON: Yes.

MACKAY: I think we really should clear up the kind of control of the periocular muscles that is envisaged in this proposed device, because if the idea is to apply local octivation rather than central innervation, then there is no evidence that you will get any central nervous system indication of the direction of the eyes at the conscious level.

So, it is only if Dr. Brodey is envisaging implanting the oculo–motor center, and giving rise to collateral innervation of the central nervous system from the neural control, that I could see any advantage in using the eye muscle, rather than the artificial motor.

BERING: The eye muscles in the normal person are such that you do not know where the muscles are pointing from the information from the muscle. You know where they are pointing because of the visual information that you are getting back.

MACKAY: That is right.

BERING: I am not talking about theirs (Brodey's and Johnson's); I am talking about the ultimate system. If you are getting useful visual information as a result of the use of the oculo–motor muscles, you would then learn with experience where they were, and it would be useful, and it would be giving you information because you were directing it.

MACKAY: That is an argument in favor of proceeding with the development of a camera which could be coupled to the cortex, or something like that, but not necessarily this active, magnet-like device.

BRODEY: There are two systems we have been talking about. One is the loop system without connections to the screen. The other is with connections to the screen.

For the purposes of the blind, we are interested in the one with connections to the screen. For other purposes, we are interested in the other pattern, and the other path.

MINSKY: I do not understand why they (Brodey and Johnson) are proposing this in connection with visual prosthetics, since the magnet-hunting device is only good for one thing at a time, and therefore it misses the goal of a visual prosthetic, namely, restoring or providing a person with an ability to handle a larger number of data at once, including the relative ones.

If you have a motor action that will find only one thing, it will not be so useful as a prosthetic device. If this device is to be used, you had better know what features it is picking out. It has to have a way of telling you.

JOHNSON: The argument is one that we have had many times.

MINSKY: We have never had that argument.

JOHNSON: Let us make it very clear that we are not interested exclusively in the area of prosthesis. We are interested in ways of organizing the user's behavior with respect to visual space.

MINSKY: It has to know something to say that, and you have to answer to criticism.

BACH-Y-RITA: May I point out you have other muscle systems. You have the neck muscles. They have very fine feedback; and if you mount the camera, or whatever it is, on the head, you can point it wherever you wish, which is much better than having it point itself.

LOEB: I appreciate the research nature of Dr. Brodey's investigations; however, some of us are very much concerned with the very real problems of visual prosthesis, and trackers require a great deal of hardware. We do not have a great deal of room. I want to know if anybody has any evidence to indicate trackers would be necessary over and above the extraocular hookup?

BRODEY: What sort of editing device you are planning for this "Cadillac" model, so you can choose what nature of picture to present is one of the questions.

MINSKY: Most of the papers are about how the experiments on what kind of preprocessing must be done.

BRODEY: It is not only preprocessing. It is sort of letting the person into the loop to get the kind of preprocessing you want.

MINSKY: This is true; you have to; but still you have to set the preprocessing.

BRODEY: We are not talking about the errors; we are talking about getting the person into the loop so they have some control over the preprocessing that occurs, and the editing, and that is where, essentially, we feel the direction we are headed has some usefulness.

MINSKY: Surely, it does, but probably you cannot do the whole thing at once. As with many complicated things you have to study what kind of stimuli work, and what kind of gradients, and it is only knowing what kind of pre-processing has to be done that will let you guess how small the technology of today can make it.

JOHNSON: If I may add one comment to those of Dr. Brodey, we have been asking questions here directed toward finding out, in each piece of research that has been reported, where the man is in the loop; how he can modify what is being transmitted to him. Every question we have asked has been directed in this way, and most of the answers have shown no such self-referenced behavior referred back to the man for his modification.

MINSKY: I think that any kind of visual prosthetic would have an oculo–motor type of control. Is there anybody here that does not?

VAUGHAN: It may possibly help a bit to consider what ocular motility is generally used for in vision. There are, perhaps, three functions that we can identify.

The first is receptor orientation. We respond to certain stimuli which appear in the periphery of the visual field, frequently stimuli whose nature cannot be identified. We respond to movement; to brightness. We also respond to non-visual stimuli, such as loud noises with orienting movements of the eye. It should not be too difficult to build a sensing system which would orient to peripheral stimuli.

The second function is what could be called "scanning for detail." When one fixates voluntarily on a point, this does not necessarily eliminate eye movements. These continue in the usual pattern of fixation drifts and saccades. The eye moves in a pattern centered around the fixation point so that the retinal image is never actually stabilized. We do not now understand why the eye does this. It would seem that there is a necessity for shifting the pattern of retinal exci-tation to maintain a visual response. The visual system becomes refractory to a sustained input, so that a stabilized retinal image rapidly fades.

The third mechanism is one that Dr. MacNichol has already referred to, and this concerns the stabilization of external space. I have discussed this briefly in my paper.

It is not clear at this point that preprocessing in terms of specific pattern detectors is going to be necessary. There is not now enough data as to what specific transformations would be useful.

I know there are those here who have a very heavy investment in preprocess-ing, and I think this is fine. It may well turn out that this particular concern can make a substantial contribution to prosthesis implementation, regardless of whether it is with a cutaneous or a cortical input. But, at this point it is not possible to specify in detail the nature of the preprocessing required.

PREPROCESSING IN RELATION TO
LEARNING AND OTHER MATTERS [1]

VAUGHAN: While you may be given a very unfavorable topography of phosphene screen, and assuming that this is a stable phenomenon, how can you handle that information? How can you preprocess it in some way which will make use of this rather unfavorable phosphene screen?

STERLING: I really see very little evidence that the primitive perceptual field of a Brindley-type phosphene screen can be changed by learning. I see no evidence for it. I see no evidence against it, particularly. However, I would think it would be fatal to hang on to the notion that when we produce some screen we can just go ahead using it in the hope that the nervous system will make sense of whatever images appear on it.

POLLACK: Regardless of the amount of preprocessing or rearrangement we think can be done practically, there is an assumption of adequacy of input. You talk about a maximum of preprocessing. We have to have an adequate amount of information presented for preprocessing, regardless of how badly aligned it might be.

For expansion of the field there must be available some minimal amount of information for the preprocessing mechanism to expand upon. It is unfair at this point to talk about the Brindley screen as the ultimate amount of available input regardless of the preprocessing.

BRODEY: I just want to relate an anecdote which is relevant to preprocessing and to the point just made.

I was asked to take my television equipment out to a riding ring. One of our

---

[1] The following exchange articulates well the differences in opinion concerning preprocessing. Similar exchanges appear sporadically in the transcript.

colleagues thought that this would be an interesting thing to do. It turned out that it was at night and there was only one very poor floodlight.

The girls and the fellows were going over the jumps. After the jumping was over, and everything settled down, I went back over the tape. There were these sort of "blobby" shadows which, as far as I am concerned, meant there was nothing on the tape. Then the girls who had been going over the jumps came over and said, "Let's see the tapes."

I said, "Well, you know, you don't want to see that; it is just awful."

They said, "Let's see it."

I turned it on. One girl said to me, "My god, there I am going over." And then she was talking and jumping over the thing on the horse in her mind, and the next one said, "Oh, there's me!"

They were actually picking themselves out and talking about their style. It was very shocking to me, because as far as I was concerned, there was no image there. As far as they were concerned, within the kinesthetic and other sensations that were there for them, already, there was a great deal of information present, and in some ways, it became a kind of augmentation of their memory of things that had happened through other channels.

BACH-Y-RITA: There is a lot of discussion about the value of preprocessing, the necessity for preprocessing. We feel that if the information is presented through a normal receptive surface, such as the skin of the back, that any information from there to the brain will have to go through the normal relays in which some filtering and some processing is undertaken. We have found in our studies, in which we have compared, on a rudimentary basis, preprocessing versus no preprocessing, that there was absolutely no advantage to preprocessing in the context in which we studied it; and I think the more computation and filtering that you allow the central nervous system to undertake through its normal channels and its normal relay stations, as well as its normal cerebral interactions, the better it will be.

STERLING: Dr. Bach-y-Rita says that preprocessing is not necessary; in fact, it is detrimental. However, what do I find Dr. Collins telling me?

He says that under some conditions the subject discriminates things better than under others. We live in a world in which we are always divided between our need for computers and our distaste for them. But we should not allow our prejudices to carry us away. I think the fact is that if you (Dr. Bach-y-Rita) were to simulate your system using a computer, making use of techniques as those Dr. Stockham has suggested, or those which you yourself have seen to be useful, you could enhance the output of your very fine research by a considerable margin.

BACH-Y-RITA: First of all, there is a slight difference in the way I said it. I did not say preprocessing was unnecessary. I said it may be necessary. I would not be willing to say at this point that preprocessing will not at some future time aid us in our development; but there is a possibility that it will never aid us.

BLISS: On the preprocessing question, our experience I think is a little bit different from Dr. Bach-y-Rita's and Dr. Collins'. We tried three kinds of pre-processing; the white-on-black series, the etched-sharpening version, and something very similar to delta modulation, where the image that is presented is the difference between the new image and the previous one.

We found in those situations that there were circumstances that we could contrive in the laboratory in which each instance of preprocessing was more beneficial than no preprocessing. However, we also found situations in which a particular form of preprocessing was not beneficial. It is my opinion that something closer to the kind of preprocessing which Dr. Stockham has talked about, in order to solve the dynamic range problem, a general-purpose pre-processing, may be very difficult to obtain, and what we did may really need a repertoire of preprocessing schemes that the subject can have at his demand.

MINSKY: There is a very large gap between looking at objects in cluttered context and objects in a clean background, even if there are one or two or three objects overlapping. I guess in this discussion of preprocessing I am mostly concerned with that. When you have a really cluttered scene then you may have to do something artificial to separate out the objects.

On the other hand, nobody has done very well at that in the computer visual systems yet, except in some of the most complex, slow, large programs. I do not feel right now that you could make a practical realtime scene analyzer that would handle scenes and produce a fairly clean diagrammatic input to prosthetic devices. There is a real difference between clear background scenes and anything else.

I.5 SYSTEM DESIGN

DESIGN OF A PROSTHETIC SYSTEM

H. Schimmel and H. G. Vaughan, Jr.

Our earliest studies of the feasibility of a prosthetic system, completed in 1965 and 1966, convinced us that the balance of anatomic and electro-physiological data favored the investment of a substantial effort in the development of a prototype. The system which we concentrated upon is fundamentally similar to that employed by Brindley, but it is far more sophisticated. For reasons we have already given (see Dr. Vaughan's paper), we decided that we would have to complete a system which, if our basic hypotheses regarding cortical stimulation were correct, could serve as a working prosthesis for the first volunteer human subject.

In this review of our work to date, we shall first describe the basic system and its components, including some information on earlier designs, partly because the history of the experience may become important, and partly because it may still prove necessary to return to some of these earlier designs. Then we shall summarize a number of experimental and theoretical studies which have guided our design. Finally, we shall describe the current status of system and component development and plans for further work.

The System and its Components

The definition and evaluation of the prosthesis to be developed was given as follows in our report of 1966:

> The function of the prosthesis is to deliver spatially and temporally differentiated electrical patterns to the visual cortex of a blind human subject.
>
> The development of a compact prosthetic device involves a complex optical-electronic system capable of meeting the electrophysiological requirements, still unknown, of visual perception. In its essentials, such a prosthetic device can be envisioned as consisting of three major system components:
>
> (1) An optical electronic camera in which a visual scene would be projected onto 1000 to 10.000 light sensitive elements;
>
> (2) An electronic stimulus encoding generator system which would use the information contained in the light sensitive elements to deliver a pattern of stimulation to the human visual cortex;
>
> (3) A multiple electrode permanently implanted in the occipital region overlying striate cortex. This electrode would contain as many leads as there were photosensitive elements (1000–10,000) and would reproduce in an appropriate electrical stimulus pattern the light pattern observed in the camera.
>
> In evaluating the technological feasibility of the project, these three major system components were considered in the order of their apparent difficulty. Thus, the multiple electrode with its requirements for biological compatability and effectiveness clearly presented the major problem upon whose solution rested the entire project. The next component, the stimulus encoder, although complex, requiring more knowledge of physiological stimulus parameters than is currently available, is clearly a development within the current state of microelectronics. The photoelectronic camera was known to be under development in similar form to that required for prosthetic application by several NASA contractors, and was therefore not necessary to consider as a unique problem [1].

It was also planned that the prosthesis would provide for a simple topological transformation of elements in the visual field to corresponding electrodes implanted over the cortex. Different light values would be translated into different patterns of electrical pulses. Figure 1 shows the transformation.

Two different small areas of the visual field are sensed by elements E1 and E2. The light values L1 and L2 at these elements are converted to voltage V1 and V2 which are transmitted to separate stimulators S1

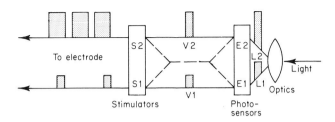

Fig. 1. Transformation of light pattern to electrical stimulus pattern figure.

and S2. The values V1 and V2 determine the parameters of the stimuli which are generated. In this simplified case the higher light value L2 is converted to a voltage signal V2 higher than V1. These are passed on to the stimulators S1 and S2 where they control the stimulus pattern. In this hypothetical case the larger voltage V2 has resulted in a stimulus of higher voltage, longer duration and faster repetition rate.

Note the joined dotted lines over which V1 and V2 can be transmitted. This is to indicate that it is not necessary to have 4000 separate leads from the photosensing field to the stimulators. The light values might be scanned serially and then transimtted serially to the 4000 stimulators instead of in parallel. Each stimulator then must include storage so as to correct for the different times of appearance of the voltage signals if the stimulus system is to act independently of the temporal scanning pattern of the visual field.

Our conceptualization contemplated some interaction between the light values in adjacent fields. For example, the limitation of the total amount of current flowing into adjacent areas is considered (see below and the discussion of Libet's results). We also considered the transformation of light values to enhance edge effects (see Fig. 2). Macro- and microscanning features would be included, either mechanically or elec-

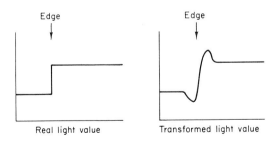

Fig. 2. Transformation to enhance edges (see text).

tronically. Although we realized that some major topological transformations might be necessary, we placed principal reliance on the learning capability of the user to correct for field distortions. To quote our 1966 report:

Requirements for stimulus encoding will be further defined during the course of the human studies, which are envisaged in three stages.

(1)   The effects of systematic variation of stimulus parameters on perceptual experiences of the subject will be determined. The effects of basic stimulus parameters such as pulse amplitude, duration, and repetition rate upon intensity and other aspects of the percepts; the spatial projection and extensity of the percept as a function of stimulus position and number of contacts activated; and the effects of simple patterned stimulation with and without attempts to enhance edge effects will be evaluated. The computer will be employed to control the sequence of each experiment series of stimulation and to produce the required stimulus transformations.

(2)   While the first stage may yield substantial guides as to what is effective stimulation, it is possible that the subject will not be able to develop percepts for even elementary geometric figures without some form of learning. In the second stage the subject will control stimulus presentation for elementary objects. Tactile and kinesthetic feedback will be provided so that learning may take place (cf. [2]). The visual experiences resulting from electrical stimulation may thus be consolidated into stable visual percepts. Although stimulation will be controlled by the subject during this stage, the effects of systematic variation of stimulus parameters will continue to be studied.

(3)   In the third stage it is expected that the stimulus pattern will be controlled by a real visual field. The subject will be ambulatory and the electronic stimulus pattern will be based on the optical input of the electronic camera and encoded on the basis of the knowledge gained during the first two stages. This stage will still involve learning and may guide further adjustment of stimulus parameters to yield more effective stimulation.

Though our basic design provides for a passive multiple electrode with 4000 separate leads, we recognized that a great simplification in design is offered by a combined parallel–serial approach. In our 1966 report we put it this way:

The complexity and cost of the stimulus encoder would be substantially reduced if it were possible to address each of the stimulating electrodes serially rather than simultaneously. A serial address system could activate each electrode utilizing column by row scanning, thus requiring only 128 inputs to the electrode. It is not believed that serial scanning of the entire array is feasible due to the required pulse durations and repetition rates. Thus, with 100-μsec pulses, scanning of the entire array would require 6.4 msec whereas it is likely that repetition rates as high as 1000/sec may be required. It would therefore, be necessary to reduce the pulse duration by a factor of 10, with a concurrent 10-fold increase in stimulus current, which would be undesirable. By subdividing the electrode into 16 $\times$ 16 arrays, the desired pulse duration and repetition rate could be achieved and the total number of stimulators reduced from 4096 to 256. If this type of operation proves feasible in the experimental prototype system, then subsequent electrode designs could be substantially simplified by reducing very substantially the number of leads passing through the skull and connecting the electrode to the stimulating circuitry. Certain other design simplifications might also be achieved since the photoelectric camera systems considered for the prosthesis also employ scanning for transmission of the sensed photic information.

The major features of the present design remain the same as those of 1966. As we anticipated, serious problems were encountered in making the high density thin film platinum/Teflon electrode of 4000 points. Success in this has eluded us, in spite of industrial assistance and what seemed like imminent solution of the problems involved in its fabrication.

Our initial electrode design was made with the assumption that adhesion of the electrode to the cortex due to scar tissue formation would occur, and that this would not permit removal of the original electrode. This assumption led us to specification of extraordinarily high reliability and long life for it. These requirements also virtually eliminated the possibility of incorporating any active circuit elements within the electrode array. The design also stipulated leads passing through the skull and skin to a stimulator. Rapid progress in microcircuity led us to explore again the possibilities of incorporating the stimulating circuitry into the electrode array. In our talks before 1967, with Westinghouse Corporation, we were told that the device we planned should not be seriously contemplated for two to three years; and that the specification of ". . . indefinite life with failure rate of less than 2% per year . . .." was not likely to be achieved for a period considerably longer than that. But we understood that the progress anticipated at that time would permit us to consider installing the stimulator under the skin, and to expect to replace it in a few years.

A system design based on this thinking is shown in Fig. 3. We had decided, before Brindley and Lewin's report, that the stimulus code would be transmitted either serially or by a multiplex technique through the skin via one or more antennae. How to transmit sufficient power to operate the required number of stimulators through the skin safely is still under study.

Brindley has shown that, in chronically implanted baboons, adhesions do not develop between the electrode and the brain. Instead, a membrane less than 80μ thick grows over the electrode surface, adhering to it, but not to the brain. This finding makes it possible to consider removal of the electrode when it wears out and/or fails, and to consider replacement by an improved version. If we can accept a more limited life expectancy of

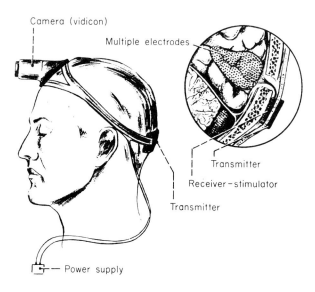

Fig. 3. Diagram of the prototype visual prosthesis. The miniature camera and encoding circuitry are external to the body and can be readily removed. Receiving and stimulating circuitry are implanted beneath the skin and the multiple contact electrode overlies the visual cortex.

some two to five years, we can then consider the use of active microcircuitry in the electrode. We are now exploring this option again in view of the difficulties encountered with the passive electrode and its large number of leads. It appears now that if one is prepared to accept a combination of serial/parallel stimulation, as described above, the required electrode density can be reached. This is particularly so since we require only that transistor switches and isolation diodes will be included along with the multiple electrode. The number of stimulators required is relatively small and can be placed either directly with the electrode or remotely (see Fig. 3).

Efforts regarding the optical component (an electronic camera) have been limited to following the substantial progress made by the electronics industry. A miniature Vidicon, equivalent to a matrix of 100×100, or 10,000 points, is capable of repetitive scanning at a rate of several hundred frames per second. This appears to be a more than adequate frame rate. Its output information is delivered through a wire pair. This stands in sharp contrast to the 4000 electrode points that must be separately activated by this output. Since we began our studies, there has been great progress in the development of photosensitive matrix

devices by the American Telephone and Telegraph Company, Westinghouse Corporation, and Radio Corporation of America. These efforts
are likely to yield a miniature electronic camera suitable for the final
prosthesis, and with a small number of leads (for an $N \times N$ matrix, only
$2N$ leads are required, that is, 200 for a 10,000 point matrix). Its possible
additional features, including adjustment of the visual field, macro- and
microscanning movement, mechanical or electronic, and utilization of
oculomotor information, are relatively modest problems compared to the
development of the other elements of the prosthetic system: the implanted
multiple electrode and the encoding–stimulating system.

Mathematical and Physical Studies

The design of components and of systems is highly dependent on the
size and number of electrodes in it, and on the range of stimulus parameters to be taken account of (e.g., voltage or current, duration, and time
pattern). It is therefore necessary for us to anticipate the effects of changing the ranges of parameters. For example, we have been concerned
about the possibility of excessive temperature rises due to current flow
from the beginning. Preliminary calculations, based on what we thought
were suitable variations in parameters, showed that temperature rises
would not be excessive. Brindley and Lewin's subject, they reckoned,
required currents and voltages three to five times larger than our calculated values. These larger values would result in temperature rises
10–25 times greater than we had anticipated. We have had to review our
original temperature study with care, and we shall present our results
below. First, however, we would like to consider some of Brindley and
Lewin's results, and other physiological data, which are relevant to
stimulus parameters [3].

THE PLATINUM–SALINE INTERFACE

The platinum–saline interface is extremely complex. Its nature depends
upon local metallurgical or chemical conditions with their own prior
history. Experimental study also gives varying results depending on the
surface conditions at the moment of examination. It cannot be described
by passive linear electrical circuitry, particularly at low voltage levels.
The interface has been studied for us over a wide range of voltages,
durations, saline concentrations, and electrode sizes that one might consider in a prosthetic design, by Mr. Victor Klig of Albert Einstein Medical
College, and by Dr. Robert Schoenfeld of Rockefeller University. Figure
4 gives some typical data from their study. It shows data for a 5.0-mil

(0.125 mm) diameter electrode immersed in a 0.05 normal sodium chloride solution; the other electrode is large, remote, and made of platinum. There are six curves for each of the four slides; these correspond to pulse voltages of 0.1, 0.5, 1.0, 5.0, and 10.0 V. The curves are in corresponding ascending order. They indicate that the lower the voltage, the more rapid the decay, and the greater the overshoot. In (a) and (b) the current enters the cathodal electrode; in (c) and (d) the current leaves the electrode.

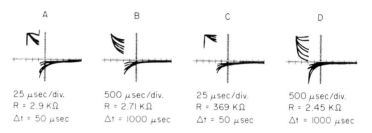

A	B	C	D
25 μsec/div.	500 μsec/div.	25 μsec/div.	500 μsec/div.
R = 2.9 KΩ	R = 2.71 KΩ	R = 369 KΩ	R = 2.45 KΩ
Δt = 50 μsec	Δt = 1000 μsec	Δt = 50 μsec	Δt = 1000 μsec

Fig. 4. Variation of normalized electrode current (i/i peak) as a function of time and pulse voltage and duration. See text for further details.

We can see readily from Fig. 4, that the data cannot be interpreted in terms of passive linear circuitry. Consider, for example, (a): at the end of 50 μsec, the current of a 0.1-V pulse has been reduced by half; now an examination of (b) will show that at the end of 1000 μsec it has been reduced to about 0.25. Under the assumption of passive linear circuitry, the current would have been expected to be reduced to 10^{-7}.

Anodal stimuli behave somewhat differently, but still not linearly. Curves taken at concentrations of up to 0.2 normal concentrations, for the same size electrode, cathodal current, and anodal current, all show similar patterns.

These data conform to the results of Le Blanc's classical experiments, showing that using large platinum electrodes the voltage must exceed approximately 1.7 V before direct current will flow. The largest part of the difference observed can be accounted for by the EMF required to dissociate hydrogen and oxygen (i.e., 1.2 V), the balance used for rate-limiting processes or equivalent counter EMF generated at the electrode surface. The rate of development, and the size, of the counter EMF varies with the condition of the electrode, current density, salt concentration, and polarity. The error introduced by considering only the passive resistance involved is smaller for short pulses and high voltages and for durations under 50 μsec, and intensities over 5.0 V, the error is less than 10%. For

long durations and higher voltages the current can be estimated by sub-
tracting one or two volts from the impressed voltage.

Electrode Size, Electrode Density, and Field Penetration

One of our earliest studies dealt with the question of the depth of the
cortex which would be penetrated by a differential field pattern. If we
put aside the complex questions of timing and phase effects, the question
can be put simply: If a multicontact electrode is placed at the surface
of a homogeneous conducting volume, at what distance from the surface
will the effect of individual electrodes disappear so that the currents would
seem to be due to a single continuous surface electrode? And to what
extent will the result be influenced by the size of the electrode?

A good estimate can be obtained by inferring from the case of an
infinite two-dimensional equally spaced array of square electrodes,
positioned in the $z = 0$ plane, and centered at all positive and negative
integral values of x and y. This arrangement corrensponds to a rectangular array with an interelectrode distance of unity. Table 1, below repro-

TABLE 1. Maximum and Minimum Field Intensity as a Function of Depth and
Electrode Size; Infinite Rectangular Electrode Array

Depth	Edge size = 0.5		Edge size = 0.1	
	$z = 0.5$	$z = 1.0$	$z = 0.5$	$z = 1.0$
$x = 0; y = 0$	1.129	1.005	1.230	1.008
$x = 0.5$	0.909	0.995	0.876	0.993

duced from our report of 1966, gives the field intensity values at depths
of 0.5 and 1.0 interelectrode distances, respectively; and for electrode
edge sizes of 0.1 and 0.5 of the interelectrode distance. The two points
chosen for computation of field intensity are (1) $x = 0$ and $y = 0$; this is
directly under an electrode, where field intensity will be a maximum at a
given depth; (2) $x = 0.5$ and $y = 0.5$, which is a point equally centered
between four neighboring electrodes; it is also the point for which the
field is a minimum at the same depth. The field intensity is normalized
to 1 for $z = \infty$, that is, to the field intensity value at which the multielectrode appears as a single continuous plane electrode.

The computation in Table 1 shows that for an electrode whose edge
size is half an interelectrode distance, at a depth of half an interelec-

trode distance, there is about a 20% difference between maximum and minimum field intensities; at a depth of one interelectrode distance the difference is less than 2%. At the latter depth, in fact, the grid has become degraded to a single planar electrode. When the edge size is decreased by a factor of 5, and electrode area decreased by a factor of 25, the results turn out to be substantially the same: the difference between maximum and minimum intensity is about 25% at a depth of half an interelectrode distance, and about 1% at a depth of one interelectrode distance. We also calculated the outcome when the electrode size was reduced by a factor of 10 and the electrode area by a factor of 100. There was little change from the results just presented.

These calculations of field penetration are useful in helping us decide on an acceptable minimum electrode density. Thus, for a density of $400/cm^2$, the interelectrode distance is 0.5 mm. If the cortex is considered homogeneous, then the differential field effects should penetrate 0.2–0.3 mm, the distance from the surface at which the nearest neuronal bodies are located. But the cortex is not homogenous, and inhomogeneities which provide special paths between electrodes and electrically excitable regions like dendrites or cell bodies would permit a greater density to be still more effective. Not all inhomogeneities are favorable, of course, and surface fluids and blood vessels will tend to pool signals from a number of electrodes, making a higher density less effective.

The finding that the area of an electrode is not critical for depth penetration is an important one. It suggests that for a given interelectrode distance the size of the electrode disk can be large, that is, that it have a diameter equal to about half the interelectrode distance. The reason is that smaller electrodes will have higher resistances, require higher voltages, and will tend to give higher rises in local temperature, than larger electrodes. And the smaller electrodes will have stronger, possibly deleterious, electrochemical effects. Higher voltages also impose more difficult system and component design specifications.

One interesting calculation which illustrates the results of the depth penetration studies just described is given in Fig. 5, drawn from our 1966 report. Here, field intensity is shown as a function of depth when 20 selected electrodes of the infinite array are stimulated. The stimulated electrodes are organized in two 2×5 (bar) arrays. For Fig. 5a the two bar arrays are next to each other. Figures 5b and 5c show them moved away from one another by 1 and 3 interelectrode distances, respectively.

The charts in Fig. 5 show the variation of the scalar value of the field intensity and its x, y, and z components along a line parallel to the x

axis and almost at the midline $(y = 0.1)$. Computations were made for the four different depths shown. The electrodes are assumed to be point sources. The effect of individual electrodes is apparent at a depth of 0.5 interelectrode distance, but it disappears at a depth of 1.0. The separation of the bars at a depth of $z = 2$ effectively disappears when their sides are separated by a distance of 2; but it is clearly visible once again when the separation rises to 4.

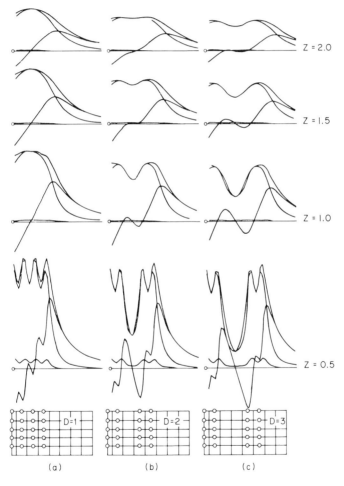

Fig. 5. Computations of current density as a function of electric arrangement. See text for description.

A Review of Physiological Stimulus Parameters

Brindley and Lewin's report [4] gives systematic observations of threshold voltages for stimulation of the human visual cortex over a range of stimuli varying in frequency and duration. We can compare these with the data obtained by Libet, *et al.* [3] for stimulation of human somatosensory cortex. Figure 6 is a reproduction of Libet's Fig. 4, on which we have superimposed computed data from Brindley's paper for comparison purposes. Note that the estimate of threshold currents in the Brindley experiment is obtained by dividing the voltage by the passive resistance of 3000 Ω. The counter EMF generated in the platinum saline interface could lead one to overestimate the currents involved by as much as 10% for the longest pulses (1000 μsec), and 5% for the shorter pulses (100 μsec). The stimulus rate for the Brindley experiment is 30 pulses/sec, which would tend to give larger values than the 60 pulses/sec of Libet's subjects. According to Libet's data, this difference could increase currents by as much as 50%, whereas in Brindley's data the increase would be limited to about 10%. Brindley has also indicated in a private conversation that the stimulus train durations are about 0.5 sec, which contrasts sharply with Libet's train duration of 5.0 sec. (This alone could account for an increase of 10 to 25%.) A final difference is found in the electrode size: 0.8 mm for Brindley, 1.0 mm for Libet. This factor would tend to reduce the currents in Brindley's experiment by a few percent; perhaps by as much as 10% (but see the discussion below of Libet's

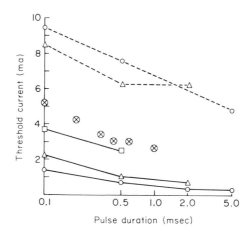

Fig. 6. Libet's Fig. 4 with superimposed data computed from Brindley and Lewin (see text).

results). All in all, it would seem that differences in experimental methods could account for an increase from as little as 10% to as much as 100% from Brindley's to Libet's data. One of Libet's subjects required about twice the current of the other two; Brindley's results give values after corrections of about this same high level. Figure 7 (our Fig. 7 is a reproduction of Fig. 3 from Libet's paper, upon which we have superimposed some data computed from Table 2 in Brindley's paper) shows that for the atypical Libet subject, the level is more than twice that of other subjects for a comparable stimulus at 60 pulses/sec of 0.5-sec duration (2.6 mA versus a range of 0.6 to 1.2 mA for seven other subjects). Brindley's data thus tend to be higher than Libet's data by a factor of 3 to 4. We can note the large variation in individual responses among Libet's subjects, but we cannot tell whether the differences between Brindley's results and Libet's are due to individual variability or to differences between the visual and somatosensory cortex.

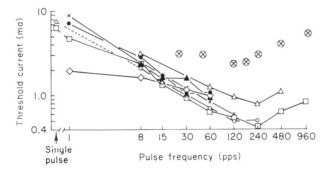

Fig. 7. Libet's Fig. 3 with superimposed data computed from Brindley and Lewin (see text).

Larger values are also suggested for Brindley's subject in Fig. 7. The computed points are based on a passive resistance of 3000 Ω, and a reduction of his reported values for 30 μsec by a factor of 9/28 (this is the ratio of voltages for 500 μsec to 30 μsec pulses in Brindley's Table 1. This correction was made for comparison with Libet's data, which are for 500 μsec pulses).

The decline in threshold stimulus as the pulse frequency was increased for Brindley's subject from 25 to 100 pps is not as large as the decline for Libet's three subjects from 30 to 120 pps, namely from 30 to 50%. But Brindley's data are consistent with Libet's data if we take into account substantial subject variability, already noted for Libet's subjects.

Libet's experiments generated some data on the effect of varying the number of stimuli in a pulse train. The threshold current required for single stimuli in two subjects required only about 9 mA for 100-μsec pulses, and about 7 mA for 500-μsec pulses (Fig. 7). In one experiment, in which the pulse frequency was 30 and pulse duration 500 μsec, when the number of pulses was increased for this subject from 2 to 4, the threshold current was reduced from 3.8 mA to 2.4 mA—or close to 40%. For still longer trains, the threshold current was gradually reduced to 1.5 mA. In a second subject who had higher thresholds, when the frequency was increased from 10 to 30 pps, the current threshold reduced from 4.3 to 1.9 mA. This large difference between the two subjects makes inference difficult, but the data do suggest that for a limited range of values, the threshold current may be reduced in inverse proportion to the number of stimuli.

Figure 8 contains some estimated parameters of minimal threshold stimuli as a function of pulse duration for long trains, computed from both Brindley's and Libet's data. Brindley's results have been used for the relation between stimulus duration and peak current, for the long trains of pulses at 30 and 120 pps; Libet's data have been used for the absolute values. Since we recognize that Brindley's current values were three to four times higher than the values from Libet's experiments that were used in constructing this figure, these data were labeled as "minimal threshold parameters."

The data on peak and mean power, and heat generated per pulse ($i^2R\Delta t$) were computed by assuming a 2000-Ω resistance for the 1.0-mm diameter electrode that Libet used. The value of the resistance R of a circular disk electrode is 0.25 ρr^{-1}, in which ρ is the resistivity and r is the radius. If we use a commonly accepted value of 300 Ω for cortical tissue, this would have given a value of 1500 Ω. The same value of ρ would give a resistance of 1875 ohms for the electrode Brindley used, but his measurements give a value almost twice as high as this. We do not know whether this difference is due to added membrane resistance in a chronic implantation, or to some defect in electrical measurements. In any event, we used the higher figure rounded off to 2000 Ω, instead of 1500 Ω, for the computations based on Libet's data.

Figure 8 shows some facts useful for system design. For long trains, peak current and peak power increase sharply as pulse duration is increased. Yet the mean current is sharply reduced, and this would correspond, for trains of similar duration, to the quantity of electricity per stimulus.

It is also significant, as these data lead us to infer, that mean power and mean energy per pulse both are affected very little when pulse

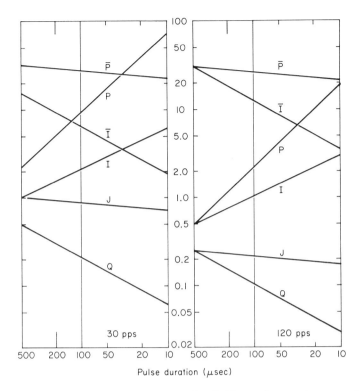

Fig. 8. Estimated parameters of minimal threshold stimuli as a function of pulse duration for (a) 30 pps and (b) 120 pps long trains. See text for basis of estimates. Peak current (mA) = I; Mean current (μA) = $\bar{I}$; Peak power (mW) = P; Mean power (μW) = $\bar{P}$; Micro coulombs per pulse = Q.

duration is changed by a factor of 50. Still more interesting is that mean power is not affected by pulse frequency, although the energy per pulse is substantially higher at the lower frequencies. In fact, the energy per pulse would be inversely proportional to frequency, in the range of 8 to 240 pps, according to Libet's data. Peak currents are increased as the pulse rate is reduced from 120 to 30 pps; the mean current is increased.

Figure 8 also suggests that a mean power of 20 to 30 μW is minimal for threshold parameters. If the pulse currents actually required were three to four times higher than this, then mean power could be increased by a factor of about 10 to 15. This would bring the total requirement within the range of 0.2 to 0.5 mW. We have included estimates on single pulses, derived from Libet's data, which suggest that in conjunction with his limited data on stimulus train length effect, it may be possible to reorganize stimuli into shorter pulse trains with the same mean power requirements. For example, the mean energy per pulse for single pulse stimuli of 100-μsec duration is about 15 μJ. If three such pulses were delivered per second, the mean power would be about twice that of longer trains. We noted earlier that one of Libet's subjects required only four pulses of 2.4-mA current for threshold stimulation. This implies a requirement of 25 mJ for four 500-μsec pulses, with the likelihood that still less would be required for 100-μsec pulses. Note that the single pulse stimulus of 500-μsec duration required 50 μJ.

Neither Libet nor Brindley has published current or voltage requirements for suprathreshold stimulation, but it is quite likely that both groups have data bearing on the question. It is not clear from the literature on animal experiments just what the appropriate stimulus parameters are that should be modified to increase subjective intensity. In the central nervous system, one common way of responding to increased external stimuli is that the peripheral sensory neurons will group their action potentials into high frequency trains without altering substantially the mean firing rate. How this affects the appropriate cortical cells is not certain, although synchronous firing by a number of peripheral neurons could result in a similar pattern of firing of a group of cortical cells. Here, the work of Landgren and co-workers [5] is particularly relevant. In the baboon, they showed that single stimuli of 200-μsec duration and 0.4-mA current delivered by a cortical surface electrode, could stimulate neurons immediately under the electrode; and that increases in current 1 to 2 mA would stimulate cortical neurons in a disk roughly 1 cm in diameter. Their result suggests that subjective conscious sensation requires the synchronous firing of a population of neurons, probably repetitively (because of the much larger currents, of about 8 mA for single pulse stimulation, required in Libet's studies). Libet's subjects also reported clearly different sensations produced by single stimuli and short trains, compared to long trains. Libet's work pointed to the larger currents required for conscious sensation in observing that subthreshold stimuli in the sensory cortex could produce motor responses. It thus appears unlikely that intense sensations would require currents more than 3–5 times larger than threshold stimuli, or mean power more than 10–20 times greater than threshold. It is also possible that much smaller increases might be satisfactory. As a hypothetical example, a train of two 100-μsec pulses at 10-mA current, with a frequency of 120 pps, might represent threshold; then a train of 10 pulses might represent maximal stimulation. In this example, there is an increase of five times in the mean power required. It is also quite possible that one might obtain increased light intensity through minimal changes in mean power, merely by changes in the train frequency.

So far, we have discussed stimuli delivered through a single electrode. When many electrodes are involved, the current per electrode is likely to be much smaller. Libet reported the effect on threshold currents of increasing the size of the electrode from a 1-mm to a 10-mm diameter. Although the area increased 100-fold, current increases range only from 1.5 to 9 times, with a mean of 4.1; currents ranged from 3.3 to 10.8 mA. One would expect the resistance to decrease inversely to radius—here, by a factor of 10. But the power consumption (which is proportional to I^2R) actually decreased substantially, for two cases, when currents were increased by a factor less than 2. In fact, for the mean 4.1-mA increase in current, the increase in power consumption would amount only to 65%.

The explanation for these results is not immediately clear. It might be that the most sensitive local group of neurons responded within the larger area. Or, there may be an effect due to spread of the electric field, reported by Landgren et al. [6]. We might also suggest a spatial integration effect in the cortex due to stimulation of many neuronal processes.

Whatever the explanation might be in detail, it appears that total current required to stimulate an area of 1 cm² at threshold level in the visual cortex might be only four times that of a single electrode. If this current were divided among 400 electrodes, the current per electrode would be 1/100 that of a single electrode. For 4000 electrodes and an area of 10 cm², the threshold current might be only six times that for 1 cm². Maximal stimulation might require perhaps a further fourfold increase in current. It is therefore possible that simultaneous maximal stimulation through all 4000 electrodes would require no more than 100 times that current required for threshold stimulation of a single electrode.

PRESENT STATUS OF SYSTEM AND COMPONENT DEVELOPMENT AND PLANS FOR FURTHER WORK

For reasons set forth in the first section, it appears to us that only a high density electrocortical prosthesis should be attempted since low and medium density systems may function well enough by mechanical or electrical stimulation of the skin. It appears that given adequate funding and necessary cooperation from industrial facilities, it is possible to build a high density prototype prosthesis within two to three years. At the present time a figure of between 4000 and 10,000 points appears to be the practical limit of a prototype prosthesis which could be constructed within three years. Technological limitations of matrix size have been significantly reduced by advances in integrated microcircuitry and further improvements are to be anticipated. Of great siginficance is the fact that costs of production do not increase in proportion to matrix size. Thus, on the basis of present estimates from industry, a tenfold increase in number of stimulus circuits (from 250 to 2500) would not quite double the cost. This is an estimate based on a modular prototype development. Actual production costs in quantity would be far lower. It may be concluded that there is no advantage to be gained either in cost or simplicity in reducing matrix size in a prototype system involving integrated circuitry. Thus, once the decision has been made to proceed with the development of suitable components, the prosthetic system may be designed to provide the maximum number of points which can be physiologically utilized, which is estimated to be 4000 on each half of visual cortex.

The discussion of system and component development which follows is limited to the two most difficult components: (1) the thin film multiple electrode containing 4000 platinum electrodes insulated by Teflon which will have the flexibility to follow the surface contours of the cortex; and (2) the decoder–stimulator microcircuit which is to be implanted outside the skull, but beneath the skin, and will receive code and power by induction.

Stimulating multiple thin film electrode: Over a year ago Westinghouse (Baltimore) had succeeded, in collaboration with us, in preparing printed circuit thin film electrodes with platinum plated gold sandwiched between Teflon. They had not then devised a method for effective exposure of the electrode contacts on a large scale basis. At that time they found it impossible to provide support for this project out of company funds and estimated that completion of a satisfactory electrode would cost in the order of $100,000.

In addition to the above work, three other approaches to thin film platinum-Teflon electrodes are being explored as possibly cheaper than the effort involved in completing the Westinghouse project, either manually exposing electrode contacts one by one, or perfecting technology for exposing the electrodes automatically. In any event, the work to date shows that for a sum of up to $100,000, and possibly substantially less, sufficient electrodes and thin film circuits to construct at least three 4000-point prototype systems can be fabricated. All electrode designs which have been developed or are still being considered are modular. Electrodes are organized from 32 to 64 contacts on 0.5 mm (20 mil) spacings at the end of a flexible Teflon tape. At the other end of the lead tape, the leads are spaced on 3-mil or larger centers, depending on requirements for bonding to microcircuitry. The corners of the tapes of the electrode ends which have been designed, both as squares and as triangles, can be welded together to cover an irregularly shaped cortical surface.

Decoder design and fabrication: Our basic designs depend upon serial transmission of a code to a separate switch for each electrode. In the simplest design each switch is either closed or open. A pattern of switch closures can be set within 0.5 to 8 msec for all 4000 switches. All switches within a microcircuit module are connected to a common stimulating source. From a combined analysis of the Brindley and Libet data, it would appear that pulses of 100-μsec duration, presented at a frequency of 100 to 200/sec, would provide optimal stimulation. On the basis of our calculations given previously maximal stimulation on a single electrode may require a peak power of 200mW and mean power of 2mW. If the Libet effect is fully present, a group of 500 electrodes will require no more than 400 mW and 4 mW for peak and mean power, respectively. If spatial summation effects are minimal, these values should not exceed 2 W and 20 mW for 500 electrodes.

One company has developed a preliminary proposal based on this approach, providing for a separate MOS flip-flop at each switch. Their proposal envisions a microcircuit module containing 128 points and connected to two 64-lead, or four 32-lead platinum–Teflon electrode tapes. The mean switching power required by this design would be between 50 to 100 mW for 4000 points. Peak power would be 20–150 times higher depending upon switching speeds. Preliminary estimates for this design shows that modules for three prototype systems of 4000 points each would cost on the order of $500,000. Other designs are being explored which are not only likely to cost less, but also allow separate modulation of the amplitude at each switch point.

One of the factors leading to higher costs of microcircuitry has been the necessity, as a result of Dr. Brindley's experiment with his first subject, to provide for higher currents than originally contemplated. We have been discussing with Dr. Brindley the possibility of his performing additional experiments oriented particularly toward establishing those maximum stimulus parameters which most affect system costs, e.g., the requirement of up to 40 V stimulation per point.

Combined electrode and switching microcircuitry: We have from the beginning of the study examined periodically the feasibility of incorporating the switching microcircuitry directly with the cortical electrode. Within the past two years, progress in MOS/FET circuit technology has permitted the preparation of small enough chips to incorporate the required decoder–stimulator circuitry within a package less than 0.5 mm thick. While such an electrode would lose the advantage of flexibility, each chip could be small enough to contact the cortex underlying it, and curvature of the electrode would be obtained at the junctions among chips. The advantage of such a design is great, since the conversion from serial input of the code to the parallel switching pattern would occur within the electrode, thus sharply reducing the number of leads required, from receivers to intracranial electrode, which would pass through the skull. Until recently these circuits have been packaged in steel and ceramic cases which could not be implanted intracranially, although they could have been coated with Silastic for subcutaneous implantation, due to their size. Recently, however, there have been apparently successful experiments in packaging these circuits in a new plastic material, which when coated with Silastic, would permit development of encapsulated chips of the required size for cortical implantation. This work has not reached the commercial stage, but has been sufficiently promising to be considered as a serious possibility for our initial prototype system. Accordingly, we are pursuing a design which would provide Silastic electrode tapes with platinum electrodes protruding from microcircuits embedded therein. Each tape would contain approximately 500 contacts and would require only six input leads. For the 4000 contact system less than 50 wires would have to be brought through the skull to the subcutaneous code and power receivers. If this design can be implemented within the time schedule set for the thin film system it would be preferable, due to its relative simplicity and the likelihood of substantially lower cost.

Other components present no major challenge. A prototype transmitter–receiver set has been constructed for measuring temperature rise of intervening tissue as a result of transmission of stimulus power through the skin. Estimated power requirements are high, and the results of these studies will be employed to insure safety of the system. Other safety studies now under way include a check on the theoretical temperature rise studies previously summarized. Under the worst conditions unacceptable temperature rises might occur in a high-density system, although the possibility of spatial summation of stimulating current (the "Libet effect—see below) would substantially ameliorate this problem by reducing the total power requirements. The theoretical analysis is now being checked empirically in animals, employing a special platinum–platinum alloy stimulating thermocouple electrode which has been developed for this purpose. The experiments, both acute and chronic, are employing rat cortex, and stimulus parameters equalling and exceeding the values predicted from the human data obtained by Brindley will be evaluated.

Final selection of the camera and its adaptation, and design of the encoder, are awaiting the completion of decisions about the thin film electrode and decoder design. During the past four years there has been substantial progress in miniature Vidicon camera (Sony) and matrix type sensing devices (Westinghouse, RCA, and AT&T). The relative merits and availability of the various sensing devices at the estimated date for prototype system completion (about two years) are being continually evaluated. Selection can be deferred for at least a year, and depends upon the rate of development of other more critical system components.

The detailed design of the encoder whch will translate output from the camera into the pulse code to be transmited through the skin (to set up the pattern of cortical stimuli) awaits final decision on decoder design. The prototype will be fabricated from existing microcircuit components rather than employing specially designed integrated circuitry, as is required for the intracranial components. This will permit maximum flexibility at relatively low cost, but will comprise a larger extracranial package than will ultimately be possible. Special microcircuitry will be fabricated only after the initial studies on the prototype prosthesis have been carried out with a human recipient.

Financial requirements and time schedules: We have presented our designs and specification to a number of the leading electronic companies. It would appear that the total project could be completed within five years, of which the first three would be required for fabrication of components and assembly and testing of the entire system. The financial requirement is of the order of one million dollars. Table 2 gives a provisional schedule based on separate electrode and microcircuit compo-

TABLE 2. ELECTROCORTICAL VISUAL PROSTHESIS SYSTEM SCHEDULE OF FABRICATION AND EVALUATION

	FABRICATION PROGRAM			EVALUATION PROGRAM
1970	COMPLETION AND REVIEW OF ALL DESIGNS FOR CORTICAL SYSTEM	SAFETY TESTS IN ANIMALS OF COMPONENTS AND ASSEMBLED CORTICAL SYSTEM	SPECIAL DESIGNS AND FABRICATION FOR SKIN EXPERIMENTS	ELEMENTARY SKIN EXPERIMENTS
	LETTING OF SUBCONTRACTS			TEST AND USE OF PRIMITIVE SKIN PROTOTYPE SYSTEMS
1971	FABRICATION OF ALL MAJOR COMPONENTS—ELECTRODE–DECODER–STIMULATOR, CAMERA, ENCODER, TRANSMITTER–RECEIVER SETS AND POWER SUPPLIES			
1972				TEST AND USE OF SOPHISTICATED SKIN PROTOTYPE SYSTEM
1973	ASSEMBLY OF SYSTEM			
1974	REFINEMENT OF EXTERNAL SYSTEMS AND DEVELOPMENT OF NEW DESIGNS			TEST AND USE OF CORTICAL SYSTEM WITH HUMAN RECIPIENT(S)

nents. If the electrodees can be directly integrated with the decoder-stimulating microcircuits, then camera fabrication would be advanced and a separate and simple prototype prosthetic would be developed for skin stimulation tests (Fig. 9).

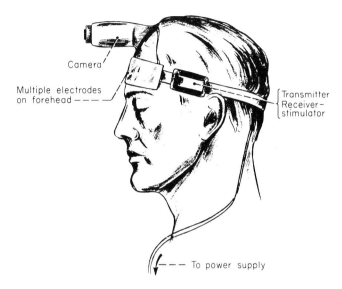

Fig. 9. An electrocutaneous prosthesis employing an electrode matrix overlying the forehead. The camera and encoding system utilize components required for the cortical prosthesis.

Appendix

SOME VOLUME, CURRENT, RESISTANCE, AND HEAT RELATIONSHIPS: SINGLE ELECTRODE

Consider the case of a single electrode at the surface of a medium assumed to be homogeneous, which has a resistivity ρ_0 of 500 Ωcm-1 (after Brindley), a heat conductivity k_0 assumed to be 5×10^{-3} W $°C^{-1}$ cm-1, a heat capacity c_0 the same as water ($c_0 = 4.2$ W $\times$ sec $\times$ cm-3 $\times$ $°C^{-1}$). Finally, assume a heat absorption factor a_0, due to blood circulation, in which $a_0 = 4.2 \times 10^{-2}$ W cm-3 $°C^{-1}$.

The basic heat flow equation has the form

$$k_0 \Delta^2 T + i^2 \rho_0 - a_0 T = c_0 \frac{\delta T}{\delta t} \tag{1}$$

where k_0, ρ_0, a_0, c_0 are parameters of the medium previously defined and estimated, T is temperature, and i is local current density.

To simplify discussion and solutions, assume a half-sphere electrode of radius r_0 instead of a disk of radius r_1, where $r_0 = 2r_1/\pi$, so that the disk and half-sphere electrode have the same resistance R_0, with an area 20% less for the latter than that of the disk electrode. If V_0 is the electrode voltage and I_0 the total current, then we have the following useful relations:

$$R_0 = V_0 I^{-1}{}_0 = \rho_0(2\pi r_0)^{-1} = \rho_0(4r_1)^{-1};$$
$$i^2\rho_0 = I_0{}^2\rho_0(2\pi r^2)^{-2} = I_0 V_0 r_0(2\pi r^4)^{-1}; \quad i = I_0(2\pi r^2)^{-1}.$$

Assuming spherical symmetry, Eq. (1) can be put in the form:

$$k_1 \frac{\delta^2 U}{\delta x^2} + b_0 x^{-3} - a_0 U = c_0 \frac{\delta U}{\delta t} \tag{2}$$

where $k_1 = k_0 r_0{}^{-2} = 1.2 \times 10^{-2} r_1{}^{-2}$; $\quad b_0 = P_0(2\pi r_0{}^3)^{-1} = 0.63 P_0 r_1{}^{-3}$; $P_0 = I_0 V_0 = I_0{}^2 R_0 = V_0{}^2 R_0{}^{-1}$; $\quad U = Tx$; $\quad x = r/r_0$.

In the above equation, the spatial dimension has been referred to the electrode radius; at the surface of the electrode, $x = 1$. We note that as the radius gets smaller, heat conduction gets more important in terms of this space unit. This is as expected and P_0 is seen to be power.

Estimates of various effects can be obtained easily from Eq. (2). First consider temperature rise ΔT during a short pulse of duration Δt. For very short pulses a satisfactory estimate can be obtained by ignoring both conduction and absorption; then the range of validity of such an estimate can be checked if necessary. Thus,

$$\Delta T = b_0 \, \Delta t \, c_0{}^{-1} x^{-4}; \quad \Delta T_{max} = 0.15 \, P_0 \, \Delta t \, r_1{}^{-3} \qquad \text{for } x = 1. \tag{3}$$

It had been noted previously that $P_0 \, \Delta t$ (the "J" of Fig. 8) is approximately independent of pulse duration at a fixed frequency. For 120 pps stimuli, $J = P_0 \, \Delta t \cong 0.2 \, \mu\text{J}$. For an $r_1 = 4 \times 10^{-2}$ cm (after Brindley) Eq. (3) gives $\Delta T_{max} \cong 5 \times 10^{-4} \, °\text{C}$. Even with a forty-fold increase in stimulating current, the temperature would rise less than $1°\text{C}$. It is, therefore, unnecessary to examine the offset realized by taking into account absorption or conduction.

In the case of continued stimulation, an estimate of the maximum temperature rise can be obtained by examining the steady state solution $\delta T/\delta t = 0$ of Eq. (2). As a first step, absorption will be ignored. Also, in place of the coefficient b_0, one must use a $\overline{b}_0$ based on a mean power, $\overline{P_0}$ which is equal to $D_0 P_0$, where D_0 is the duty cycle.

Equation (2) is readily integrated under these assumptions and the result is

$$T = \overline{b_0}k^{-1}(x^{-1} - 0.5x^{-2}); \quad T_{max} = 25\overline{P_0}/r_1 \quad \text{for } x = 1. \qquad (4)$$

From Fig. 8, we note that $\overline{P_0}$ is independent of pulse frequency and duration in the range 30–120 pps, and it is approximately equal to 25 μW. For a radius $r_1 = 4 \times 10^{-2}$ cm, we find $\Delta T_{max} \cong 1.5 \times 10^{-2}$ °C.

Thus, if current levels were increased by a factor of 10 and power accordingly by a factor of 100, the maximum temperature rise would be about 1.5°C. What is the effectiveness of absorption? To estimate it consider the ratio of the heat absorbed to the heat being generated (i.e., of the third term to the second). It is

$$3.5r_1^2(x^3 - 0.5x^2) \cong 3.5r_1^2x^3 \text{ if } x > 2. \qquad (5)$$

For $x = 3$ and $r_1 = 4 \times 10^{-2}$, the ratio equals about 0.5, indicating that absorption would tend to dominate at about this distance. Since the temperature at this distance is about 60% of the surface maximum according to Eq. (4), then to a first rough approximation, it is seen that absorption will tend to cut the maximum temperature by a factor of about 0.5. In fact, if one takes into account only absorption, the steady state solution for Eq. (2) is

$$T = 0.63 \, \overline{P_0}a_0^{-1}r_1^{-3}x^{-4}.$$

For the example previously cited, the temperature change at $x = 4$ would be only 10^{-3} °C, justifying that absorption would reduce ΔT_{max} by about half.

It is difficult to generalize these results to the case of electrodes of smaller radii, because there are no clear guides to the current and power requirements for stimulation by smaller electrodes. If neuronal bodies or processes to be affected are at a distance of the same order of magnitude or less as the electrode diameter, we can expect Libet's basic finding to hold, and less power would be required as the radius of the electrode is decreased—but only slightly. Thus, if P_0 and $\overline{P_0}$ were decreased by a factor of 0.9, while r_1 was decreased by a factor of 0.3, then ΔT_{max} and T_{max} would increase by factors of 33 and 3, respectively. This would give quite a considerable range of stimulus levels, but the range is far more restricted than for larger electrodes, particularly regarding the temperature rise during the pulse. We might then try to examine the estimate given for ΔT in Eq. (3), and ask whether it is seriously reduced by taking into account heat conduction and/or absorption. If we compare the first and third terms with the second term in Eq. (2), for heat generation, we find that for a radius $r_1 = 1.3 \times 10^{-2}$ cm, conduction would begin to remove only about 10% of the heat at the surface after a pulse duration of 2 msec, while absorption becomes effective even more slowly. In the range of pulses which we have been considering, neither of these factors affects our estimates.

Temperature Rise: Multiple Electrodes

We shall use Libet's data to estimate the temperature rise for simultaneous stimulation of the entire area A of 10 cm^2. In a first-order estimate, the problem can be divided into two parts. First, we shall deal with current flows and temperature rises up to the surface of the electrode as though the electrode were continuous. Second, we shall add an additional temperature rise due to the local currents from individual electrodes.

This situation can be approximated by considering the continuous electrode to correspond to a disk of $r_1 \cong 1.8$ cm. To this approximation we add local effects in the immediate neighborhood of the electrode. The concave curvature would tend to give higher values of current density and temperature, but this will be offset by an irregular shape and, for a first approximation, appears adequate.

In accordance with our earlier discussion of Libet's results, we shall assume that approximately 60 times as much current is required for minimal threshold stimulation as in the case of a single electrode. For a 100-μsec pulse duration and 120-pps frequency, this would require 60-mA current flow from the entire electrode (see Fig. 8). For a tissue resistivity of 300 Ω/cm, this means an electrode resistance $R_0' \cong 40$ Ω, and a driving voltage $V_0' \cong 2.5$ V. Peak power would be about 150 mW, mean power about 2 mW. Inserting these values into Eq. (3), we find that ΔT_{max} is less than 10^{-6} °C. This temperature rise is insignificant unless currents are increased by a factor of 1000.

Regarding the steady state temperature rise under conditions of continued stimulation, only the effect of absorption appears important. Integrating Eq. (2) gives

$$\Delta T = \overline{b_0' a_0}^{-1} x^{-4}; \quad \Delta T_{max} \cong 5 \times 10^{-3}. \tag{6}$$

Current levels could therefore be increased by a factor of 15, for a temperature rise of about 1°C.

Individual electrode currents would have been reduced by a factor of 0.01 for the case of the multiple electrode versus the single electrode stimulation condition. Peak and mean power would be reduced, accordingly, by a factor of 10^{-4}. We can thus infer from the earlier computations for single electrodes that corrections for local heating effects are negligible.

REFERENCES

[1] Schimmel, H., and Vaughan, H. G., Jr., Preliminary Study of the Feasibility of Electrocortical Prosthesis (Progress Report), VRA Grant No. RD-2064-5. Albert Einstein College of Medicine, New York, 1966.

[2] Hein, A., Recovering spatial–motor coordination after visual cortex lesions, *in* *Proc. Assoc. Res. Nervous and Mental Disease* **47** (in press, 1969).

[3] Vaughan, H. G., and Schimmel, H., Preliminary Study of the Feasibility of Electrocortical Prosthesis (Progress report), VRA Grant No. RD-2064-S. Albert Einstein College of Medicine, New York, 1966.

[4] Brindley, G. S., and Lewin, W. S., The sensations produced by electrical stimulation of the visual cortex, *J. Physiol. (London)* **196,** 479 (1968).

[5] Libet, B., Alberts, W. W., Wright, E. W., Jr., DeLattre, L. D., Levin, G., and Feinstein, B., Production of threshold levels of conscious sensation by electrical stimulation of human somatosensory cortex, *J. Neurophysiol.* **27,** 546 (1964).

[6] Landgren, S., Phillips, C. G., and Porter, R., Cortical fields of the Monosynaptic pyramidal pathways to some alpha motoneurones of the baboon's hand and forearm, *J. Physiol.* **161,** 112 (1962).

ADDITIONAL RELEVANT REFERENCES

Brindley, G. S., The number of information channels needed for efficient reading, *J. Physiol.* **177,** 46 (1964).

Vaughan, H. G., Jr., and Schimmel, H., Preliminary Study of the Feasibility of Electrocortical Prosthesis (Progress report), VRA Grant No. RD-2064-S. Albert Einstein College of Medicine, New York, 1965.

Vaughan, H. G., Jr., and Schimmel, H., Preliminary Study of the Feasibility of Electrocortical Prosthesis (Progress report), VRA Grant No. RD-2064-S. Albert Einstein College of Medicine, New York, 1967.

Vaughan, H. G., Jr., and Schimmel, H., Preliminary Study of the Feasibility of Electrocortical Prosthesis (Progress report), VRA Grant No. RD-2667-S. Albert Einstein College of Medicine, New York, 1968.

SOME DESIGN ASPECTS OF A
VISUAL PROSTHETIC SYSTEM

E. Marg

I shall discuss what appears to be the best practical device in the way of an indwelling visual prosthesis for cortical stimulation. In this conference the analogy was made as to whether we wanted to devise a "Cadillac" versus some unnamed low-grade automobile. I think that this analogy is not a very suitable one. We all want a Cadillac, or, let us say, a Rolls-Royce; but we have to have a 1920 Rolls-Royce before we develop the 1930, and the 1930 before we develop the 1940 and so on. Our devices cannot spring perfect like Botticelli's Venus from the shell.

The Brindley and Lewin device has been shown to work in principle. In considering the design for a phosphene prosthesis to stimulate the brain directly we can start from there, assuming their basic specifications. We have only to build upon their experiences. The problem was discussed with Dr. John E. Adams and also with experts in integrated circuitry. As you know, MOS integrated circuits comprise a very fast-moving field in which some wonderful devices are being developed. We have worked out a design for a prosthesis that I should like to present.

The prosthesis (Fig. 1) consists of two devices or two parts. There is the external device, which goes above the head, and an internal indwelling device, which would go, literally, on the brain. The external device

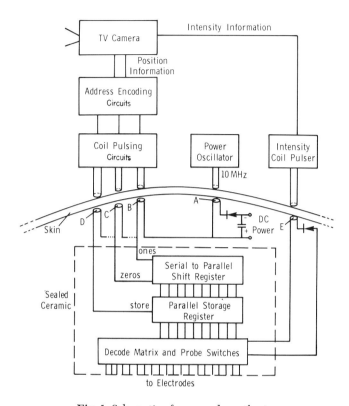

Fig. 1. Schematic of proposed prosthesis.

would consist of a special television camera which has an array of 512 silicon diodes on a monolithic silicon chip. This array would cover an area of 4×6 mm, the image area of a commercial 8-mm camera zoom lens. The resolution would be more than adequate, and the small size and low weight would be very suitable. The external device could ultimately be confined to the inside of a man's hat, with the lens peering out the front. It would provide position information, feeding to addressing and coding circuits, and intensity information going to an intensity coil pulser. A patching system to make the signals isomorphic with visual space would be necessary but is not shown in the diagram.

The signals would be electromagnetically driven across the skin into coils buried in the scalp. The pulsing circuits would feed to three coils, which would go into a serial-to-parallel shift register, giving binary signals, one or zero. When the shift register was filled, the signal would come through on another coil operating the parallel storage register. The binary number then would go to the decode matrix and probe switches, and then out to the electrodes. The power would come through the skin via a 10-MHz power oscillator. Intensity information would be pulsed separately.

This general design seems to describe the prosthesis we are seeking but there are still special problems which require further consideration. First of all, there is a problem of reliability, which in a situation like this has to be somewhat greater than the reliability we expect in our satellites and space vehicles. It is not easy to retrieve either satellites or implanted prostheses; in both, retrieval can be expensive and dangerous. Redundancy can be built into these circuits to give greater reliability.

One of the main problems, however, is that the environment of the brain is more hostile to these microelectronic circuits than that of outer space! Sodium ions, which are plentiful within the body, destroy the functioning of integrated circuits. It is essential to use some material that is impervious to sodium ions to package this device. Plastics are not, but ceramics are, and are also acceptable in regard to tissue tolerance.

A ceramic box for 512 elements or electrodes can be made about $1 \times 2 \times \frac{3}{8}$ in. It can be inserted into a hole in the cranium, replacing part of the skull.

The electronics present no major problem. In fact, they are at the state-of-the-art now, and actually the only serious problem, as far as concerns electronics per se, is money. The major technical problem is in the leads out of the device. If you will look at this integrated circuit, electronic desk calculator (Fig. 2), you will see that it consists of a ceramic slab in the center of which is a small mirror-like surface, approximately 3 mm², on which all of the electronics are contained on a silicon chip. All of the electronics in the internal prosthesis can be put on a single chip like this one. The problem is in getting the leads out of the box. In this slab there are approximately 40 leads but more than 12 times as many are needed for the prosthesis. It appears that the state-of-the-art is such that the number of leads can be increased and be spaced $\frac{1}{100}$ of an inch from center to center. Each slab could have approximately 100 leads. With five slabs stacked we could have approximately 500 leads. Such a configuration will require some development.

If we are going to go in the integrated circuit direction, the design presented seems to be a promising way to do it. Computer enthusiasts may be pleased to point out that when the prosthesis is functional there literally will be a digital computer on the brain.

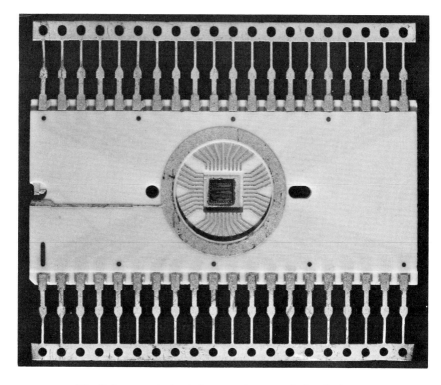

Fig. 2. Integrated circuit from an electronic desk calculator.

DISCUSSION

STERLING: Dr. Marg, why do you limit yourself to a television camera? Do we not have a variety of cameras like the sonic device, and the infrared device? In fact, if I were blinded I would like to have a sonic device because I could walk around at night and not worry about daytime.

MARG: Certainly. You can use this with filters, infrared, almost any sort of radiation you wish. There is no limitation in that respect. Using light as we do in normal vision just seemed to be the most simple and direct way of doing it.

KO: The proposed scheme looks feasible. In fact, I am surprised at the similarity of this proposal to the design efforts we are undertaking in cooperation with Dr. Vaughan's group to realize this type of blind aid.

I would, however, like to point out a few problems. The fabrication technology is here, but to assemble such a unit is far beyond the mere question of financial support. Besides the matter of manpower, I want to stress a few technical points that seem to be simple but extremely important.

One is power. If you have 500 electrodes and want to stimulate with a mosaic pattern, the peak power is very large. Based on Dr. Brindley's data, each electrode requires about 150-mW peak power, and if you have, say, 250 electrodes to be stimulated simultaneously, you are talking about many watts of transmission across the skin. The peak power transmission problem is serious.

MINSKY: It is not 150 mW.

MARG: No. It is peak power, not average power, but you have the same peak power transmitted through the skin, with the scheme proposed.

MINSKY: A tiny capacitor would have to do it.

KO: No. I am talking about several watts of peak power to be transmitted by stimulating rf channel. With the proposed scheme, the advantage of low duty cycle cannot be used to our advantage. Second, is the heat dissipation within the patient. There is a certain amount of power dissipated at each electrode. Although this individual power is small, if one multiplies with the total number of electrodes, then the resultant total dissipation of power is significant. Furthermore, the electronic circuits consume power; take 500 shift registers with two levels and calculate the total dissipation; one recognizes immediately that there is a heat removal problem.

Third is the size. Fourth is the handling of such a device, particularly the connection of electrodes to the electronic circuit and to external items.

MARG: Of course there are problems. This is why we are here. The point is that it appears that these problems can be solved.

There is one additional thing I would like to mention, and that is to put a signal into the serial-to-parallel shift register takes about 2 μsec, obtaining 10 bits in 20 μsec. A new electrode can be stimulated each 20 μsec. With approximately 500 electrodes, all electrodes can be energized serially in 10 msec with a pulse repetition rate of 400/sec for each electrode. Since these are done serially, there should not be the power limitation problem we were discussing earlier.

LOEB: I just wanted to ask if you had given any consideration to the size and shape of the electrodes and the interfacing.

MARG: We have considered it, but we have not come up with any specific design. As mentioned initially, we are fundamentally starting from the basic specifications of the Brindley–Lewin device. It works. We depend on their demonstrated basic validity. Of course, some new and different parameters can also be tested if we have the opportunity.

VAUGHAN: I would like to point out to Dr. Marg that he has in essence described our system which has been under development for several years now, and it is quite clear that what he says is correct; but as Dr. Ko has suggested the problem of reducing these concepts to practice is a very serious one. Perhaps it would be appropriate just to mention what magnitude these problems represent since we do not wish people to return to their laboratories and think they can put together this kind of prosthesis next month.

First of all, there is the problem of cortex compatible stimulating electrodes of a sufficient density to be worthwhile. It is as yet not entirely clear what the lowest useful electrode density may be, or, indeed, what the highest possible electrode density may be in terms of both the materials problem and the underlying cortical physiology.

I think, however, the best guess that one can come up with is essentially that which Dr. Brindley stated to us, a range of total of number of points on the cortex being between 300 and 10,000. Our own estimates suggest that the range can be further decreased by technological and physiological factors to a range of approximately 1000–4000; 1000 is probably close to the lower limit which is really worthwhile, to do this thing considering all of the factors that have been raised including the psychological factors, and so on.

It is quite true that a much smaller number of electrodes could provide a useful prosthetic result for certain limited purposes.

When you start talking about anything in the order of less than 400 points, the game may not be worth the candle. This may be quite a limited device, which does not warrant for prosthetic purposes the intrusion on the brain of a blind person.

We have been struggling with this dilemma for several years. As to when and under what circumstances it would be acceptable for us to go ahead and implant a system, I think that the answer to this is that when we have at least 1000 electrodes we can stimulate in connection with a suitable camera .

To this date we have not been able to solve the problem of constructing a thin-film, high-density, multiple electrode which is tissue-compatible, and which will meet reliability requirements. These requirements are not as great as we thought originally, because it is clear from Dr. Brindley's work, and some other experience that we have had, that we can remove a thin-film electrode from the cortex safely after a long period of implantation.

Yet, I am not going to be certain about this until Brindley has actually succeeded in doing it, that is, in replacing the electrode in his first patient with another, and have it work. Although we may not be faced with the reliability requirement of 20 or 30 years, a two- to five-year life, perhaps satisfactory for initial devices, will still be difficult to achieve.

When you get to the problem of packaging, and whenever you are talking of a system such as outlined by Dr. Marg, with necessary miniaturization, this is a project which is going to be extremely expensive. We are talking now in terms of sums of money which are in the order of magnitude of the entire present expenditure for research and development in the area of blindness.

This very fact, I think. gives rise to at least some of the dismay and concern among workers in the field for the blind about what we are proposing, because if it were the case that this development should replace support which now exists for other developments, I think this would be very foolish. I do not think that it will happen, but we have to realize that we are talking about sums of money which are not available in the current research and development budget for sensory aids to the blind.

MARG: First of all, I was very happy to learn of your (Dr. Vaughan's) work. I did not know of it until coming to this conference. You have put in a great deal of effort on a phosphene prosthesis, and have probably done a great deal more thinking about it than anyone else.

On the other hand, you must admit that until you actually construct and implant a device you are still in the realm of speculation. Dr. Brindley and Dr. Lewin have done us a great service, because we are no longer speculating about fundamental specifications. They have defined certain parameters, and we can start speculating from there, which is an entirely different proposition from starting de novo. Also, I do not think that the amount of money you are talking about is necessary. A device like this could be built for a few hundred thousand dollars.

VAUGHAN: That is the kind of money I am talking about.

MARG: If it is spread over four or five years, it is no more than a number of research projects require.

USE OF A MODEL OF THE PRIMATE VISUAL SYSTEM AS A VISUAL PROSTHESIS

L. L. Sutro

Five years ago we undertook to develop for NASA a device that could be placed on Mars to look around and report what it sees. It reports what it sees in far less data than it acquires in seeing. This device can do the same for the blind.

Our approach is to model properties of the primate visual system. We simulate the photoreceptor layer of the retina by a binocular television camera (Fig. 1). Contrast enhancement is achieved by a computer that will eventually be a sheet of shift registers. Stereopsis is obtained at present in the commercially-available computer, but we aim to model it eventually in a small layered computer. The distance away of edges and texture, determined by this stereopsis, can then be reported to the blind man by a tone—a low pitch for a distant edge, a high pitch for a near one. By using bone conduction we can leave his ears open. We are also studying the lateral geniculate body and the superior colliculus with a view to modeling these structures.

The advantage of this approach is that as models are completed, they can be pieced together in different combinations to assist the blind. The first combination that is needed is one that will rangefind for the blind man so that he will not bump into things. A very simple sound could tell him where the camera–computer found an object.

With the camera on his head and the computers in his pocket, the blind man can be told by the varying pitch of a sound, the distance away of objects before him. For example, as the electron beam, within the camera tube, slowly sweeps the face of the tube, he will receive a tone of varying pitch that will be like a contour map of the scene before him. A single scanned line of a scene containing a nearby post will be a low-pitched tone with a brief high-pitched peak.

As Warren McCulloch put it,

> When a man loses his eyes he loses ⅔ of his inputs. If you then use all the rest of his inputs to replace his eyes, you disable him. However, you don't have to occupy all of his earspace to provide him with a tone indicating distance away.
>
> Going directly into his brain with sufficient detail for useful images, is way off still. The first electrodes implanted into the brain in England are still producing speckles of light, but nothing else.
>
> We are not trying to make something that reads print. We need something that is mobile. Attach it to the blind man's head, making use of his vestibular system. Since he cannot do range finding, we will provide that. We can also provide color filters, changeable either manually or by myoelectric signals, that can enable him to tell the color of a traffic light.

To keep the resolution of the camera high, the vergence of the mirrors needs to be variable. Vergence control can be either manual or slaved to a muscle in the man's face through a myoelectric signal detected at his skin. The sharpness of the image can be indicated by a warble added to the steady tone. As the blind man adjusts the vergence–focus control he can tell by the warble whether focus is being improved or made worse.

The details of the shape of a scene will thus be provided by the electronics. The blind man will discover the course appearance of the scene by turning and tilting his head. To find a step, he will look not only down, but sidewards, so that the edge of the step will be more nearly vertical in the camera images and therefore suitable for stereopsis.

Figure 1 diagrams the camera, the "sheet" computer that performs contrast enhancement and an early design of the layered computer to perform stereopsis. We call the first computer "sheet" because it models a sheet of cells in the retina.

The figure shows left and right images of an object such as a rock projected by the optics onto the face of the vidicon. Converted to digital form, the signals enter shift registers (1) which move the images past computing elements (2) and (3), which represent the filtering and summing effects of living cells. The digital filter employed for level 2 is shown schematically at the upper left of the figure. It consists of a

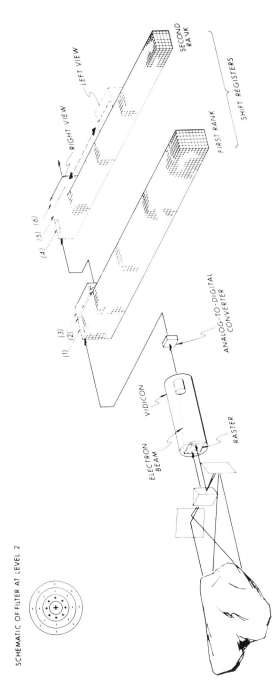

Fig. 1. Diagram of television camera (left); sheet computer in the form of the first rank of shift registers (1) that move digitized image past filter (2) and summer (3) where contrast is enhanced and the effect summoned at each point; layered computer in the form of a second rank of shift registers (4) that move contrast-enhanced data in such a way as to achieve stereopsis (5 and 6).

strongly positive central weight, less positive immediately-peripheral weights and weakly negative more-peripheral weights.

The images are advanced from left to right in the shift registers at the same rate that the tip of the electron beam in the vidicon advances. As data reach the right end of the top row, they are transferred to the left end of the next lower row. In this illustration, when the electron beam of the camera tube has swept nine lines of the raster, the shift registers in the bank are full. From then on, for each new position of the electron beam, computations take place in the box behind the shift registers, and one digital word is discarded from the right end of the ninth row of shift registers.

We estimate that elements (1), (2), and (3) of Fig. 1, built of off-the-shelf components, would occupy about 100 in.^{3}. We have not yet estimated the volume of the layered computer to perform stereopsis.

Our method of contrast enhancement is adapted from that presented by Rosenfeld and Lee [1]; our method of stereopsis, from that presented by Julesz [2]. Details of our methods will appear in a master's thesis by Jerome Lerman to be published by MIT's Draper Laboratory in June 1970.

REFERENCES

[1]   Rosenfeld, T., and Lee, F., Edge and Curve, Enhancement in Digital Pictures. Report 69–93, Univ. Maryland Computer Science Center, College Park, Maryland, p. 27, 1969.
[2]   Julesz, B., Toward the automation of binocular depth perception (Automap), *Proc. IFIPS Congress, Munich 1962,* North Holland, Netherlands, 1963.

COMPUTER-AIDED SYSTEMS FOR PROSTHETIC EXPERIMENTS

T. D. Sterling and H. Bomze

We shall talk about a system that appears to concern itself only indirectly with the problem of visual prosthesis. However, the association is much more direct than is immediately apparent. This system is conceived to investigate problems of stimulation that have to be resolved before substantial work on a practical prosthesis can continue. These are fundamental problems shared by all devices. In some cases, they are general and in others they may be more acute for particular individuals. For instance, when using a tactile device such as that described by Dr. Bliss, there may be certain ways of presenting changes in images which are easier to perceive than others. Then, too, we might find an individual whose finger sensitivity is not as acute as that of others. Therefore, in developing a general notion of how to optimize stimulation, it may be necessary to try different approaches so that their relative merit could be assessed. It is the purpose of our system to provide this facility.

Essentially, this system presents to the subject and/or his prosthesis a wide range of "perceptual" experiences. We do not really care whether it is a punctate screen embedded in the visual cortex, or something on which the subject puts his fingers, something he puts on his forehead, or something touching his back. All these devices consist of a series of points that have to be stimulated simultaneously or in sequence. To obtain flexibility and generality, arrangements are ordered to exist so that these points may be stimulated in some arbitrary fashion according to the instructions of an investigator or a subject interacting with the system. This can best be done with the aid of processes controlled by digital hardware and software. The use of a digital system offers two basic advantages over an analog configuration. In the first place, a digital system is much more flexible; secondly, initial experimentation with the help of a digital system does not mean that the final hardware would also be digital in nature. However, the useful way to proceed is to use the widest range of possibilities. Once we decide which way to go, then appropriate dedicated hardware can be built. Until such a decision is made, it is a digital system which offers that kind of flexibility.

The software required to support a flexible stimulation system must be built around a simple command structure. Those of you who have worked with computers a great deal and for a long time know that unless you have a good flexible problem-oriented language to work with, you will spend endless hours and large amounts of money in trying to produce the necessary programs to do what you want to do. Very often a research effort may be held up endlessly because of some program debugging problem, especially when the available language for describing the procedure is not well suited for that purpose. To solve this problem, we are working on an appropriate command structure that will enable the investigator to operate conveniently. For instance, by using simple terms, he can describe the image he wants to show, the angle at which he wants to show it, or the sequence in which he wants certain points stimulated. Furthermore, we want to be able to operate on the display, filter it, enhance it or modify it some other way, all by means of a number of simple statements.

As far as the hardware part of the system is concerned, we are in a peculiar dilemma. To create this convenient software, this powerful yet simple command structure, we are stuck with large computers. The more flexible we want this package to be, the larger the computer we must use. This results in a serious cost problem. There are two solutions as far as we can see. One is to use a large computer to prepare programs for small ones. The other is to try the experiment through the large computer, which is then used on a shared basis. This presents problems of transmission and buffering of the display device which are not inconsiderable.

The basic system currently proposed will use the IBM system/360 computer as the basic data processing device, with an 1827 data terminal for obtaining the output. This output will then be transmitted to what we call a "transducer addresser," which will allow us to address approximately 1000 points in any form of desired sequence. Since each point has an individual set of coordinates, it can be turned on or off by appropriate commands. In addition, the entire display can be cleared.

Although we were talking in terms of simultaneous stimulation, it turns out that in many cases it is easier to address the points sequentially, since computation usually occurs that way. Because of the high speed of the computer, the output is simultaneous for all practical purposes. With something on the order of a LINC computer that can produce a 12-bit word every 3 μsec, we can achieve a range of just under 1000 points in

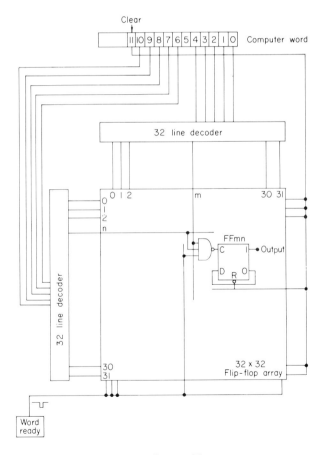

Fig. 1. Transducer Addresser.

2 msec. As far as the sensory system is concerned, this array of points would appear to be produced simultaneously. Furthermore, it is highly doubtful that we would want to use all of the points in an array for a given frame.

The transducer addresser will be buffered to any number of output devices. Based on present considerations, these will include a tactile display such as Dr. Bliss's and a light board. These can either be worked together with the light board displaying the same picture as a tactile display or the addresser can be partitioned in some manner and the light board and tactile display may operate completely independently. This would give us a chance to investigate the possibility of enhancing the display with other modes of sensory input.

In the future, this same addresser could very well be hooked up to stimulating electrodes which could possibly be used in some implantation. With this system, it is possible to explore the basic effects of simultaneous stimulation of a number of points, as suggested by Dr. Minsky in his paper. Furthermore, a very wide range of advanced tests can be constructed and performed to examine human perceptive and processing mechanisms at a great many levels.

The transducer addresser (Fig. 1) consists of an array of D-type flip-flops whose outputs are used to turn on or off the individual points of the display. For the purpose of controlling the flip-flops they are arranged in a 32 × 32 array. Two groups of five bits in the computer word are used to address the flip-flops. These are translated by two 32 line decoders which inhibit the clock pulses to all but the selected flip-flop. Each time a flip-flop is clocked the output is complemented; this allows individual points in the display to be turned on and off without having to clear the whole display. The computer is used to signal when a new word is ready and clocks the flip-flops. There is also a clear input which clears the entire array simultaneously. The highest possible repetition rate of this device is approximately 3 MHz.

Part II
OTHER POSSIBILITIES

Introduction

In a larger sense, a visual prosthesis is any device that translates "optical" stimulation to some kind of input for a substitute sensory system. Until the phosphene was suggested as such a sensory mode, these inputs were predominently auditory and tactual. Although the conference was concerned primarily with phosphene type prosthetic devices, two questions formed part of the background of the first conference and also of this one. Were there other promising devices sufficiently superior to a phosphene implanted visual prosthesis so as to create more desirable alternative goals? Then, if investigations for a phosphene based prosthetic device were to compete for funds with ongoing efforts, what other developments stood in danger of being neglected? One may question the validity of these concerns. The existence of other promising developments does not mean that work on some visual aids should be neglected; nor does it necessarily follow that the work using phosphenes would be supported at the expense of other work. Nevertheless, these were important questions and their discussion was included in the conference. It was well that this was done.

Three areas are presently used for sensory substitution—the finger, the back, and the forehead. The finger stimulating device (developed by Linville and Bliss), being more modest in its aim to provide a direct reading machine for blind individuals, appears to be eminently successful in allowing blind persons to read a wide variety of type fonts at rates of up to 60 words a minute. The use of the back (Bach-y-Rita and Collins) and use of the forehead (Starkiewicz and Kuprianowicz) give only rudimentary recognition of objects or letters in very well-defined situations and then only after long periods of learning.

Substitution of sound for optical stimuli was demonstrated by two different types of devices. One was a distant obstacle probe—a device responding to the echoes of a high frequency emitting probe (demonstrated by Mann). The others were reading machines that translated letters into their spelled equivalents and into computer-generated speech (demonstrated separately by Ingham and Murphy). Unfortunately, none of these devices were really as good as the state-of-the-electronic arts makes practical in other instances. For example, the computer generated speech demonstrated by Ingham and by Murphy falls far short of what is now routinely possible over telephone lines for interactive programming purposes in some university computing centers. Similarly, the sonar probe shown was a far cry from the infrared and high frequency devices used by the armed forces and space agency for diverse purposes.

Conspicuously absent was discussion about the two most successful sensory substitution devices the blind person uses, i.e., the cane and Brailled reading material. This was a regrettable shortcoming of the conference. Certainly, the blind person obtains more sensory input from a cane and is able to tell more about the environment from this device than from any existing electronic aids. Indeed, existing electronic aids tend to compete with other sensory input that comes from the environment and has a much richer information content than the buzzing and warbling that these electronic aids are presently capable of giving to the human ear. In this respect, too, the superiority of the Brindley type of implant is apparent.

A READING MACHINE WITH TACTILE DISPLAY

J. Bliss

I would like to talk a little bit about general systems ideas. Approximately eight years ago some of my colleagues and I began thinking about visual prosthesis, only we did not call it by that name then. The quest, however, was basically the same: How do you present a three-dimensional spatial image to a blind person?

The distinction between the points you need in a sensor and the number of points you may need in a display has not always been clear. Perhaps I can help by describing a very simple system.

A great deal of what we have seen and talked about has involved this simple system because it is the place to begin. We have a binary array of photoreceptors. The simplest system would be to have a similar binary array for a display, with a 1-to-1 connection between arrays. The display could be anything from a Brindley screen to tactors to what-have-you, including even an array of light for a visual display.

I agree that, given preprocessing and pattern recognition, we might be able to do a tremendous job of compression so that the number of required display points may be much less than the number of sensors. But first let us look at how many sensors we would need in the simple 1-to-1 system and try to relate this to some kind of measure of visual acuity.

A simple rule of thumb can be obtained by relating the number of sensors to measures like 20/40 vision or 20/100 vision. The maximum degree of vision given an N line system is 20 by the quantity $2400\theta/N$, where θ is the field of view in degrees and N is the number of rows in a two-dimensional array of rows and columns of photosensors.

To understand what degree of visual acuity might be adequate, let us take the definition of "legal blindness" and see how many photosensors we would need if we were at the threshold of legal blindness (20/200). If say that $\theta = 30°$ and we find that we need an N of at least 360 or a total number of points in the field of 360^2 or approximately a hundred thousand. Thus, the visual prostheses discussed here are several orders of magnitude away from the threshold of "legal blindness."

Realizing that this large *number* of sensors is merely a starting point in terms of providing two-dimensional patterns to a blind person for mobility, we decided to look for an easier visual problem. Such a problem is reading, which has a constrained input; the input patterns are inherently binary and you can manage with a much smaller field of view.

In fact, if the field of view is a letter space, you only need a 20×20 matrix, or 400 points. My point, however, is that while we are interested in a visual prosthesis, the reading problem is the place to start. That a number of people have realized this is indicated by the fact that one of the first things shown on the simulated Brindley screens are letters of the alphabet.

We have been interested in trying to develop a reading aid to the point that it is a practical system which can be given to someone for use in practical situations. This has involved considerable engineering development and careful attention to many details.

One type of tactile stimulator which we have found to be particularly useful for displaying two-dimensional tactile images is the piezoelectric bimorph. Figure 1 illustrates how we use this element to make a tactile stimulator. The piezoelectric reed is cantilevered at one end and a short 10-mil diameter wire pin is fastened to the free end. Such reeds, constructed of two slabs of lead zirconate, are commonly used as generators in phonograph cartridges. The upper and lower surfaces, as well as the middle, are conducting and serving as electrical terminals. Under application of voltage of proper polarity, the upper slab contracts longitudinally and the lower one extends. As a result, the reed flexes and the end deflects upward. Voltage of opposite polarity has the opposite effect.

The upward deflection of the free end of the reed drives the wire pin through a 40-mil hole to impact the skin. The most intense sensation is felt when the rest position of the skin is slightly above the rest position

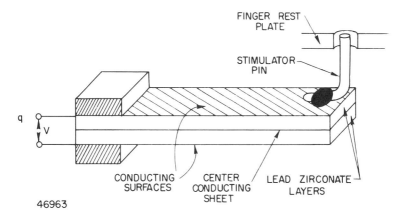

Fig. 1. Optacon reading device.

of the pin tip. Under this condition, the bimorph tip impacts the skin and contact between the skin and the pin is broken during each cycle of bimorph vibration.

One advantage of this unit for tactile displays is that many such units can easily be arranged to obtain a small dense array of stimulators. We have constructed many such arrays for studying tactile pattern perception. Some of our arrays have been connected to a computer for on-line pattern presentation, while others have developed into portable, stand-alone systems.

Figure 2 shows a typical array of tactile stimulators. The piezoelectric reeds in this array are driven near their resonant frequency of 200 Hz. Our psychophysical tests have indicated that the tactile sense has better spatial and temporal resolution at this frequency than at lower frequencies. The 24 × 6 array of 144 stimulators shown in Fig. 2 fits on a single finger, spanning the distal and a portion of the middle phalanges. The top of the pins and the perforated surface are curved to fit the finger.

This array is a key part of our reading aid. It produces a tactile image from printed material, making virtually any printed document readable by a blind person. We now have three of these units in every day use by two college students and a professional computer programmer. Our best reader reads at a typical rate of 60 words per minute with the device and it is her sole connection with much of the printed material from her college course work. This reading aid (Fig. 3) has an integrated silicon array of 144 phototransistors in the hand-held probe. This is small enough so we only need an optical magnification of one. The phototransistor sig-

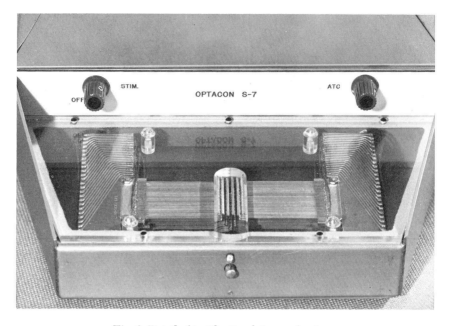

Fig. 2. Detail of tactile stimulator mechanism.

nals are then coupled, one-to-one, to an array of 144 tactile stimulators which are in the electronics unit.

To illustrate what can be done with this device I have a short movie. In the movie you will also see a light box, in which a light gets turned on every time a tactile stimulator is turned on. Thus, you will able to observe the tactile stimulation that the person is getting on a fingertip.[1]

Obviously, by changing the input lens from a "microscope objective" to a "camera lens," one can experiment with the same device as an environment sensor. We have, indeed, done that by building a very similar device in which the input was environmental scenes.

Of course, the resolution is very poor, but our experience has been that we can set up situations in the laboratory in which subjects can easily distinguish between such patterns as squares, circles, and triangles when they are allowed to manipulate the optical problem.

There have also been experiments in which the subject had to track a moving point of light that is being projected on a background of pattern noise. Subjects can learn to track this very satisfactorily using the tactile array.

---

[1] The movie is shown in which the subject is reading an English text.

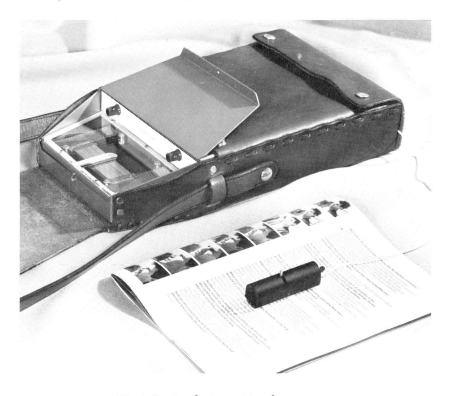

Fig. 3. Sensing device positioned over text.

We have developed a 144-channel system that is portable and battery-operated (Figs. 1–3). The aspect of this system that is immediately apparent in use in the environment is how often the output pattern appears to be nothing more than a noise. Resolution is just so poor in relationship to the complexity of the visual world that very little information is obtainable. Worse than that, it is impossible to tell when the information on the display is worth attempting to interpret, and when it is too difficult to process.

DISCUSSION

MACFARLAND: Dr. Bliss did Candy [2] have an opportunity to read that article (referring to the movie) prior to reading it on a machine? That is in the National Geographic isn't it?

BLISS: Right. She saw that article for the first time when we took the movie, but I think we had about three shots of the movie and I am not sure which one was actually used in this edited copy. However, her reading was not sufficiently different in any of the three takes.

MACFARLAND: That was faster than 50 words per minute.

BLISS: She has had the device in her home for some months and we have not recently checked her reading rate. Her reading rate of 50 words per minute was obtained around April, 1969, and it would not surprise me at all if she is doing better than that; in fact, she feels she is improving all the time.

FRANK: I would like to ask you a question about this. If one were exploring this environment with his fingers, you would couple the movement of his hand and his arm with his impression of space around him. If you let that little cradle in which Candy's fingers are reclining, move with her hand, but let the pattern that is displayed on it be the pattern that it would be following if it were following an enlargement of the page image, would it not be a more natural way of feeding this information back into the frame?

BLISS: That is a possibility and, in fact, every time I talk about this someone asks me that question. Up until now we have attempted to make the probe as light in weight and with as low inertia as we could so it would be easy to manipulate. Technically, it would make it more cumbersome to put the tactile stimulator on the probe.

However, we are reaching the point technically that it will not make much difference. It is my own opinion that this kind of transformation is something you can learn to compensate for in the matter of an hour or so, and after that there is very little difference in performance. Therefore, I think with someone like Candy it would make very little difference whether the tactile simulation was on the probe if she were moving, or whether it was on the other hand. I think she has learned the transfer very satisfactorily.

INGHAM: How much of the printed material was available under the fingers at a given instant?

BLISS: A little bit less than the width of the letter space and little bit more than the height of the space. The area on the page approximated 170 mils by 60 mils.

---

[2] Miss Candy Linville, for whom the first reading machine of the type described by Bliss was built.

INGHAM: She was getting less than a letter at a time?

BLISS: Just slightly less; certain letters fit on.

INGHAM: When she was doing such words as "Southwestern" was that exhibiting her experience? Or, was she guessing, as we do in Braille when we read rapidly?

BLISS: She tends to guess quite a bit, and if she gets a few letters she can guess the rest of the word and will say it.

Unfortunately, the light box in the movie did not show up very satisfactorily, and I do not know whether all of you could see the letters on it, but if you did, you noticed that there is a delay between when she said the word and when she has been stimulated with it.

COGAN: Why did you use just a portion of one finger rather than the whole palm? Or, a lot of area that you could have used?

BLISS: The fingertip is the place where you have more acuity, and its pattern perception appears to be better, particularly by people reading Braille who have had a lot of experience with the use of the fingertip for this kind of tactual pattern perception. It is a more natural thing. The two-point limen, even though it is a bad measure, is less on the fingertip than any other place on the hand.

TACTILE VISION SYNTHESIS

C. C. Collins

Introduction

I take the position that, given sufficient points of contact, geometric optical information taken from a television camera in its raw unprocessed state can be successfully conveyed through the tactile modality by point-for-point image projection employing a form of energy to which the skin is sensitive. Free directional control of the camera and kinesthetic feedback of camera position to the subject are very important for success. Recognition is poor if only the experimenter moves the camera. Although coding of visual–tactile input information is apparently not necessary, the image quality and detail may be enhanced if a satisfactory coding algorithm can be devised.

To support this contention we have developed a system to provide a blind person with a dynamic pictorial display [1, 2]. As he directs the television camera, a 20-line video image is applied to an array of 400 vibrators spaced at ½-in. intervals on the observer's back so that he perceives a vibrating facsimile of the television camera's field of view. I shall describe this passive tactile television system and discuss our continuing studies to develop a high resolution, portable sensory substitute [3]. We have found that projected tactile images can be perceived, recognized, correctly identified, and interpreted as visual [4].

However, the limited capacity of existing apparatus does not allow high resolution pictures to be presented.

One of the first requirements of a mobility aid is provision for a sufficient amount or bandwidth of information to define the shape and position of objects. The complex processes such as recognition, orientation and mobility require a vision aid providing a rich sensory input. We believe the most direct route in dealing with visual loss is presentation of the information in the same format as encountered by the retina, as nearly equivalent to vision as possible. Since it is not always feasible to define unambiguously what constitutes relevant information when devising a preprocessing algorithm, we have depended upon the central nervous system to operate on the raw information directly as it does in the case of the eye. Although the visual and tactile neural pathways are not the same, our experiments indicate that the required information reaches the central nervous system and is effectively processed and interpreted as visual [4]. Our congenitally blind students have developed many of the same visual introspections as sighted people, and have learned to assess a number of the fundamentally important features of space.

Preprocessing of visual information may not be necessary in human modality substitution systems since such information is less extensively preprocessed at the peripheral retinal level in man than it is in lower animals. In man the bulk of visual information processing, such as edge detection, orientation, and directional selectivity, occurs at the central level [5]. The skin, the brain, and the eye are all derived from the same tissue layer, the ectoderm. Hence, it is not surprising to find the retina and the skin innervated with receptors arranged in two dimensions in space, each capable of detecting and transmitting dynamic pictorial information. Thus, in searching for a modality to replace vision one finds the skin to be the most natural substitute for the retina.

Numerous prosthetic devices using tactile input have been evolved, including active electromagnetic and ultrasonic energy radiating systems. We shall be concerned here with passive, ambient light, imaging systems with tacile output displays. Since the original investigations of Noiszewski in 1897 [6], many experiments have been performed to determine the feasibility of using the skin as a receptor of images normally perceived by the visual system. Starkiewicz and Kuliszewski have described a 120-photocell array witht transistor energized solenoids for producing mechanical images on the forehead [7]. Kuprianowicz reported the recent progress on this project [8].

Bliss, who has probably done more work in this field than any other investigator, has assembled a 144-photocell array driving piezoelectric stimulators for reading printed text with the fingertips [9]. With Gardiner he has employed a hand-held optical detector system permitting a subject to scan objects in the surround [10]. Linvill and Bliss have achieved remarkable results in the tactile communication of printed text, permitting the blind to read at rates up to 30 words per minute with an 8×12 array of stimulators [11].*

For the past five years our work has been directed primarily toward the transmission of pictorial information through the skin. Many millions of points would be required to match the capabilities of the eye. For transmitting images of commercial television quality, many hundreds of thousands of points are required. However, the fovea of the eye (sub-serving the central two degrees of clear detailed vision) is made up of a matrix of approximately 34,000 light receptor cone cells (i.e., an array approximately 200 cells across [12]). It is within this highly mobile two degrees (1.2 mm diam.) foveal region that almost all of the visual infor-mation permitting reading and recognition is funneled. A 20-line sys-tem should be capable of transmitting pictures with $\frac{1}{10}$ the linear resolution of the human fovea; in our laboratory this has proven to be adequate for the recognition of human faces, common objects, and words.

In the design of a tactile image projector, either mechanical or elec-trical stimulation of the sense of touch can be employed. The thermal and chemical senses of the skin respond too slowly for practical utility in a dynamic pictorial display. As with other investigators, our early pro-totype devices have employed mechanical vibratory stimulation. How-ever, where others utilize a mosaic of photosensitive elements each re-quiring a separate driver amplifier to control a corresponding mechanical vibrator, we have taken a slightly different approach embodying some of the principles of commercial television. The optical image is scanned by a television camera tube and an electronic switch allows the bright-ness at each picture element to control the stimulus at corresponding points on the skin. Thus, only a single video amplifier is required, thereby permitting considerable economy when a large number of picture ele-ments are to be processed.

Our first prototype tactile projection unit employed a 3×3 vibrator array driven by a television camera [1]. This apparatus established the feasibility of using the skin as a pictorial communication channel. Sub-jects were able to resolve stimulator points spaced at 10-mm intervals on the back [13, 14] compared with a 68-mm two-point limen previously

---

* *Ed. note:* Bliss has reported more recent reading speeds of 60 words/minute.

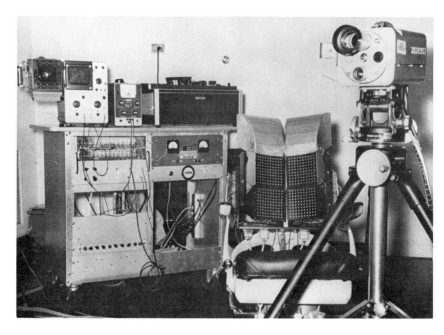

Fig. 1. Tactile television hardware comprising the vision substitution system. The digitally sampled television camera with zoom lens is seen at the right; the electronic commutator and control electronics with monitor oscilloscope and videotape recorder are on the left. In the center, the 400-point two-dimensional tactile stimulator matrix array is shown mounted in the back of a dental chair for projecting mechanical television images onto the skin of the back of blind subjects.

established [15].* Of more practical interest, blind and blindfolded subjects were able to determine the position of visual objects, their relative size, shape, number, orientation, direction, and rate of movement by scanning the camera [1].

Our second tactile television unit has employed 400 electromechanical stimulators permitting 20-line televised mechanical images to be projected onto the skin [2]. This unit is fixed in a heavy dental chair, and is consequently immobile (Fig. 1). The schematic drawing (Fig. 2) illustrates the operation of this electromechanical image converter. A zoom lens focuses an image on the face of a vidicon camera tube which is scanned in a stepwise point-by-point fashion. Synchronized electronic switching circuits steer the binary video signal to the corresponding 60-Hz solenoid stimulators in a 20×20 array contacting the skin with

---

* Ed. note: But the standard measuring technique for two-point limen is quite different from that employed by Collins and Bach-y-Rita.

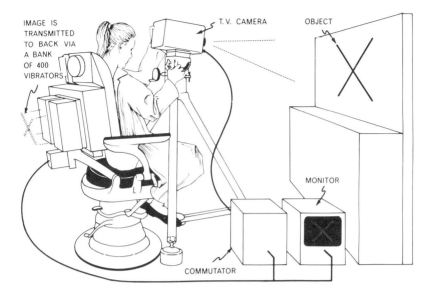

Fig. 2. Schematic drawing of the vision substituting system.

1-mm diam plastic tips spaced 12 mm on center. This matrix acts as a mechanical image projector to impress a two-dimensional vibrating facsimile of a visible object onto a large continuous area of skin.

Binary stimulation is employed; shades of grey are not presented as variations of intensity of the tactile stimulus. This all or none stimulation is achieved by electronically selecting a threshold illumination level above which the vibrating stimulators are turned on and below which they are turned off in the corresponding areas of the projected tactile image. However, noise modulation in the signal integrated over time produces the equivalent of a time duration modulated signal resulting in shades of grey being perceived. The field of view of this system's zoom lens can be varied from 6 to 30° providing a resolving power of approximately 15 min of arc. Further field size variation can be achieved by varying the amplitude of the deflection signal (electronic zoom) or by using different lenses.

In order to achieve sufficient resolution to appreciate image detail with a mobility aid, many points must be utilized to present a fine grained representation of images. We have chosen 400 points in a 20-line system which has proven adequate for the recognition of familiar objects and human faces. To present this fairly large amount of information, a relatively large unbroken area of skin is required. We have avoided the hands

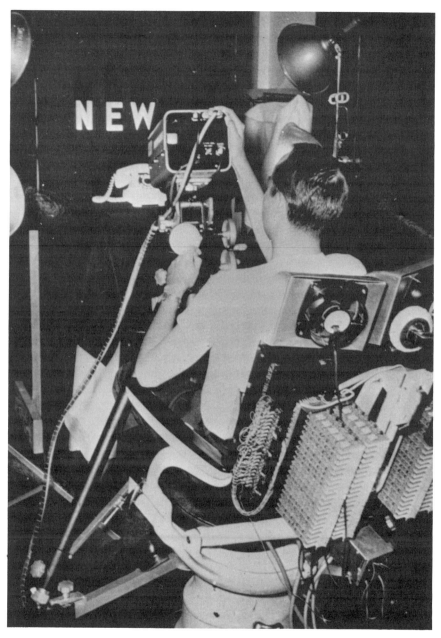

Fig. 3. Tactile television camera and mechanical image projector seen from the rear. A blind subject is directing the camera at a familiar object on the table. Block letter words can also be read by subjects using this apparatus.

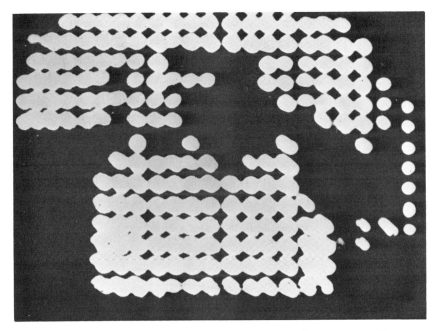

Fig. 4. Appearance of the telephone of Fig. 3 as seen on the experimenter's monitor oscilloscope. Approximately half of the 400 tactile stimulators are activated in this instance. Subjects do correctly recognize this tactile stimulus array as a telephone. (Visual perception of this type of display is sometimes aided by squinting the eyes to blur the image.)

or fingers which display reasonably high tactile resolution simply because they are useful and necessary in the performance of other tasks. We felt the skin of the face was a cosmetically unacceptable location for a tactile stimulator array. The skin of the back was chosen as the largest relatively flat continuous area of exposed integument on which to project haptic images. It is essentially unused for other sensory inputs and permits full use of the functions of other parts of the body. Tactile acuity to vibrating stimuli on the back has proved to be adequate for this application, being less than ½ in. for experienced subjects [13, 14]. The back will also be a practical and convenient location for a portable stimulator matrix which we propose can be worn as a sweater or vest.

Figure 3 shows a rear view of the tactile television mechanical image projector with a blind subject directing the television camera at a familiar object on the table. Block letter words are placed on the screen beyond the table. Figure 4 shows the appearance of a telephone as converted into a 400-point digitized representation of its continuous tone picture in Fig. 3. Note that approximately half of the tactors are actuated in this display.

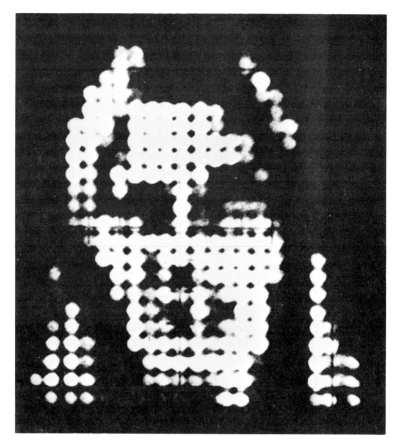

Fig. 5. A digitized representation of a woman's face as seen on the monitor oscilloscope of the tactile television system. This tactile presentation utilizing approximately 200 of the 400 available tactile stimulators can be recognized as a woman's head by experienced blind subjects.

Figure 5 is a digitized representation of a woman's face. It is sometimes of help to squint or otherwise blur the vision, thus causing the individual stimulus points to coalesce and form a more continuous tone representation.

In this prototype system we have made every effort to demonstrate the feasibility of haptic image projection. We have not attempted to make the apparatus portable since such additional demands at this early stage might have reduced the probability of success of our main objective. This philosophy has paid off; our initial efforts have been rewarded by seeing the blind successfully recognize environmental objects and faces, perceive movement in depth, and read block letter words at rates up to 50 letters a minute.

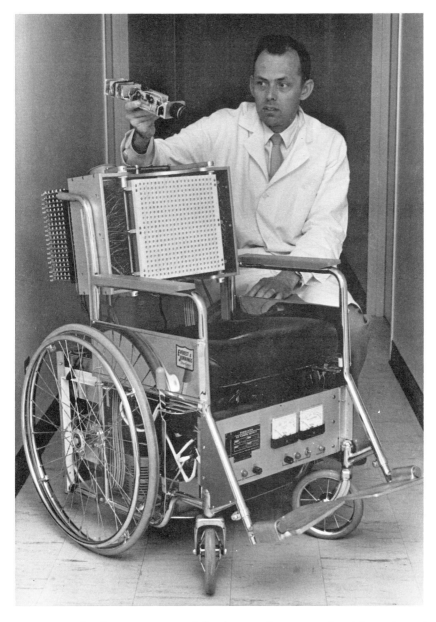

Fig. 6. Tactile television system with head-mounted camera and mobile mechanical image projector mounted on wheelchair.

We have recently completed a third tactile television unit employing 400 mechanical vibrators mounted in a wheelchair to allow subjects a degree of mobility (Fig. 6). The electronic control and switching cir-

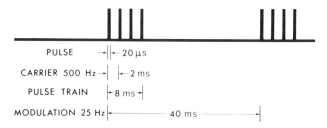

Fig. 7. Electrical pulse-train stimulus waveform used to evoke the painless tactile sensation of mechanical vibration.

cuitry is essentially unchanged. A lightweight head-mounted television camera employing an electrostatic vidicon and a plastic Frenel lens with a 30° field of view and operating with available light has been completed for use with this mobile unit. The speed and freedom of directing this camera is expected to produce a marked improvement in the accuracy and latency of object recognition by blind subjects.

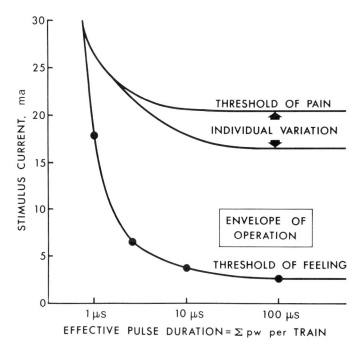

Fig. 8. Stimulus–response characteristics with the electrical stimulus waveform of Fig. 4. Note the threshold of feeling is about 2 mA and the threshold of pain is above 15 to 20 mA. The tactile television system can be reliably operated in the 6–10 mA region as shown in the enclosed block.

To achieve an adequate back-mounted portable tactile television display system, it would appear that electrical stimulation will be more practical than mechanical from the standpoint of reduced weight, cost, and power consumption. Gibson [16] has reported painless electrical stimulation with 10-mm diam contacts on the skin. In our preliminary studies, an extension of Gibson's work, we have found it possible to employ 3-mm diam electrodes by choosing appropriate electrical stimulus parameters [3]. Stimulation with the waveform shown in Fig. 7 results in the painless sensation of mechanical vibration or touch. The thresholds of sensation and pain occur at approximately 2 mA and above 20 mA, respectively, as illustrated in Fig. 8. As with mechanical stimulation of the skin of the back, the threshold of sensation occurs at a power level in the reign of 50 μW. With most subjects, it is possible to stimulate the sensation of vibration reliably by using a stimulus of 1 mW per electrode.

Projection

Our current efforts are being devoted to developing a high resolution, economical, portable, tactile television system to be worn by the blind. Initial experiences have been encouraging and indicate the feasibility of constructing such an apparatus with a weight of approximately five pounds (including batteries for eight hours of operation). Electrical stimulation would be applied via a matrix of electrodes extending through a flexible garment worn against the skin, with an eight-ounce headmounted camera facilitating the control of the direction of view. It is possible that the electrotactile display might be made directly on the scalp.

Of primary concern in the transmission of pictorial information is the resolution capability of the integument. Tactile communication bandwidth is limited by the spatial and temporal resolving power of the skin. We have found that experienced subjects can resolve stimulator tips spaced between 5 and 10 mm on the trunk [3], and closer elsewhere. This indicates that over 10,000 points may be available on the approximately 4000 cm^2 area of skin of the trunk. This would permit 100-line television picture projection, providing a relatively high resolution display.

According to Goff [17] the flicker fusion frequency of the skin is approximately five times greater than that of the eye, exceeding 500 Hz. Consequently, the input capacity of the skin of the trunk could theoretically exceed 5 MHz (10,000 points times 500 Hz), which is comparable to that of the fovea (34,000 cone cells times 100 Hz). The actual obtainable bandwidth can only be determined by direct investigations such as those being pursued in this and other laboratories. It may be possible to

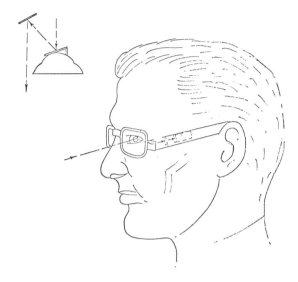

Fig. 9. A scleral contact lens fitted with a mirror may permit the wearer to direct the angle of view of the tactile television system by his own eye movements. A spectacle mounted fiber optical system transmits the image of regard to a small television camera carried elsewhere. An angled mirror on the spectacle frame relays the contact mirror image to the objective lens. Development of very small imaging devices would eventually allow the camera to be mounted in the earpiece of the spectacles.

trade the extra frequency response for improved resolution by proper preprocessing techniques.

Finally, by the application of contact mirrors to the otherwise adventitiously blind eyes it may be possible for a subject to control the direction of view of the input camera sensors by the use of his oculomotor muscles, thus permitting the reestablishment of the vestibulo-ocular and other oculomotor reflex arcs. Figure 9 is a sketch representing this concept. Looking to the future, it appears that miniaturized direct photoelectric converters are a distinct possibility. Such input sensors could be conveniently mounted on the frames of a pair of glasses with 8-mm optics and 45° mirrors to direct the optical axis of the camera at the eyeball mounted contact mirrors such that the eyes control the vertical and horizontal angle of view of each camera.

We do not yet know the level of capability of the tactile image perceptual system. Performance scores of our blind subjects continue to increase and it is tempting to speculate that a continuously worn personal system may permit an approach to the calculated theoretical information transmission bandwidth of the skin.

ACKNOWLEDGMENTS

I wish to express appreciation to Mr. Gordon Holmlund, Mr. Robert Acker, and Mr. Jack Shore for their contributions to the final design and fabrication of the apparatus, and to Mr. Jules Madey who was responsible for the design of the head-mounted camera. Many others have contributed to this project to whom we owe our sincere thanks.

REFERENCES

[1] Collins, C. C., Tactile image projection, Nat. Symp. *Information Display (abs)* 8, 290 (1967).

[2] Collins, C. C., Tactile television: mechanical and electrical image projection. *IEEE Trans. Man-Machine Systems* (in press, 1970).

[3] Collins, C. C., and Saunders, F., Tactile television: electrocutaneous perception of pictorial images. *Proc. Neuroelec. Conf. 1969* (in press).

[4] Bach-y-Rita, P., Collins, C. C., Saunders, F., White, B., Scadden, L., Vision substitution by tactile image projection. *Nature* **221,** 963 (1969).

[5] Michael, C. R., Retinal processing of visual images. *Sci. Am.* **220,** 104 (1969).

[6] Noiszewski, K., "Gazeta Lekarska" Vol. IX, Chap. 24, Ser. II, p. 1018–1022, 1889.

[7] Starkiewicz, W., and Kuliszewski, T., Progress report on the elektroftalm mobility aid, *Proc. Rotterdam Mobility Res. Conf.,* 27 (1965).

[8] Starkiewicz, W., Kuprianowicz, W., and Petruczenko, F., this conference.

[9] Bliss, J. C., A relatively high-resolution reading aid for the blind. *IEEE Trans. Man-Machine Systems* **MMS-10,** 1 (1969).

[10] Bliss, J. C., and Gardiner, K. W., An optical-to-tactile image converter. *Proc. Intern. Conf. Sensory Devices for the Blind,* 299 (1967).

[11] Linvill, J. G., and Bliss, J. C., A direct translation reading aid for the blind. *IEEE Proc.* **54,** 40 (1966).

[12] Ruch, T. C., and Fulton, J. F., "Medical Physiology and Biophysics," p. 435, Saunders, San Francisco, California, 1960.

[13] Morris, A., Collins, C. C., and Bach-y-Rita, P., Factors influencing cutaneous perception studied with a video-tactile display system. *West. Psych. Assoc. Meet., San Francisco, May 5, 1967.*

[14] Eskildsen, P., Morris, A., Collins, C. C., and Bach-y-Rita, P., Simultaneous and successive cutaneous two-print threshold for vibration. *Psychonomic Sci.* **14(4),** 146 (1969).

[15] Weber, H., cited by Sherrington, T., *in* "Textbook of Physiology" (N. Shafer, ed.) Edinburgh, Pentland, 1900.

[16] Gibson, R. H., Conditions of painless electrical stimulation. Report No. 42, ONR Project NR 140-598. Univ. Virginia (Psychology Lab.), Charlottsville, 1960.

[17] Goff, G. D., Differential discrimination of frequency of cutaneous mechanical vibration, Doctoral dissertation, Univ. Virginia, 1959.

A TACTILE VISION SUBSTITUTION SYSTEM BASED ON SENSORY PLASTICITY

P. Bach-y-Rita

Introduction

For more than five years, a tactile television system (TVSS) has been under development in our laboratory [1–7]. The concept and details of the instrumentation were discussed by Collins in the previous paper. This paper will be concerned with a presentation of some of the results obtained to date, together with some theoretical neurophysiological considerations.

Methods

The TVSS in operation at present includes 400 solenoid stimulators arranged in a 20 × 20 array built into a dental chair. The stimulators, spaced 12-mm apart, have 1-mm diam 'Teflon' tips which vibrate against the skin of the back. Their on–off activity can be monitored visually on an oscilloscope as a two-dimensional pictorial display. The subject manipulates a television camera mounted on a tripod (Fig. 1). The camera can

Supported by DHEW, Social and Rehabilitation Service Grant No. RD-2444-S; USPHS Research Career Award No. 5 K3 NB-14,094; Rosenberg Foundation Grant; USPHS General Research Support Grant No. S01 FR 05566; T. B. Walker Foundation; and Trust in Memory of Beatrice and James J. Ingels.

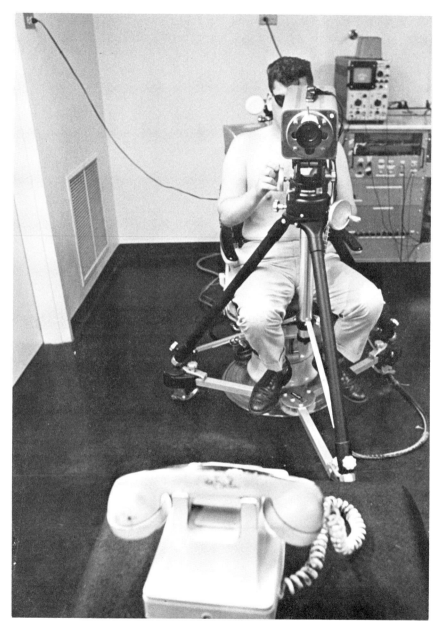

Fig. 1. A blind subject is pointing the television camera at a telephone. The subject is leaning against the 400-point stimulus array which is mounted on the back of the dental chair. At the upper right, the oscilloscope monitor is displaying a 400-point representation of the telephone. The same image is displayed on the skin of the subject's back through the Teflon-tipped solenoid driven tactors.

be used to scan objects on a table in front of the subject, or can be directed at a back-lit screen on which slides or motion pictures can be presented. Additionally, the subject can aim the camera, with its zoom lens, at different parts of the room, locating and identifying objects or persons.

Six blind subjects have undergone extensive training and testing with the TVSS. The first of these subjects—a psychologist who has been blind since the age of four—has had over 150 hr of experience in the chair and has contributed greatly to the training of other subjects. The remaining five subjects are college undergraduates, blind since birth (retrolental fibroplasia), who have been selected for their verbal abilities, motivation, and general adjustment. Their experience in the chair ranges from 20 to 40 hr of training. While these six subjects provided the major results to be presented, additional studies have been performed with 25 other blind subjects. As controls for some studies, six sighted persons were included.

Results

After being introduced to the mechanics of operating the apparatus, subjects were trained to discriminate vertical, horizontal, diagonal, and curved lines. They then learned to recognize combinations of lines (circles, squares, and triangles) and solid geometric forms. After approximately 1 hr of such training, they were introduced to a "vocabulary" of 25 common objects: a telephone, chair, cup, toy horse, and others. For each object, placed on a table several feet in front of the subject, the trainer first directed the subject's analysis of the object, pointing out its parts, their relationships, and the object as a whole. After each object had been so analyzed, the trainer presented one object and asked the subject to identify it, recording the time to correct response and giving such feedback as he thought appropriate. Recognition times were between 5 and 8 min per object for the first few presentations. After 10 or more hours of training, the subject became more familiar with each object and with its different possible orientations. As his techniques of visual analysis developed, the recognition time fell to 2 to 20 sec. Recognition time for new objects also fell markedly [3].

As the blind subjects became more familiar with objects, they learned to recognize them from minimal or partial cues. This skill permitted them to describe with accuracy the layout of several objects on a table, in depth and in correct relationship, even though the objects were overlapping and only partially visible. For example, a telephone could be located even though only its cord was showing. As the latency or time-to-recognition fell, the student discovered visual concepts such as perspective, shadows, shape distortion as a function of view-point, and apparent change in size as a function of distance.

The techniques and concepts of visual analysis thus developed were then used for recognition of letters, for perception of moving stimuli, and in the exploration of other persons standing before the camera. The subjects could learn to discriminate among individuals, to decide where they were in the room, to describe their posture, movements, and individual characteristics such as height, hair length, presence or absence of glasses, and so on.

Our subjects spontaneously report the external localization of stimuli. That is, sensory information seems to come from in front of the camera, rather than from the vibrotactors on their back. Thus, after sufficient experience, the vision substitution system seems to become an extension of their sensory apparatus.

Recently, the first steps have been made toward testing and quantifying the perceptual acuity of the six experienced blind subjects, and comparing their ultimate efficiency with that of sighted subjects viewing the oscilloscope monitor. The quantitative studies undertaken to date include the following:

(1) The orientation of parallel lines: Grills of parallel black and white lines were prepared at five levels of difficulty, containing four, six, eight, ten, or twelve pairs of lines. These stimuli were presented vertically or horizontally in a random sequence by photographic slides. The subject was asked to detect the orientation, and his response latency was recorded (Table 1).

(2) Detection of slant utilizing monocular cues: a portion of a large checkerboard was photographed at an angle of $70°$ from the perpendicular, so that a slide was filled with slanting, converging black and white squares. The ratio of convergence was 2:1, with a total of 60 white squares. By rotation of the slide in the projector, the direction of convergence could be presented to the top, bottom, left or right. A random series of 20 presentations per testing period was given, with the trainer recording the latency and accuracy of the response.

Table 1 shows that the two groups did not differ significantly in detecting the orientation of the parallel lines. On the checkerboard slant task, the sighted group was more accurate (97.5% to 82.9%, $P < 0.01$), and latencies of the sighted group were significantly shorter (2.8 sec to 8.4 sec, $P < 0.001$) than those of the blind group.

The blind subjects, restricted to manual manipulation of the camera, were somewhat slower in exploring the image than were the sighted sub-

TABLE 1. Response Accuracy and Latency for Blind and Sighted Subjects on Judgments of Line Orientation and Checkerboard Tilt

	Accuracy	
Subject	Line orientation	Checkerboard tilt
Blind $N = 6$	99.6%	82.9%
		$\sigma = 10.4$
Sighted $N = 6$	100%	97.5%
		$\sigma = 1.5$
Significance	Nonsignificant	$P < 0.01$

	Latency (sec)	
Subject	Line orientation	Checkerboard tilt
Blind $N = 6$	1.2	8.4
		$\sigma = 2.9$
Sighted $N = 6$	1.1	2.8
		$\sigma = 0.7$
Significance	Nonsignificant	$P < 0.001$

jects who visually scanned the monitor, thus perhaps explaining the difference in latency. (In subsequent testing and training, three of the blind subjects have attained a criterion of 100% accurate discrimination [3].)

(3)   Block capital letters on individual photographic slides were presented in a random sequence. The subject scanned the letter and responded verbally. The trainer told the subject whether his judgment was correct or incorrect; in the latter case the subject responded again. The latency to correct response was recorded and averaged over 26 letters. For six subjects, the initial mean latency to correct response was 52 sec; this latency fell to 17, 14, and 10 sec on three successive testing periods, respectively. In later studies the latency for individual letters was as short as 3 sec. When letters were joined into words, the speed of recognition increased [3].

(4)   Detection of a hole in a three-in. circle. A target was placed alongside a solid circle of the same size. With the camera placed 4 ft from the circles, the subject was requested to determine which one was the target. The holes in the target circles were centered and varied in size from 1½ in. down to ¼ in. The mean accuracy for five experienced subjects was as follows: 1½ in., 100%; 1 in., 99%; ¾ in., 97%; ½ in., 92%; ¼ in., 66%. Chance level was 50% and we considered 75% as cri-

terion for success. The range in accuracy for detecting the smallest hole
was 45–100% among the five subjects.

(5)   Data for form recognition, using the same subjects. Each subject
had earlier reached 100% accuracy for recognition of three geometric
forms (circle, square, and triangle) each having an area of 9 in.² In the
present task, the forms to be identified had an area of 1.6 in.², and the
targets were placed 4 ft from the camera. For external form recognition,
a solid form was utilized. For internal form recognition, the form was
embedded in the center of a 5-in. white square. Thus, in the latter task,
the target represented a silent area within an area of stimulation. Results
on these tests were as follows: external form recognition: mean 72.0%
accuracy; internal form recognition: mean 55.3% The range of accuracy
was 66.7–76.7% for external, and 33.3–80.0% internal. While internal form
recognition was significantly more difficult than external, it could be
achieved by the better subjects.

Analysis

In the present studies, we have utilized the receptors of the skin of the
back despite the insensitivity of this cutaneous area relative to other areas
of the body. This site was most amenable to the contingencies of instrumentation design and suited our wish to utilize a receptor surface least
likely to interfere with other tasks. The highly sensitive skin of the hand
was eliminated as a possible receptor surface on the basis of these guidelines.

The TVSS interface at the receptor surface of the back consists of
tactors separated by 1.2 cm. Reports of the two-point discrimination
limen of more than 6 cm [8] were evaluated in our laboratory and
seemed to constitute a skin acuity measure which was inapplicable to the
TVSS. The validity of this interpretation has been demonstrated both by
our results [5, 3] and also by the recent work of Vierck and Jones [9]
who have shown a similar inconsistency with the two-point discrimination limen. The latter investigators have shown that if relative size judgments are measured, the acuity of a skin area is greater by a factor of
10 than that shown by the two-point limen studies.[1]

The cutaneous receptors, activated by the 20 × 20 array of vibrotactile

---

[1] *Ed. note*: It is unfortunate that here Bach-y-Rita ignores the method by which
the two-point limen is a statistically defined point. The two-point limen *was* tradi-
tionally measured by the distance that could be detected 50% of the time between
two hairs that touched the skin under application of a standard pressure. This is
quite different from using distances between vibrating tips and calling the limen any
detectable distance.

stimulators, produce a pattern of neuronal impulses which is carried to the brain via the afferent nerves from one or both of the receptor types present: hair follicle receptors and free nerve endings. The morphology and distribution of these cutaneous receptors has been discussed by Sinclair [10]. If the concept of receptor specificity were interpreted strictly, it would be expected that stimulation from the tactors would produce cutaneous sensations such as touch. However, after several hours of training, the sensation produced during a perceptual task is not cutaneous: the cutaneous receptors are mediating telereceptor pattern information and in that sense the sensation is comparable to a visual one. The blind subject, using the TVSS to explore such objects as a telephone or a stuffed animal, perceives what a sighted subject sees when looking at the same objects on the oscilloscope monitor. This includes depth information, obtained by "monocular" cues such as occlusion and elevation in the visual field when perceiving spatially distributed arrangements of objects. Thus, the neural pathways are carrying pictorial information from the TV camera (which functions as an artificial retinal receptor surface) and the tactile receptors are relaying this information to the brain.

The evidence that vision substitution can be provided by cutaneous stimulation raises theoretical questions of interest to neurophysiologists. For instance, what mechanisms allow information arriving by cutaneous channels to be subjectively interpreted as "visual"? How are visual concepts such as the two-dimensional representation of three dimensions, size-constancy and linear perspective mediated by central nervous system regions normally used for surface-contact information? Which central nervous system areas participate in information processing?

Some insight into these questions may be found in the theory of phase interference. Thus, if sensory information is holographically distributed throughout much of the brain, as has been discussed by various authors (including Pribram [11]), incoming sensory information should interact with other afferent inputs arriving via the same or other modalities. In this way, both percepts and motor responses to them can be the products of instantaneous afferent input modulated by memory and previous experience. The latter could integrate newly arriving information and produce centrifugal impulses which modify afferent information arriving at the receptor and at the relay nuclei. It would also be of great interest to know if centrifugal afferent receptor mechanisms can be developed for efficient handling of the information arriving at the cutaneous receptors as "visual" information.

Pribram [11] has discussed the influences exerted by the association cortex areas on the content of the sensory information that reaches the brain. He suggests that somewhere between the receptor and the cortex the inflowing signals are modified to provide information already linked to a learned response. Desmedt [12] has demonstrated that central structures can modify incoming information at the receptor level. We have considered these factors, as well as the descending influences involved with motor performance related to perception, in developing methods of training blind subjects to use the TVSS. There is a great difference in the speed of learning when the movement of objects is by a passive video-tape presentation as compared to the subject's control of camera movement and zoom and aperture settings. However, in the latter conditions, not only are the descending regulatory influences related to experience and to motor movements involved, but valuable proprioceptive information is also gained by controlling all camera movements.

Alternatively, if the primary sensory cortex is the principal receiving area for "visual" information carried by the cutaneous sensory system, is the portion of the sensory homunculus representing the skin of the back sufficiently extensive to mediate complex "visual" tasks, or will the representation of this region on the sensory homunculus be modified? Desmedt and co-workers [13] have shown that the late components of the cortical evoked potential recorded over the somesthetic sensory cortex change when the subject concentrates on a tactile stimulus. It is possible that changes will occur in the somesthetic cortex of a blind subject undergoing training with the TVSS as the pattern stimulus becomes more meaningful.

A final point to consider is the mode in which information is presented to the receptor. Is it necessary, or even desirable to encode the output from an artificial receptor in order to reduce the amount of data delivered to the skin? The (subsequently stated) view of White *et al.* is pertinent to this point:

> In the past many efforts at providing information to the blind have been based upon somewhat old-fashioned ideas about the way perceptual systems work. In early psychology, there was a distinction between sensation and perception. The former had to do with stimulation of end organs, which sent their messages to the brain where they were synthesized and correlated through long experience until a percept emerged. Many efforts at creating sensory aids are still restricted by this evaluation, and set out to provide a set of maximally descriminable sensations. With this approach, one almost immediately encounters the problem of overload —a sharp limitation in the rate at which the person can cope with the incoming information. It is the difference between landing an aircraft on the basis of a number of dials and pointers which provide readings on such things as airspeed, pitch, yaw and roll, and landing a plane with a contact analog display. Visual perception thrives when it is flooded with information, when there is a whole

page of prose before the eye, or a whole image of the environment; it falters when the input is diminished, when it is forced to read one word at a time, or when it must look at the world through a mailing tube. It would be rash to predict that skin will be able to see all the things the eye can behold. However, we might never have been able to say it was possible to determine the identity and three dimensional layout of a group of familiar objects if this system had been designed to deliver 400 maximally discriminable sensations to the skin. The perceptual systems of living organisms are the most remarkable information reduction machines known. They are not seriously embarrassed in situations where an enormous proportion of the input must be filtered out or ignored, but they are invariably handicapped when the input is drastically curtailed or artificially encoded. Some of the controversy about the necessity of preprocessing sensory information stems from disappointment in the rates at which human beings can cope with discrete sensory events. It is possible that such evidence of overload reflects more an inappropriate display than a limitation of the perceiver. Certainly the limitations of this system are as yet more attributable to the poverty of the display than to taxing the information-handling capacities of the epidermis. [7].

Conclusions

TVSS research has focused upon discovering whether congenitally blind subjects can learn to identify a variety of objects, make fine discriminations between similar objects, and use the monocular cues of vision necessary to judge position and distance of familiar objects. Results with 30 blind subjects to date indicate that such techniques are learned within 20 hr of training. Of course, each new object or pattern requires additional learning, but the bases of analysis are learned in this period of training. As many as 10 objects have been placed together, some partially occluded, and were still identified by their distinctive features; their relative positions were noted, and accurate distance-judgments were made. The bright college students serving as subjects learn the monocular cues rapidly, and the less intelligent or less spatially oriented seem to respond favorably to raised-line drawings used as demonstrations of the needed concepts. We have been limited to distances of 20 ft by laboratory confinement but our findings to date suggest that freedom of mobility, provided by a portable system, would enhance the development of the ability to locate desired objects and to avoid hazards and would permit more independence.

Easy access to printed material is considered by the blind to be a prime necessity. We have demonstrated, with the present TVSS prototype, that it is possible for the blind to read block letter words and slide presentations of upper and lower case letters. We do not approach the reading performance level of the subjects training on Dr. Bliss' reading machine, but this may be due largely to the cumbersome reading arrangement necessary with our present prototype.

Our studies have demonstrated that the blind can successfully scan slide presentations of patterns, photographs, and drawings, as well as oscilloscope displays. Experienced subjects are able to detect a quiescent space one-tactor wide in the midst of a mass of stimulation with the present system (Scadden, in preparation). This target-space represents ¼ in. in the display 4 ft from the camera, and is achieved with a lens setting of 3° visual angle after an average of 40 hr experience with the apparatus. Our subjects perform significantly better on this task with 400 tactors spaced ½ in. apart than with 200 at twice the spacing.

ACKNOWLEDGMENTS

The author wishes to acknowledge the valuable editorial comments of Mrs. Betty Hart and Drs. Jane Hyde, Arlen Slusher, and Forbes Norris.

REFERENCES

[1]   Bach-y-Rita, P., Sensory plascity: applications to a vision substitution system. *Acta Neurol. Scand.* **43**, 417 (1967).

[2]   Bach-y-Rita, P., Neurophysiological basis of a tactile vision substitution system. *Tactile Display Conf.* (in press, 1970).

[3]   Bach-y-Rita, P., Collins, C. C., Saunders, F., White, B., and Scadden, L., Vision substitution by tactile image projection, *Nature* **221**, 963 (1969).

[4]   Bach-y-Rita, P., Collins, C. C., White, B., Saunders, F., Scadden, L., and Blomberg, R., A tactile vision substitution system. *Am. J. Optom.* **46**, 109 (1969).

[5]   Eskildsen, P., Morris, A., Collins, C. C., and Bach-y-Rita, P., Simultaneous and successive cutaneous two-point thresholds for vibration. *Psychon. Sci.* **14**(4), 146 (1969).

[6]   Scadden, L., A tactual substitute for sight. *New Sci.* **41**, 677 (1969).

[7]   White, B. W., Saunders, F. A., Scadden, L., Bach-y-Rita, P., and Collins, C. C., Seeing with the skin. *Perception and Psychophysics* (in press, 1970).

[8]   Myers, cited by Mathews, B., "The Physiological Basis of Medical Practice," C. H. Best and N. B. Taylor, eds., p. 1141. Williams and Wilkins, Baltimore, Maryland, 1961.

[9]   Vierck, C. J., and Jones, M. B., Size discrimination on the skin. *Science* **163**, 488 (1969).

[10] Sinclair, D., "Cutaneous Sensation." Oxford Univ. Press, London. 1967.

[11] Pribram, K. H., The neurophysiology of remembering. *Sci. Am.* **220**, 73 (1969).

[12] Desmedt, J. E., "Neurophysiological Mechanisms Controlling Acoustic Input in Neural Mechansms of the Auditory and Vestibular Systems" (G. L. Rasmussen and W. F. Windle, eds.). Thomas, Springfield, Illinois, 1960.

[13] Desmedt, J. E., Debecker, J., and Manila, J., Mise en évidence d'un signe électrique cérébral associé à la détection par le sujet, d'un stimulus sensoriel tactile *Bull. Acad. Royal Med. Belgique* **5**, 887 (1965).

DISCUSSION

BERING: What size do your letters have to be? How small?

BACH-Y-RITA: That would depend on how close you would get to the camera. If you have a focusing mechanism you can use them straight off the page, and actually we have done that.

BERING: How large, or how small, can you make one on the simulation back?

BACH-Y-RITA: We use pretty much the whole array per letter, the whole 400. You may have one letter in the middle, and parts of a letter on either side, as it proceeds across, but generally we have one letter at a time.

I may say we are not at the point that Dr. Bliss is in reading directly from pages where the letters are quite close together. We have not spent much time on this because of our bulky system.

MANN: As I understand it, your experiments are conducted in high contrast. What would happen with the types of photographs Dr. Brody and Johnson showed?

BACH-Y-RITA: We are working with photographs. These are quite difficult because of the shading and high amount of very intricate detail. Our blind subjects can work it out but it takes more time.

COLLINS: At present we have only a 400 point display compared with the fovea containing 40,000 receptors. As we increase the number of displayed points to 10,000 or so, we expect faster recognition of continuous tone pictures.

DOBELLE: Are these congenitally blind patients?

BACH-Y-RITA: We had seven or eight subjects all of whom are congenitally blind. We wanted a population in which there was no previous visual memory.

DOBELLE: I am wondering what would happen if somebody had a previous memory. If you did the experiment on yourself and presented yourself with an object, what would happen? Let us take a disk as an example. Would they recognize it as a rotated disk?

BACH-Y-RITA: We have trained some previously sighted blind subjects. Dr. Reed could probably tell you about the reactions of a naive sighted subject.

DOBELLE: (To Dr. Reed) Does it present any great problem?

REED: No. I think it is an unfair question because I apparently have unusual depth perception, or some such thing. I was able to identify one of the most complex objects without ever having seen it or known anything about it. I described it very satisfactorily and then, from this description, I was able to tell the size, shape, and what it was.

DOBELLE: You say it takes several seconds to recognize these objects?

BACH-Y-RITA: In part, because they have to move the camera, it is very awkward.

DOBELLE: How long does it take to discriminate something like a telephone?

BACH-Y-RITA: It depends on the subject. It may take a few seconds.

DOBELLE: But it could be longer than that?

BACH-Y-RITA: It could be longer if it were partially blocked or had never been exposed previously.

DOBELLE: As you go to increasingly complex items do you attempt to calculate the increased time versus the complexity? Do you get an idea of how complex a scene you can transmit to the subject as a function of speed?

BACH-Y-RITA: No we do not. Not all subjects at all times will identify the telephone in a few seconds. The same subject, for some reason, may take more time. In other words, it is not always immediately recognized as a telephone. He might go over it two or more times before he recognizes it.

DOBELLE: So, actually, we are talking in terms of a number of seconds for pretrained simple objects.

BACH-Y-RITA: Yes, especially in combination with other obejcts on the table.

BLISS: I think there is a logical trap, both in some of the things that Dr. Bach-y-Rita and I presented, as well as in the Brindley screen sort of thing. The image that you see visually may not be anything like what the person is perceiving tactually or with the Brindley screen by phosphenes. The fact that it is very different is even brought out fairly strongly by the statement that the tactile performance, in which Dr. Bach-y-Rita's subject moved the camera was only 50% recognition accuracy. On the other hand, we did not have any control over the camera in the experiments we reported here, and we did recognize the pattern visually. I think this illustrates that you should not make the logical jump that what you see in a 400-point visual picture is comparable to the information the subject is getting tactually, or with the Brindley screen, or what have you. The subject may not be able to get that much information to you. He may not have the pattern processing gear to process that information.

Also, I would like to challenge the statement that the temporal resolving power of the skin is five times that of the eye. It is true that you can feel a 60- or 100-cycle vibration while you cannot tell that a 60- or 100-cycle light is flickering. However, it is not true that you can tell which of two sequentially applied points came first any faster tactually than visually. In fact, if you do that type of experiment, it turns out that you get the same result tactually, visually or auditorily. Very recently, we have done the experiments not using two points, but three points, four points, five points, and six points. It turns out that as you increase the number of points and you ask the subject to order those in time, that tactual performance grows progressively worse than visual performance, as the number of points increases. What happens is if you give the subject two points and ask him which came first, he can do this with a 75% accuracy at 20 msec both visually and tactually. If you give him three points, it takes a longer interstimulus time to achieve this performance level tactually than is required visually. If you go to four or five points, the temporal separation that you need visually is much, much less than that needed tactually.

COLLINS: I would like to rebut the challenge on flicker-fusion frequency. The eye seems to fuse at approximately 50 cps or 100 cps, apparently, depending on intensity level. Goff has quoted 500 cycles to the skin. Darling, through experimentation, indicates that the tactile images presented on the skin can be tracked faster than those presented to the eye.

BLISS: I disagree with the tracking. I have done many tracking experiments and there the skin does not do as well as the eye. I do not think flicker-fusion is an appropriate measure of how fast you can transmit information, because the perception of the stimuli is as a tone. You cannot change that tone any faster tactually than you could visually for sending say, morse code.

COLLINS: That is true as far as the rapidity with images is concerned. However, the bandwidth should be there for preprocessing information such as color, or other information. The skin will perceive these higher frequencies, and we should be able to make use of that bandwidth for coding and other information.

BLISS: I do not think it could be done if the patterns were relative, rather than parallel.

COLLINS: Only in so much as we can project almost raw video information to the skin, and it picks it up.

BLISS: That last statement is where I object. How do you know it picks it up?

COLLINS: What is the objection?

BLISS: It seems to me you are doing an experiment with a visual person, and the person does it visually, and you ask some person to do it tactually, and move the camera, and he can recognize it after a period of time with lower accuracy.

If you do it under static conditions, and present patterns tactually, you say recognition falls to 50%. So, it seems to me there is a great difference between what the person does tactually and what you do visually when shown a 400-point pattern.

COLLINS: Static images are nonphysiological. A fixed retinal image fades out. The same is true of projected tactile images. The eye moves to change the picture and to perceive detail at many points in the surround; the subject moves the tactile television camera over the object to appreciate more details as well.

SIMMONS: I am interested in items concerning lateral inhibition. In any one incident of time for a particular image, how many points were actually transferring information? In other words, what is the redundancy of the system?

BACH-Y-RITA: I guess it is somewhere around half of our points; approximately 200 points.

PROSCIA: I think I am the only blind person here who has had a little experience with the vision substitution system. I sat in the chair last September for about an hour and a half and examined objects. As I recall, I did not recognize objects, but I did recognize shapes or parts of shapes.

When we did get to looking at letters, however, I was able to make intelligent guesses as to the actual letters themselves. I did not recognize the telephone, or the water can, as objects, but I could recognize the various shapes or an edge of scanning associated with the objects.

60-CHANNEL ELEKTROFTALM WITH CdSO₄ PHOTORESISTORS AND FOREHAND TACTILE ELEMENTS

60-CHANNEL ELEKTROFTALM WITH CdSO$_4$ PHOTORESISTORS AND FOREHAND TACTILE ELEMENTS

W. Starkiewicz, W. Kuprianowicz, and F. Petruczenko

From the physiological viewpoint, a certain analogy is felt to exist between the formation of ordinary visual perceptions and the formation of space orientation in the blind by means of multichannel elektroftalm. The mechanism of formation of ordinary space visual perceptions is based upon the creation of so-called optic localization reflexes [1]. This term is applied to all kinds of movement of the whole body or its parts provoked by the optic stimulus. Optic localization reflexes (e.g., the movement of an animal toward the food, movement of the infant's arm toward the milk bottle, etc.) are formed in human beings after birth only, as so-called "conditioned reflexes." In animals these reflexes are, to a great extent, unconditioned, i.e., they are congenital. An example may be provided by a chicken which, just after being hatched from the egg, pecks at minute yellow specks against a grey background with great precision. Upon noticing that an animal displays the optic localization reflexes, we say that the animal "sees." This also refers to man's vision. The space optic localization reflexes are originated by linking the optic stimuli falling upon the eyes with tactile and kinesthetic ones operating throughout the optic stimulus action. If, for instance, straight in front of the infant's eye appears an object of importance to him and it irritates the macula lutea, at the moment he touches it with his hand, the optic stimulus links up in the cerebral cortex with the tactile center of the fingers as well as with kinesthesia of arm muscles stretched in front. After several conjunctions of this kind the macular stimulus itself instantaneously provokes the forward movement of the hand. Then it is said that the child "sees."

The role of the muscular system in the formation of optic perceptions has not been fully appreciated in spite of the fact that records on this subject are encountered in papers of 19th century physiologists. The role of touching in this process has till now practically not been taken into consideration at all.

The congenital absence of vision, i.e., the lack of the optic stimuli receptor, excludes the possibility of forming the optic localization reflexes. Loss of sight at a later age prevents a man from making use of these reflexes although they had previously been formed. When this occurs in an animal, other adaptive mechanisms are created to secure the possibilities of localizing objects that are vital for them. Most frequently cited is the example of a bat which catches minute airborne objects in its snout, with great precision, taking advantage of the ultrasonic localization by means of its ears. It should be emphasized that the main factor facilitating the bat to engage the echolocation is its high speed and agility. Therefore, the example of the bat cannot be resorted to when appliances for the blind are designed.

Space orientation of the blind without technical aid has been the topic of many works. At the present time, however, the greatest success is expected to come from technological developments which aim at converting the optic stimuli into other perceptible sensory stimuli.

Apparatus for the blind constructed to date can be divided into two groups: devices enhancing space orientation and those facilitating the recognition of prints and drawings. Space orientation may be further categorized as obstacle detectors, light detectors, and devices for performing professional work.

The obstacle detectors fail to perceive the light and color of the surrounding objects. Many of the obstacle detectors are single-channel ones. Thus a blind person, who turns the apparatus in different directions, gets at any moment the unidirectional perception of distance at which the obstacle is located. It is only by moving the apparatus that he is given a chance to be oriented, in an extremely inexact and slow way, as to the size and position of the obstacle. The most popular device of the general type is Kay's ultrasonic apparatus [2].

All one-channel detectors of obstacles and lights are of little practical use; Leonard [3] wrote in 1964:

> In practice . . . almost all devices which have got beyond the breadboard stage have been narrow beam, single-channel affairs. With such devices one perceives the environment in a manner analogous to a person having gunbarrel vision. It is well known that persons with telescopic vision field, even if their sight preserves the full acuity, behave practically in the same way as the blind persons do.
>
> I am not yet convinced that the information which the Kay device can gather is of more use than that which could be obtained by intelligent use of the cane.

The multichannel obstacle detector of Nelkin [4] should be highlighted. It is composed of nine ultrasonic transmitters and receivers. This apparatus provides tactile information to nine areas of skin on the blind man's chest. The light detectors are, as a rule, simple one-channel devices transforming the light-ray beams into auditory or tactile stimuli. The prototype of these devices was the single channel elektroftalm of Professor Noiszewski [5]. The blind subject set such a device in various directions, being in this way oriented by turns where the light was. Noiszewski felt that it was possible to create a thermo-tactile image on the forehead composed of 400 points, and even of 40,000 points. Such an image would be the reflection of the optic picture formed on a complex selenic photocell placed at the bottom of the optic camera which was kept on the head of the blind man. In 1956 Prof. Dembowski [6] elaborated on an analogous apparatus. Unfortunately neither Prof. Noiszewski nor Prof. Dembowski could realize their concepts.

In 1958 Prof. Starkiewicz described an analogous apparatus [7]. The multichannel elektroftalm we constructed is applicable in a variety of ways: It serves for space orientation, it is used to decipher large letters and various figures against a dark background and, finally, it is applied for setting white elements into various figures and signs; the latter function is thus analogous to writing and drawing under the control of sight. Execution of the technical side of the elektroftalm project was undertaken at first by T. Kuliszewski of Wroclaw Technical University [8, 9] and it is currently being carried out in our department.

The structure of our multichannel elektroftalm is as follows: On the head of the blind man is mounted an optic camera, on the bottom of which there is, instead of a focusing screen, a mosaic of 60 photoresistors of cadmium sulphate. Previously, we had also tested the function of germanium and silicon photoresistors, but is has been found that the cadmium photoresistors are most appropriate, since their light sensitivity is most similar to that of the human eye. An elastic plate with 60 electromagnetic tactiles is put on the forehead of the blind person. Over his shoulder is suspended a box containing a transistor amplifier. Current is supplied by means of a cable kept above the user's head. Every mosaic photoresistor is included in the composition of one optic–tactile channel. The optic image of the surrounding objects falls upon the mosaic of the photoelements, while the user detects it on his forehead in the form of tactile image.

We carried out experiments with earlier types of multichannel elektroftalm on several blind subjects. The exercises were performed several hours daily over the period of some weeks. They were performed in a special hall whose walls were painted dark and the floor was covered with a dark linoleum. On the ceiling there were incandescent lamps providing a light intensity of 300 to 400 lx. Pieces of furniture inside the hall were painted white and there were special models in the form of gates, human silhouettes etc. Also, geometrical figures and letters measuring 20×40 cm were used for conducting the exercises (the strokes were 7 cm thick). The exercise of a blind patient consisted in moving among the objects, in touching, pushing, etc. This was done in order to obtain a collection of optic–tactile localization reflexes analogous to optic localization reflexes formed in people with normal vision. In this way the skin of the forehead becomes an organ similar to the retina. In fact, after some weeks of training the blind person equipped with the elektroftalm began to be oriented as to the distance and shape of surrounding objects. He managed to move upon a white path painted on the floor, he recognized big white letters against the black background, and he was even able to assemble white elements into letters and figures.

At present we have made an improved model of elektroftalm. With the former models it happened quite often that the reflection of the surrounding images on the forehead were not exact. We have also constructed an apparatus for the blind subjects to distinguish color. The description of the first apparatus of this kind was presented by Starkiewicz in 1959 [7]. The essence of the device is based upon the application of three photocells, one of which reacts solely to the red rays, the second to green or yellow, the third one to blue. It is obtainable either through sensitizing the photocells to appropriate wavelengths, or by placing a proper filter in front of each one of them. As soon as such an apparatus is directed to the red surface, only the photocell with the red filter begins to act, evoking skin vibration of the compressor with a pointed ending. The apparatus directed onto the green field provokes skin stimuli being moderately blunt. The blue rays give rise to blunt skin stimuli. In this way the blind person may recognize the color of the surface on which he

sets the device. In the future we want to provide our multichannel elektroftalm with a number of threefold compressors of the described type.
This will enable the blind subject to distinguish not only the shape of the
objects but also their color.

A similar apparatus for recognizing color by the blind was described
by Bishop in 1965 [10]. The device was not actually constructed, but a
description covered its functioning, which is found to be somewhat different as compared with our apparatus. The Bishop apparatus originates
vibration in the first finger whenever the apparatus is directed onto the
red field, in the second finger when green, etc.

The scope of our work on the elektroftalm was widened by the studies
on tactile feeling in the blind. In these studies, various shapes (letters,
circles, hooks, etc.) were touched by subjects to determine recognition
rates. In general, this ability in people is developed extremely poorly.
A man does not distinguish a big circle from a square applied to his chest.
In real life only numerous single, point localization, skin-to-skin reflexes
are originated. (For example, we perform an accurate finger movement
toward the irritated point of the skin.) In our blind subjects we were
able, after some days of training, to obtain the faculty of distinguishing
the letters measuring 9×5 cm being placed upon the skin of the abdo-
men and the thorax. It may be expected that longer training will lead to
better results.

REFERENCES

[1] Starkiewicz W., "Psychofizjologia wzroku." PZWL, Warsaw, Poland, 1960.
[2] Kay L., *Proc. Rotterdam Mobility Res. Conf.* 3–7, **VIII**, 9 (1965).
[3] Leonard J. A., *Res. Bull.* **7**, 1 (1964), Am. Found. for the Blind, New York.
[4] Nelkin A., *Proc. Rotterdam Mobility Res. Conf.* 3–7, **VIII**, 17 (1965).
[5] Noiszewski K., "Gazeta Lekarska" Chap. 24. Ser. II, Vol. IX. pp. 1018–1022, 1949.
[6] Dembowski J., "Psychologia zwierzat." Czytelnik, Warsaw, 1956.
[7] Starkiewicz W., Polskiej Akademii Nauk Warszawa, **IV**, 11–12, 1958; Zaklad Narodowy im. Ossolinskich, Warszawa-Wroclaw 1959, pp. 138–161.
[8] Starkiewicz., W, and Kuliszewski T., *Proc. Intern. Cong. Tech. Blindness* **VI**, 18 (1962).
[9] Starkiewicz W., and Kuliszewski T., *Proc. Rotterdam Mobility Res. Conf.* 3–7, **VIII**, 27 (1965).
[10] Bishop W. B., *Proc. Rotterdam Mobility Res. Conf.* 3–7, **VIII**, 30 (1965).

PROGRESS IN MOBILITY AID DESIGN

R. W. Mann

I want to emphasize the role of time and urgency in the mobility situation. When one travels in any environment one cannot avoid being profoundly influenced by it. The capacity to respond to temporal aspects of the surroundings has a much more profound influence on the traveler than on the reader.

A very important point contrasting reading and mobility is the consequence of a mistake. A reading error means misinterpretation or loss of speed. For the traveler, however, the hazards may be very, very great. While the reader can afford to be casual at his task, a blind traveler cannot.

This involvement of the human with the task provides another contrast between reading and travel. The reader rarely divides his attention between reading and some other action. Conversely, the traveler would prefer not to commit his complete attention to mobility.

Thus, mobility is a much more difficult, unconstrained, unpredictable, hazardous, multidimensional, time-shared operation as contrasted with reading. If a visual prosthesis purports to be a "general prosthesis," it must anticipate and provide for these realistic considerations in addition to those which can be conveniently displayed via stimulation and computer preprocessing.

Given the void between normal sight and realistic assessment of future potentials, we need strategies which capitalize on trade-offs between present cold reality and utopian prospects of a true substitute for the eye. In our laboratory we have chosen to commit our developmental and evaluation resources to what we believe to be a good interim solution and to devote our research capability to the delineation of the means by which to study blind mobility in more general terms and thereby define the necessary and sufficient characteristics of effective mobility aids.

The Pathsounder [1], an ultrasonic mobility aid invented by Lindsay Russell, has been under study at our Center for Sensory Aids Evaluation and Development since the early sixties. Based on our cumulative evaluation experience and the redesigns of the instrument, a Pathsounder Training Manual was prepared and the current model replicated in a modest lot of 15. The response of most of the blind users and their trainers has been encouraging; there are now several blind travelers who use the aid routinely in their travel, in one case now for over a year. The next logical step would be engineering redesign using integrated circuits and other space-conserving features to substantially reduce its volume, thereby making its use by the blind less conspicuous and reducing the manufacturing costs. (We are also exploring the potential effectiveness of a novel, cutaneous display using the ultrasonic ranging detector of the Pathsounder instrument.)

A more ambitious research question is the study of the mobility of the blind per se, with an eye toward defining the specifications for mobility devices [2]. We have studied the feasibility of a computer based mobility simulator which would in principle perform much like the display simulators described at this conference by Carr, Knowlton, and Sterling. The blind traveler would carry what he thought was a mobility device; however, the device detection characteristics would, in fact, be simulated by a computer program, which at every instant would know the location of the man by means of a surveillance system. When the blind man's position was such that the simulator indicated the presence of an obstacle, the computer, through telemetry, would cue a physical tactile and/or auditory display on the human, assessing him of the hazard.

Such a scheme would permit:

(1) the rapid alteration of the characteristics of potential sensory devices, obviating the need to build all of the experimental types,

(2) the collection and assessment of quantitative data on the performance of a blind traveler,

(3) the assessment of the respective capabilities of blind travelers, thereby elucidating individual differences, and

(4) the experimental basis on which to begin to develop a general theory of mobility.

It is perhaps not unreasonable to compare this conference's earnest desire to give the blind man the enormous concomitants of vision to a Presidential aspiration of a decade ago to put a "man on the moon in the sixties." In my view the scope and scale of the visual prosthesis is vaster, more challenging and more humane.

REFERENCES

[1] Russell, L., Travel path sounder, further results, *Proc. Intern. Conf. Sensory Devices for the Blind*, Dunston, New York (1966).

[2] Mann, R. W., Evaluation and simulation of mobility aids for the blind, *Res. Bull.* 11, Oct. 1965, American Foundation for the Blind, New York.

[3] Mann, R. W., Mobility aids for the blind-environmental detection, information processing and substitute sensory modality display, *IEEE Intern. Conv. Digest,* (1969).

COMPUTER AIDED GENERATION OF
SPEECH DISPLAYS

K. Ingham

I define "preprocessing" as the transformation of the information from the surroundings into a suitably coded form for presentation to the nervous system, including peripheral systems such as the ear or the skin. In this sense, Braille is an excellent form of preprocessing; and, in that light, before I go into the auditory material, I would like to make a few points which may not be obvious to everyone here, sighted people particularly.

In the Braille area, there are at least two principal transcribing organizations in the country, numbering more than 3000 transcribers, who provide material which allows me to read at five times the rate of the proposed visual prosthesis. The only problem remaining in the production of Braille is that of quick delivery, and thanks to ongoing research, devices are now becoming available which could be placed into the hands of service organizations.

One of these, for example, is a successful prototype at MIT in which a computer translates Braille onto a Model D IBM typewriter at reasonably high rates. This system can be put into use for under $10,000, with cost effectiveness being even better in a time-sharing environment.

On the other hand, there is another presentation display for the nervous system, namely the auditory. A comment was made earlier about the number of points one could use in coding different stimuli on a screen. Clearly, the number of stimuli available in Webster's Unabridged Dictionary is far greater and far more effective as a medium of information transfer.

What I am going to play for you now is a recording of computer-generated speech. This is a time shared computer-based system where the blind person operates a $100 keyboard, typing in from his office or his home over the phone line. He receives his replies and information back in voice. The recording will begin with my typing a message at pick-and-peck speed.[1]

This particular voice output is on a Mitre computer system coupled with an information retrieval program, and the voice speaks what I direct by means of a series of commands. One of them is a dash-R command, which allows the user to type various messages, with the computer composing replies or echo messages for the user to hear.[2] The speed of this is governed strictly by my typing speed.[3]

I am going through this exercise mainly to show you that I could choose to listen to my typing to make sure I am not making a mistake; this could easily be done. Now, it will come back in message form. The program will compose the message and return with a cross between spelled speech and whole speech.[4]

There are two ways one can generate speech. One of them is a technique you have just heard, that of compiled speech. You store sound representations of words or letters, or parts of words, or whatever you desire. When a particular word does not exist in the data base, it is spelled out.

I would like to illustrate some whole speech used in the presentation of rehabilitation files of the Commission for the Blind. Here an entire repertoire of questions or queries are supplied to the counselor, giving statistical information about a particular client, ranging from address to summary reports, medical reports, and so on. The answers are obtained by phoning and querying the computer. Again, the speech here is being

---

[1] Author demonstrates typing method.

[2] Author demonstrates typing of F-T-H-E-I-B-M.

[3] Author demonstrates typing of 1,8,00, C,O,M,P,U,T,E,R, S,A,Y,I,N,G, O,U,T, T,H,E, W,O,R,D,S, A,N,D, L,E,T,T,E,R,S.

[4] Computer returns the message T,H,A,T, I, T,Y,P,E. (Output speech: "This is the IBM 1800 computer S,A,Y,I,N,G, out. The W,O,R,D,S, and L,E,T,T,E,R,S out I, T,Y,P,E.")

presented without any control over the spacing, intonation, and so on. Consequently, these are somewhat primitive, but clearly it is already an effective sensory aid.[5] Now here the system is spitting out individual pieces of information about a given client, in this case, a fictitious client, as you can tell by the social security number. The beep signals the end of the message. If there is not a personal reply before the beep, there is none recorded.

There are four basic ways in which one can code or present language, given some sort of input. In one of these, you can sit at some sort of a console and enter phonemes, stress marks, and so on, using full intuition as to how you think the machine ought to work; there are essentially no rules involved here. The second approach is to direct such activity by a set of rules. The third is to enter English letters and do no preprocessing at all, but simply translate them using some computational dictionary approach to determine the appropriate sound. The fourth and final course is to take the English letters or other characters and do some linguistic analysis (e.g., parsing) thereby producing prosodic features. What we have heard thus far is the result of the third type of processing, namely, entering English letters with no preprocessing.

We shall now listen to an example of the second approach in which the operator types in phonemes and stress marks.[6]

These are obviously successful displays with respect to translating information. The quality may not be what we, as blind people, would like to have all the time, but there is plenty of room for work and improvement.

I am a researcher and not, in any sense, against research, especially with respect to sensory aids. Although brain research is important, I do not think that calling it research in sensory aids is correct. Functional solutions, such as those described by Dr. Hallenbeck, supply all that I need, and, I maintain, all that most blind people need. The approach of treating the blind person as a raw subject, trying to drive into him as violently or strongly as necessary, the information, I do not think is appropriate. It is not socially relevant research.

The synthesized example that you just heard required 8000 18-bit words of storage on a POP-9 computer. This includes both program and data.

[5] Author demonstrates. (Computer-produced auditory output: "The value of the social security number is 777-77-7777. Beep. The value of the client's last name is L-I-T-T-L-E-W-O-O-Z, Beep.")

[6] Author demonstrates the recitation of "Little Miss Moffett" using synthesized speech [1].

The compiled speech was stored in delta encoding on a 23-lever-type disk pack. The capacity of this unit is such that it could accommodate a vocabulary of 12,000 to 15,000 individual English words.

REFERENCE

[1]   Walter, L. Edna (ed.), Mother Goose's Nursery Rhymes, A & C Black, London, 1924, p. 78.

SOME THOUGHTS ON VISUAL PROSTHESES

E. F. Murphy

The total problems of blindness are indeed serious; substantial numbers of people are affected, each to a considerable extent. Therefore, serious efforts are justified on moral, sociological, and economic grounds.

It is salutary to realize that blindness or visual handicaps, both here and especially in some areas abroad, may also result from poverty of the individual or society. Hence, the value of money urged for research must be compared with the effectiveness of comparable sums spent on prevention. Likewise, much functional and legal blindness might be overcome by greater expenditures for known remedies—ophthalmic surgery, better refraction, magnifiers, counseling on best use of existing aids, etc. Also, even for the irreparably visually handicapped and blind, known methods of rehabilitation would be more effective if more funds were available for wise investments in them.

Nevertheless, there remains a strong case for the wisdom of expenditures on research and development on a broad spectrum of aids for the blind. There is more than enough challenge for all; coordination and cooperation are needed. Systematic teamwork of many disciplines as well as of related agencies is needed to help each individual client to attain the optimum service and rehabilitation commensurate with present knowledge and to benefit promptly from new research results. To this

end the Veterans Administration has specialized multidisciplinary rehabilitation centers and has established unique teams at outpatient clinics
throughout the country to provide a meeting of skills capable of helping
each blinded veteran to reach his greatest potential.

The Veterans Administration research program on aids for the blind
has brought a laser cane and two types of direct-translation reading aids
(plus screening and training programs) to the advanced stage of clinical
application studies and has other, more advanced aids in earlier stages of
development. Work under the sponsorship of the Veterans Administration has been going on at a number of laboratories on various types
of reading machines for the blind, in a gamut of approaches from very
simple direct translation devices of the optophone type (translating the
shape of the letter into sound) through a potentially inexpensive recog-
nition-type machine that detects individual letters. These are being developed by Mauch Laboratories, with working prototypes already built.

The work at Haskins Laboratory is of the type described by Dr.
Ingham, with speech-like output obtained from a special processing
machine. The three major possibilities are: Compiled speech from a dictionary of approximately 7000 words, speech synthesized by rule, and a
somewhat intermediate version called reformed speech which attempts
to store the "skeleton" of the word rather than the complete word.

We are going to demonstrate the intermediate type of work done by
Metfessel on "spelled speech" which Mauch Laboratories is generating
as the output of a recognition type reading machine.[1]

The selections on the tape were produced by using a prototype reading machine which operated from typewritten text at a speed of roughly
75 words per minute.

In addition to these developments of the devices themselves, considerable attention has been given to psychological problems of selection,
training, and acceptance. Progress reports are published in the literature,
including the *Bulletin of Prosthetics Research* and by occasional mailings
to a list of several hundred specialists. The Veterans Administration also
attempts to keep informed of the work of other agencies and their con-
tractors or grantees. Plans for increasingly broader clinical studies on
veterans, including development of teaching facilities, will hopefully be
coordinated with development programs for children and for nonveteran
adults.

On a longer time scale, the Veterans Administration is interested in
the possibilities of more elaborate visual prostheses. Possibly these might

[1] Author gives taped demonstration.

make use of analogous experience in other fields of prosthetics and of electrodes for cardiac pacemakers.

Most people flatly reject the possibility of long-term intrusion through the integument, but a few consider that past failures and infections can be at least partially explained on the basis that the stress concentrations at the margin between a stiff rod, tube, or cable and the more flexible skin tend to tear open attempted scarring attachment. Thus, more ingenious designs with better materials and subtle transitions of stiffness (such as tapered collars) might possibly allow longer resistance to infection and extrusion.

The ASTM Committee F-4 (surgical implants) has studied metal used in orthopedics and some day will presumably reach electrode materials. There are problems of ion migrations, polarization, pulse shape, and other factors related to building of fibrous tissue and increase of impedance over long periods of time.

There is a temptation to demand proof of a major solution before anything is done, but we believe progress can be made by a series of steps, each directly beneficial to the subjects involved and each building as far as feasible upon previous accomplishments. We consider that even six operating implanted points are enough for the Braille code, already very valuable to a minority of the blind. Nine points allow the binary "map" proposed in tactile form (by Witcher) for output of a scanning-type mobility aid—three sectors of left, ahead, and right, each having three distance zones of awareness, attention, and avoidance. It might be possible to experiment with such a map in the very near future.

A few people can already read slowly with Mauch's eight-element Visotactor or nine-element Visotoner. Electrically lighted signs of only 35 lamps in five-by-seven arrays allow blocked capitals and numerals to be interpreted. Bliss and Bach-y-Rita, reporting at this conference discussed success with tactile stimulators.

Thus, increasingly complex input devices are *already* in existence, at least in a few copies, to allow relatively simple trials in conjunction with subjects in whom rather modest numbers of electrodes have been implanted. In our opinion, neither the experimenter nor the subject need wait for a television-quality presentation before expecting sufficiently useful and directly practical display of information to motivate the subject, allow meaningful practice and experiments—and fan enthusiasm. Cautious optimism regarding usefulness of long-range, persistent, carefully controlled experimentation and dogged development seems reasonable.

Part III

THOUGHTS ON PROSTHETIC
EXPERIMENTS ON HUMANS

Introduction

Little or no risk exists for humans who may volunteer for early implantation experiments. The risk to their lives is small and if nervous tissue would be destroyed, it would be tissue which is presumably useless for a blind individual. (The same would not be true for sighted volunteers. However, it is unlikely that sighted volunteers would be used for implantation experiments.)

Debate on the use of human volunteers predominantly turned around two issues.

It is likely that the first experiments could create enough damage in the visual cortex so as to preclude the volunteer from enjoying the fruits of his daring. This then leads to the demand that enough should be known to make sure the implant used for early volunteers is replaceable or is good enough to serve as a rudimentary visual aid. Perhaps this problem of ethics in science illuminates how close we may be to a workable visual prosthesis.

The second problem was one less well understood by the visual scientists since it is rather newly created—finding its origin in new advances in automated instrumentation. When a human preparation is made, it is not sufficient to use it to provide information on a few crucial points of inquiry. Rather, experimental conditions should be arranged so that as much information as possible can be learned from a human volunteer. However, to do that requires a technical preparation of the highest order of equipment sophistication as well as of those technological necessities which are summed under the name of "software." The issues are well represented, both by discussion and by the next position paper, that of Marvin Minsky.

DEVELOPMENT OF A FACILITY FOR
VISUAL PROSTHESIS EXPERIMENTS ON HUMANS

M. Minsky

This paper discusses the problem of efficient and humane management of experiments on humans who have been given direct cortical implants for visual system stimulation.

The problem is this: We do not yet know very much about how a pictorial image should be presented in order to elicit a useable image from a low-resolution array of stimulator points on the cortex. There is no really conclusive set of experiments that can be performed on animals in advance of the experiments on humans, because the interpretation of the animals' image qualities would be so ambigious. Correct animal responses could be based on all sorts of not-very-useful properties of the stimuli. Thus meaningful experiments on image processing have to be done on humans.

I consider it quite unlikely that a simple intensity modulated display will give acceptable results, even with correction for varying sensitivity of the different implant stimulator points. Of course, this is the first area that should be explored, in any case. But we must expect that some sophisticated image feature extraction and recoding will be needed.

The experiments that will have to be done are rather complex, and involve presentation of thousands of experimental patterns. There are at least two classes of parameters that must be explored: Electric-and-temporal qualities of the point-stimuli and spatio-temporal qualities of the image-processing encoding apparatus. Fortunately, it is likely that these two classes interact only moderately; experiments that yield acceptable images of single line segments might define conditions that allow us to build figures that are made of several line segments.

Before the experiments are done, a computer laboratory should be constructed with equipment for real-time control of stimulus patterns to be presented to the electrodes. The programming should be completed, and operators trained so that any of the patterns discussed below can be compiled and presented within a very few minutes. The laboratory must be as complete as possible, including high-quality real-time display equipment.

A reasonable basis for such an elaborate setup would be to combine this with the initiation of a laboratory for the general study of visual perception and for biomedical picture processing. This would justify both the programming effort for the set of programming languages outlined below, as well as the powerful hardware facility, and make it possible to recruit suitably talented staff.

Stimulus Exploration

A set of programs must be written to explore the effects of stimulation of single electrodes, and small groups of closely-spaced electrodes. The operator must be able to vary quickly parameters such as intensity, repetition rate, duty cycle, alternation between pairs, direction propagation along the array, etc., so that he can determine sets of elementary stimulus patterns that produce useful and nondistributing subjective events. The exploration system should include the following features:

(1)   complete automatic recording of all transactions and comments by the operator;

(2)   sequencing for automatic stepping through the experiments for all points and groups already supposed to be functional;

(3)   the stimulus parameters should be made as independent as possible, change in repetition rate should not affect mean intensity; and

(4)   for each parameter, we should perhaps provide a logarithmic-search hill-climbing program, operated directly by subject's responses. Thus the subject can be asked to select the most comfortable intensity for some pattern by a sequence of two-way selections, very quickly. Needless to say, he might also do this by simply turning a proportional control.

Spatial Field Mapping and Interpolation

When some usable stimulus parameters have been selected, the visual field must be correlated with the stimulus point. This poses a fascinating new problem in metrical geometry. One can begin with a rough subjective pointing by the subject to spatial directions, but these must be corrected, presumably, by information about eye direction and head position. For the long blind or congenitally blind, the problem is more abstract. In any case, once one has a rough mapping of the points, it can be refined by asking about triples of points, whether the middle one is left-or-right of the (vertical) line defined by the end points—and similarly for horizontally disposed triplets. The resulting information defines the local geodesic field. Then one must reassign the global locations in accord with the answers to questions about longer straight lines, etc., using as much of discernible geometric imagery as available. Obviously, there is interaction between this phase and the earlier stimulus exploration phase.

The result of the field mapping should be an assignment of stimulus points to visual space that is compiled into a program used by all successive phases in relating to the external world. Generally, desired stimulus points will probably have to be assigned to the nearest actual electrode, and only experimentation will determine whether some kind of interpolation is feasible; for example, representation of an inbetween point by a weighted combination of its neighbors. Offhand, it is unlikely that this will do much good. However, because our presentations are so different from normal physiological stimuli, especially in their simplicity, there is always a chance that the subject can learn to make suitable interpretations of such combinations.

Homogeneous Picture Processing

The system should contain a programming language for homogeneous picture processing—to apply local operators uniformly over the area of a picture. Local operators recognize configurations in the neighborhood of each point and can be used to produce various effects of image, contrast enhancement, and feature emphasis. They could serve, for example, to perform local gradient emphasis, reciprocal inhibitions, and other jobs that might be required to obtain a usable image on the low-resolution "retina," such as selecting the boundaries and corners in a scene. The effect of Mach boundaries can be simulated at this level. There exist a very wide variety of schemes and whole systems for such purposes; of course, they have never been evaluated with regard for our purposes.

There are known also a variety of not-quite-so-local procedures for boundary-finding. These procedures usually first find points that (locally) seem to lie along boundaries and then attempt to link or "cluster" those points into curves, rejecting "noisy" boundary-like points that do not so link up to others. Some such procedures should be provided at the start. There is some question about how much a role they will play in the long run, since it is plausible to hope that much of this linking-up function can be supplied by the cortex as a lower-level cognitive process.

It is reasonable, at this level, also to consider the role of color. At all stages of the stimulus exploration process, the subject should be instructed to report any and all interesting visual events, including senses of color, motion, and even texture. Accordingly, the prepared system should be able to exploit any such effects, and the optical input facility ought to have at least a set of easily engaged filters for making color measurements.

Accordingly, the homogeneous processor should be equipped to handle combined inputs of two and three pictures, from the same source with different color sensitivities, to produce output pictures whose "points" are actually specifications of stimulus macrooperations, including the possibilities of those stimulus sequences that have been found to elicit the special color or motion sensations.

Image Preparation Language

For efficiency and accuracy, the laboratory should be equipped with a library file of basic visual scenes, stored in digital form, ranging from the simplest geometric forms and alphabetical characters through more complex scenes of simple objects to real-life scenes of fair to poor visual quality. These can be quickly called to test hypotheses about what processing techniques will make different kinds of scenes easier to analyze. But more important is the ability to test interactions between parts of scenes even when the parts are individually perceived adequately. To explore such problems, one needs to be able to synthesize scenes quickly allowing for superposition of one object over another, and to control the simulated lighting conditions. (Programs already exist that can do this for fairly complicated geometries.)

The system should also be able to acquire real external scenes, and store suitable parts of them in memory when desired. Our own experience with computer image processing tells us that there are many unanticipated problems for particular scenes, even when a system seems to have some generality on the basis of its performance with a few recorded scenes. It is then necessary to go over the offending stimulus and try to find out just what is the disturbing feature, and to do this the operator has to have a good filing system.

This picture preparing system should also be able to handle sequences of images to experiment with various motion techniques. Since it is difficult to anticipate much about the form such sequences ought to take (frame-by-frame, or local motion cues?) the important emphasis here ought to be on programming flexibility, and upon the availability of a large primary high-speed memory to make the experiments easy. Almost certainly, as discoveries are made, the computational and memory strain on the central computer will decrease, but it is vitally important the processor begin with an unusually large speed and memory allocation to make the research phase efficient and speedy. These requirements are important also in virtually any image-processing facility, anyway.

Eye Tracking Facility

The limitations of forseeable implants and the normal modes of visual scanning combine to suggest that to achieve anything like useful vision will require integration of many successive images. The physiological way to accomplish such integration is presumably by making the stimulator inputs depend properly on the intentional eye motions; most blind persons presumably retain good control over this motor system, and could use it in conjunction with the system's inputs. There now exist on-line eye tracking devices that operate remotely—by watching the subject's face from a convenient distance. With such a device one can learn more about the mechanisms of vision, and prepare the scientific background for a much more natural visual prosthetic device. Our own laboratory is planning to explore this area and we may be able to contribute more information about it later.

DISCUSSION

FOULKE: I wonder if someone would comment on how "ticklish" this problem (of cortical implantation and stimulation) is likely to be involving human subjects with the kind of experiment that will have to be performed in order to demonstrate the feasibility of this approach?

VAUGHAN: This is, of course, a major consideration, and has led us into what is for us a difficult philosophical problem.

DOTY: There is at the moment only one known difference between effects of brain stimulation in man and monkey: There are areas of the human cortex which are silent to electrical stimulation, whereas in the monkey none have been found.[1] Whether the difference here is that the monkeys have been trained whereas no human beings have been trained to respond to electrical stimulation of these so-called "silent areas" is not known. There is, however, no reason to suspect that man would not be able to utilize them.

Another interesting aspect to this is that monkeys trained to respond to stimulation in Area 17, and then asked if stimulation of Area 19 is anything like that, reply, in essence, "No. I have never been stimulated this way before." In other words, he does not respond when Area 19 is stimulated after being trained to respond to stimulation of Area 17. Here is a further illustration of what could be asked of a human subject in an afternoon but is going to require many years to ask of the monkey.

JOHNSON: In this stimulation of Area 17 and Area 19, is the monkey involved in stimulating himself; or, are you presenting it? He is receiving it passively and then responding?

DOTY: The latter is correct. I have a minor historical note on this particular point. The paper which I ultimately published [2] on electrical stimulation of the cerebral cortex in the monkey and which was intended to pave the way for investigations such as those of Brindley and Lewin, was originally submitted to the *BRAIN*. Lord Brain, then its editor, wrote back that while these were very interesting experiments they could not have been done in Great Britain, and he was thus unable to publish them there.

I am, therefore, rather amused that while we could not publish the monkey experiments in *BRAIN*, the experiments on man could be done there, in Great Britain, and they in turn probably could not have been published in this country.

BERING: How much of the needed research might possibly be done on animals and what can only be obtained from humans?

DOTY: I could get into a rather lengthy discussion there, but let me just say immediately that Dr. Brindley showed two extremely important things which would have taken us years of difficult experimentation to ask of the monkey. The first of these is that immediately upon cessation of the stimulation, the phosphene disappears at most points. You would have to design some very ingenious and difficult experiments to ask such a question of a monkey.

The other thing Brindley found was that when the patient moved her eyes, the phosphene moved in space, whereas when her head and eyes were moved

---

[1] Doty, R. W., *Ann. Rev. Pschol*, **20**, 298 (1969).
[2] Doty, R. W., *J. Neurophysiol.* **28**, 623 (1965).

passively, the phosphene appeared to remain stationary. Again, it would be exceedingly difficult to question a monkey on this point; indeed, I have abandoned many question of this kind, knowing that it will be so much more efficient to answer these kinds of things in man rather than monkey. Simply to ask the monkey, "Can you process the information from two points concurrently in the visual cortex?"—is very difficult; but in man this can be asked and answered immediately. Therefore, I think human experimentation is absolutely essential. And while I am talking, perhaps this is the time to raise the plea that we somehow get a different climate toward experimentation on human subjects in this country.

There have been abuses which have now led to the point where investigators are having, I think, undue difficulty. My personal position is that I now know enough from my work on monkeys to ask meaningful questions by electrical stimulation as a purely experimental procedure in man, and for the past few years have offered use of my own cerebral cortex to begin the research. I see no moral or technical reason why, following a long tradition in experimental physiology, that the investigator should not be permitted to follow such procedures on himself, or on knowledgeable colleagues. Such experimentation on individuals who are fully aware of the significance and technical details, as well as the dangers, is far better than using patients whose lack of full comprehension (and, often lack of descriptive abilities) may seriously limit the scope and reliability of the observations.

There is a great problem in using information from sighted individuals. Since the input to the visual cortex will be quite different from normal in patients with loss of retinal responses, it is conceivable that there may be differences between the responses of blind individuals to cortical stimulation, particularly in those who have been blind for a long time, and sighted individuals.

SIMMONS: I am sorry, but I missed the point here of how the sighted person would be a less effective participant?

VAUGHAN: Not less effective. The problem is that the physiology of the visual system in the blind individual may be different.

SIMMONS: In terms of cortical perception?

DOTY: The electroencephalogram of the blind is very bizarre in many individuals. Dr. Sakakura and I now have experiments in blind monkeys which show extraordinary changes in the EEG of the striate cortex. Therefore one must assume that striking physiological changes accompany this alteration of background activity.

BERING: The physiology of the EEG is not known. The statement you are making, really, is that there is a change of the state of the cortex.

DOTY: Yes, the cortex is in a different state if it has a different EEG.

BERING: Which means it has a changed input.

VAUGHAN: This is the point—the input is different. For example, if one enucleates a monkey, or patches the eye, the afferent information arriving at the visual cortex will be altered and the EEG changes.

DOTY: I think it points up a very real physiological point. As Dr. Bering has said, we do not know the full significance of these changes, but their magnitude certainly suggests the possibility of greatly altered function.

JOHNSON: May I suggest that whatever device is interfacing with the visual environment, delivering information to the system providing the stimulus to the cortex, be under the effect or control of the subject; that is, if the subject can move it around to produce a change in the way it is looking, then you might as well use an animal subject and observe his changes in the use of visual space, which I think is the whole point of the devices anyway.

VAUGHAN: That is only part of it, because the visual prosthesis would be a general purpose device capable not only of use in mobility, but also for reading.

In terms of its utility for reading, I think one has to think in terms of either some sort of a coding system other than the usual spatial coding system, which would be difficult to study in animals, or in a display which is topologically similar to normal vision.

As Dr. Doty has pointed out, that kind of thing is very difficult, if not impossible, to study in animals because it is very difficult to know what the cues are that are being used for discrimination.

JOHNSON: The experimental evidence cited earlier as being indicative of the need for human subjects was, for example, that on cessation of stimulation the phosphenes disappeared. This is the kind of information to which I am referring. You would know very well that it had disappeared in the animal because he would simply stop using the prosthesis.

DOTY: I think you are "daydreaming" if you are going to have a hookup of a monkey and use this as a prosthesis and know what you are doing.

VAUGHAN: The critical questions are not whether or not the phosphenes disappear, but rather how fast. You see, there is every difference between a phosphene which persists for 50 msec, and one which persists for 3 sec, and that is the kind of difference about which we are talking.

HALLENBECK: I see no intrinsic problem in designing very simple experiments to determine that kind of thing in animals. I am not convinced that the distinction is very clear between what needs to be done and what might be done, let us say, in animals.

VAUGHAN: Although you can do it in animals for almost any single question that you want to ask, the questions that have to be asked are not single questions. If you have 1000 electrodes, you have to ask these for each electrode.

We are being asked to retreat to the pre-Brindley era when there was still a question as to whether a spatial matrix of cortical stimulation would produce a display which would conform to the topography of the retinal–cortical projection. This has now been demonstrated. We must now obtain detailed data concerning stimulus parameters, and the combinations of stimuli that will be effective in maximal transmission of visual information.

INGHAM: You can take a normal person and expose him to all sorts of flashing lights, and all sorts of hallucinatory effects and reactions will occur. I cannot imagine that some of the things possible with this device, even the simple things, would not cause similar or even more serious effects.

VAUGHAN: I disagree. I think it is true that excessive stimulation, whether it is through a normal sensory channel, or direct stimulation of the brain, will produce a disruptive effect. However, we are talking about the minimal levels required to achieve an appropriate visual display. That is quite different than driving the brain with an intense stroboscopic flash, at a rate of 10 per second —a very disturbing stimulus, that will induce seizures in some individuals.

INGHAM: I was not referring to the contrived situation, where you deliberately harass the subject to uncover effect, but where you have the average individual who is simply fatigued and is experiencing psychic fatigue. What happens in this situation?

STERLING: I do not think we have an answer to that. However, it is a point well taken, and the only thing we have to say is we shall see what is "traded off" under various conditons.

BRODEY: There seems to be a funny action going on here. In the first place, there is what I call a "skull taboo." "Skull taboo" says that you should not open the skull regardless of the physiology. This is not an anthropological kind of affair. It is a mythology that exists among us that the skull is sacrosanct, that if you open it up and fool around inside of it that you are committing a crime of enormous proportions.

This does not have much to do with the actual damage to be done physiologically—damage to be done perhaps psychologically in an actual person. So, that is one value structure that is problematical, the "skull taboo."

The second problem that we should get at is whether a person has a right to decide, when they are well-informed, about the level of risk that they wish to take for themselves. This is, again, a matter of values. On one hand everybody who looks on a person who decides he is going to take such a risk says, "You know, isn't it marvelous; such a hero!" On the other hand, there is the consideration that they might become a victim of the same quality, and the difference between "hero" and "victim" is so often very small.

I am suggesting here that as I see the situation, the person does have a right to make his own choice as to what contribution he wants to make with his body, or with his mind, or with his actions. The blind have been used as victims for a long, long time, and that they resent being victims is, I think, very natural.

Until we start to conceive of experimentation of this sort as being useful to all people, blind and sighted, and useful in trying to learn more about vision itself, and how to enhance our own vision, I do not think we can get away from this "blind victim" type of problem.

STERLING: I think we have two opposing approaches, two conflicting, divergent points of view. Dr. Brodey refers to a "skull taboo," that has as its basis the fear that we might do some real damage, we might deprive an individual of something. We might deprive an individual of some of his creative ability by interfering with the nervous system

On the other hand, there is the immutable logic of Dr. Doty's point that there are some things we just have to learn. If we are going to use a prosthetic device we are going to have to get in there and learn something about the things that take place. I do not see any way out except, of course, that some people will do experiments and other people will not.

SCHIMMEL: Dr. Brodey, wouldn't you agree that in part you meet these criticisms by having the blind person in these experiments be a sophisticated collaborator?

BRODEY: I, myself, feel that in this kind of experimentation the old concept of "subject" simply does not fit, and that it is, as Dr. Vaughan has stated, a matter where this person must be a collaborator not for reasons of ethics but for reasons of practical utilization.

SCHIMMEL: Right.

BRODEY: The old days of objective science where there was a subject in the traditional psychological experiments are passed. Now, since the person who is the primary individual in the loop, is having the experiment done on him in a sense is a part of the whole information exchange. There is none of the old objective because the thing is too complex.

MACKAY: I think we have to distinguish between the surgical risk involved in the operation and the possible trauma of going through the experience with all sorts of hopes being raised and then being dashed.

Although, if we are correctly informed, the surgical risks are small. The primary justification in the case of Dr. Brindley's patients is the hope of doing the patient some good, and this could not begin to apply to a normal person who already had sight.

I think that the trauma might usefully be compared with the sort of trauma that people went through in trying to learn to use the optophone, and similar devices. What we have to ask is whether the risk of possible disappointment is outweighed by the patient's hope of gaining some benefit. I would have thought there was much less justification for doing such experiments on normals than on blind people who were motivated sufficiently, and still less justification for doing experiments on animals. We will get far more of the kind of information we need out of suitably-motivated blind persons than you will out of an animal.

Part IV

WHY OR WHY NOT A
VISUAL PROSTHESIS?

Introduction

Visual prosthesis has been controversial from its very inception. It would be too much to expect that all the participants at the conference would agree on the purpose, the urgency, the aims, the strategy, or even the justification for producing this device. Obviously they did not. Our intent, then, is to give a fair and balanced view of the discussion regarding the motivation for further work.

DISPLAY CONSIDERATIONS IN
VISUAL PROSTHESIS DESIGN

C. E. Hallenbeck

I would like to preface my discussion with three points of more general importance in visual prosthesis research: The meaning of blindness varies more widely than is generally recognized; our view of the nature of technology helps shape our actions; and we must beware of what I shall call the "iconic trap" in this area of endeavor.

The Meaning of Blindness

Dismissing "secondary gain" as a complication which takes us too far afield, it should not be difficult to reach agreement that blindness is a negative, limiting, and undesirable human condition. Efforts to correct that condition, therefore, are positive and worthy things to do. However, the diversity which exists within these broad ground rules is generally not appreciated. For some, blindness is a social and economic problem, which requires the allocation of community resources to minimize its cost and promote the general good. For others, it is an unwelcome, but acknowledged, fact of their daily lives, constituting a colossal inconvenience in some activities, and fading into irrelevance in others. There are many for whom blindness is a terrible and tragic potential threat, bringing with it complete helplessness, abject dependence, and total emasculation. What we choose to do, if anything, about blindness depends upon that meaning blindness has for us as individuals.

The Nature of Technology

We live in an age of tools in which our chief concern is to devise better ways of making and doing things. What we can do today was beyond our reach only a few years or decades ago, and what we cannot yet do we shall manage before long. Invention, once an individual act of heroes, is now thoroughly institutionalized. It is not only possible but necessary to examine our credulous commitment to the technological, and that doing so may make us wiser designers and users of tools.

We have at least the following choice of views on the nature of technology. We may regard it as essentially unbounded by anything outside itself, capable of supplying increasingly statisfying solutions to human problems, providing only that we state those problems correctly and pursue their solutions with sufficient energy and imagination. On the other hand, we may view technology as ultimately limited by boundary conditions which are not amenable to technology-based solutions, no matter how diligent our efforts or how clever our algorithms. This choice of views is important in visual prosthesis research for two reasons. First, motivated by the former view, that of an unbounded technology, we may attempt more and thus achieve more, than if motivated by the latter view. Second, motivated by the unbounded view, we may persist in spending time and talent in areas which are intrinsically unproductive for reasons which we cannot recognize. The way in which this issue applies in visual prosthesis research is a question we must resolve for ourselves, and will play an important role in determining what we regard as potentially possible and, consequently, what we attempt.

The "Iconic Trap"

I would like to describe a model of behavior employed by Brunswik some years ago to elucidate several aspects of the behavorial disciplines. The model is based upon the simple convex lens, situated between two focal points. Light energy emitted from one focus falls on the lens and is bent as it passes through, converging as it leaves the opposite side to come together at the opposite focus. The lens establishes a correspondence between points at the two foci, just as the organism establishes a correlation between stimulus and response events which are external to it.

Brunswik distinguishes between distal and proximal events on both sides of the lens (or organism). The distal stimulus is located at one focus, while the distal response is at the other. Proximal stimuli, or cues, are distributed over one lens surface, while proximal responses are spread over the other. Internally, he distinguishes between peripheral events and central ones. The peripheral events are aligned internally along the lens surfaces, and those toward the stimulus side are separated from those toward the response side by the region of central processes. The model is shown in Fig. 1.

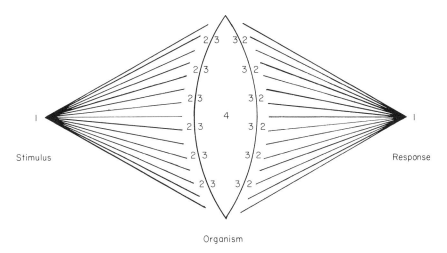

Fig. 1. The lens model of behavior. Numbered areas of the figure are interpreted as follows: 1. distal events, removed from the organism, 2. proximal events, in direct contact with the organism, 3. peripheral processes or events, and 4. central processes or events. This model adapted from Brunswik, E., "The Conceptual Framework of Psychology, Univ. Chicago Press, Chicago, 1952.

This model can be related to blindness by showing a section of the surface of the lens on the stimulus side as opaque. Proximal stimuli impinging there (the retinal image) do not produce the usual internal peripheral events, and the disturbance is propagated centrally like a shadow. It is possible to locate the various efforts to deal with blindness at different positions within the model. The opthalmologist, for instance, is concerned with the opaque boundary itself. The special educator deals instead with the remaining transparent portion of the lens surface. The parapetologist concentrates on relationships between the distal response and proximal stimuli in the transparent region. The guiding aim of all is to minimize the consequences of the opaque boundary on those correlations which the organism is able to maintain or establish between the distal stimulus and the distal response.

This model of behavior permits us to place in perspective a perennially popular topic in blindness research, the role of visual imagery in the absence of normal visual experience. Its place is indicated in the model as a concern primarily with the central region within the organism. It is an interesting problem, to be sure, but one which encompasses a relatively small part of the total problem of blindness. I believe there is a significant danger that workers on visual prosthesis may become so intrigued by the prospects of restoring the visual image to the blind that this portion of the total problem may come to dominate the scene. This is what I would like to call the 'iconic trap." It takes the form of establishing normal visual experience as the criterion of performance for visual prosthetic systems rather than adhering to the broader, though less dramatic, criterion of effective functioning. All things being equal, there is no doubt that it is better to have visual experience restored than not, but that is really only a part of the total problem. What bothers most blind persons about their blindness is quite likely not the fear of the dark, or the lack of visual experience, but the inconvenience, inefficiency, and awkwardness of doing certain kinds of things which are easily done with sight. The true value of the visual experience may well lie in what it makes possible. The iconic trap is that we shall adopt as our goal the restoration of the visual experience for its own sake, and that in doing so we shall lose sight of other goals which are perhaps more fundamental.

Summary of Display Alternatives

The remaining points bear more directly on display considerations. Any artificial perceptual system which views the organism as the passive recipient of signals, raw or digested, iconic or abstract, is bound to perform poorly. The organism seeks and participates in its perceptions. Perceptions are created by, more than received by, the perceiving organism.

The complexity of an artificial perceptual system may be reflected in the rate at which it must generate information. One method of generating complex displays while reducing information rates is by employing, wherever possible, displays whose elements have "infinite persistence," rather than "zero persistence." Such elements are "turned on" and remain "on" until "turned off." This principle is applicable to tactile, auditory, and quasi-visual displays. It requires more complex hardware, but may be applicable where a real limitation exists on information generation rates.

The degree of resolution desirable in a quasi-visual display, whether implemented by plasticity of a tactile system or by cortical electrification, ought to resemble that of ordinary television displays. This may at first seem to be an unrealistic requirement and, indeed, it may not be realizable. However, efforts to emulate the performance of the normal visual system indicate that this degree of resolution should be a minimum goal. The man of artistic temperament and experience would regard himself as functionally blind if his contact with the treasures of the Louvre, for instance, were limited to that obtainable by a television tour. The selection of goals for system performance is a very difficult problem.

Existing travel aids (the laser cane, the Kaye sonar probe, the Lindsey sonic aid) utilize mixed mode stimulation in most instances. Many devices are being made obsolete as soon as their development is stabilized by the phenomenal pace of technological innovation. Systems for acquisition and display of reading material must balance complexity against expected performance. Normally sighted persons who read well, read at a typical rate of 300 to 500 words per minute. Listening to orally read material proceeds typically at 175 to 250 words per minute. A good Braille reader may read 100–200 words per minute. These figures are rough estimates of the upper bound to be kept in mind in designing artificial perceptual systems, since they derive from large amounts of daily experience of both blind and sighted readers. The "cost-benefit" principle of decision-making is applicable.

The curious thing is that, in my experience blind people are not much interested in visual prosthesis in the classic sense of an implanted stimulator designed to restore visual experience. The question which I have attempted to deal with is one of the display of information. It is vitally important, of course, that some decisions or plans be made about what we intend to do with a visual prosthesis once it is implanted and working. I frankly have had some difficulty in coming to terms with this because what one would like to do with a visual prosthesis is a highly individual matter. For myself, I would very much like to read; other people have other needs. I am afraid that there will probably not be much uniformity in talking about questions of display.

The problems of blindness are really the problems that all of us have in terms of doing things in daily life—getting around; satisfying our needs; our being an effective person in various ways. For most of us, sight plays a very important role in these things; for others of us the lack of sight presents an unusual problem. We have made some accommodation to this. We have found other ways of doing things. Many of us who are blind, for instance, read Braille.

We have learned to rely on other people for some things. Airline travel is a particular convenience for a blind person. There is absolutely no way to get lost on an airplane.

I think the number of successfully employed blind people who are members of professions of various kinds is probably much larger than people realize. There is an important reason why that is so. The kinds of things that are particularly difficult for a blind person are most common in other groups. That is, areas of employment which involve simple, repetitive, routine physical types of things are particularly difficult for a blind person to do.

The substitution of, let us say, an intellectual kind of task for a more physical one is something which is of particular advantage to a person who is blind. Thus the number of blind persons, let us say, in teaching professions, in the service professions, as in science, technology, and so on, is probably larger than among others in general, not because the blind are more talented, or have innate gifts, or have some compensating kind of positive quality to make up for their handicap. That is not the point. The point is that most things which permit greater degrees of substitution are the ones where solutions have been worked out most satisfactorily.

This is all related, I think, very importantly, to the problem of visual prosthesis, and also to the problem of display, because the fact is that blind people do not need a visual prosthesis. The fact, however, is there are other ways of doing things. I am not prepared to say that a visual prosthesis would not be of benefit, because I can imagine the situation in which a very safe and not risky kind of procedure could be employed to install a brain stimulator, and the devices could be miniaturized and made automatic, and so on, to the point where a blind person could be given the ability to see his environment and therefore read and do other kinds of things that other people do with vision. These things would, perhaps, be more efficient, let us say, than reading Braille or using a cane, or using the kind offers of others as aids in travel.

So, there may be degrees of efficiency, let us say, which could be enhanced; but I think the context is clear: Whatever is to be derived from visual prosthesis needs to compete with other systems. A visual prosthesis offers another way of doing things for blind people, which means that we also need to consider what ways are used now.

I, for lack of a visual prosthesis, do not do without reading. I do get things read, not as quickly as I would like, and not as efficiently as I would like, but they do get done.

Blind people use canes to travel or use dogs as guides. Some blind people travel without canes or dogs. The question is to place this visual prosthesis problem in its context as a competitive scheme for doing things.

DISCUSSION

INGHAM: A comment was made which essentially removed from the group of blind people who would benefit from visual prosthesis those who are professionally rehabilitated, such as Dr. Hallenbeck. I felt upside-down when I heard that question, and I wondered for whom the device is good if they cannot help these people, and if they cannot help them, why?

What is being said about the rest of the blind population, about rehabilitation, for example, and what is being said about the device that would take it out of usefulness on the part of the rehabilitated blind? I would like that issue to be clarified.

STERLING: Dr. Hallenbeck feels, as indeed many of us do who have some sort of handicap which we have overcome (and such handicaps may include being deaf, blind, or black, or Jewish)—that once we have overcome this handicap and have made a success in spite of it, we have also managed a fairly good personal adjustment to life around us. We have accomplished something over severe obstacles and we may end up feeling that ours has become the best of all possible worlds; consequently, we may actively fight all change.

I would accept such opposition as data that there are a number of successful blind individuals, especially some of those who are in professions today, who do not wish personally, themselves, to become experimental subjects for such a device and do not see a particular need for such a device.

I do not think it reflects on rehabilitation. It reflects purely on the fact that some people have made a successful adjustment to their immediacy and they are not interested in a different world.

INGHAM: The point that Dr. Hallenbeck made, which I am surprised nobody had replied to, was the statement that the blind do not need the device. He was very inclusive there, for the whole population; and I cannot help but agree with him from all the people I know, including those who are not rehabilitated, who would not touch this thing with a 10-ft pole.

MACFARLAND: I think you are generalizing here about the blind as though they were a homogeneous group. The problem here is much more complex. I think the device could ultimately be beneficial to a blind person in a profession; but the problem of obtaining a volunteer is really one of economics. I daresay any of you would think twice before you left your profession and gave up salary to become the subject of an experiment, especially an experiment which is in the rudimentary stages.

I think that such an experiment could be beneficial to a blind person but he must be in thorough agreement and able to adjust to it. I, for one, having a family dependent upon me, could not take a year out for experimentation if that experimentation were going to be pin-pointed toward determining whether or not I could see a few phosphenes, get direction from the light, and so forth. This would not be terribly meaningful to me. I would have to be shown how this would, in some way, substitute for the salary I am getting on which my family depends. It is just as simple as that.

There is another historical problem here that I think permeates the whole attitude of a blind person, a rehabilitated blind person, and an intelligent blind person, and that is the long and fruitless experimentation that has taken place in some other fields. For example, in the Forties, someone talked about an electronic cane that would give a great deal of information to a person, that would substitute for the feeler device that Hoover invented. This is approximately 25 years ago. We still do not have that kind of cane that gives the information and gives it continuously, and in a manner on which we can depend. And so, the fact that some of these devices have not proven out I suppose gets back to the old adage about "once bitten; twice cautious."

When you encounter problems of the electronic devices that have been developed, e.g., the ultrasonic device that Kaye developed in England, and you find it is useful in certain areas, but it is not useful for depth, the subject using such a device could come upon an excavation, suddenly drop out of sight, and the researcher would go, I guess, to the next subject. This kind of experimentation is not appealing to the individual who has made an adjustment and who is making a living.

HALLENBECK: This I think encompasses what I meant by my remark that the blind do not need a visual prosthesis.

MACFARLAND: I need one, but it has to be better than the phosphenes.

FOULKE: I would agree, with some reservations, that the blind do not need a visual prosthesis. Those blind who have made a successful adjustment and who have developed successful alternative methods of obtaining information from their environment do not need a prosthesis. I have had some experience in talking with a group of blind veterans from the war in Vietnam. It is quite characteristic of these people that many of them were not making the effort to find alternative solutions to their problem in the fond hope that some prosthesis would shortly become available which would make that effort unnecessary.

So far we have talked about a visual prosthesis in terms of its ability to pro-vide visual experience to the blind, and whether or not blind people feel they need some prosthesis, or would be willing to participate in research in which the efficacy or the feasibility of such a prosthesis was demonstrated. It might very well turn out that it could provide useful information to them. So, I think that is one reason why one might be interested in a visual prosthesis.

It strikes me, however, that there is another important reason for being interested in it. It would provide a really fascinating opportunity to observe the acquisition of perception. As a blind person, I do not find myself, for instance, particularly yearning for visual experience because I think I have found alternative solutions to the problems created by the absence of visual experience. If the only reason for being interested in a visual prosthesis were to provide sight for the blind, I think I would probably not be particularly interested in becoming involved in research of that sort. But frankly, because of the fascinating opportunity it provides for studying the general process of perception, I think this is what would motivate me to become involved in experiments of this sort.

We have talked about what we mean when we use the term "visual pros-thesis." Are we talking about an alternative means of providing a visual illu-sion or, are we merely talking about a way of obtaining information that can replace the information that is normally obtained visually? I am not really sure that there is much of a conflict here. Any prosthesis, if it is going to be of any value at all, of course is going to have to obtain information; and if it does obtain information it may subsequently turn out, as I think Dr. Paul Bach-y-Rita has noticed, with respect to the display he is using, that the perception of the proximal stimulus changes to the perception of the distal stimulus. I think this is what you would be talking about when you talk about a visual illusion. I think this transformation is a fascinating process, and is one of the things I would personally be quite interested in observing were I participating as a researcher or as a subject–researcher in experiments of this sort.

MACNICHOL: I want to ask whether the visual prosthesis might be particularly useful to the deaf–blind who have much less ability to get around than the people who are only blind. I wondered if anybody would comment on this.

MINSKY: How many are there?

BERING: I cannot remember, but within the group of legally blind there are many who are deaf as well as blind. The total number of children that are born deaf–blind is smaller, but it is a fair number.

There is one thing, however, that has not been said by the various blind people that have been making statements, which John Dupress, who was blind, used to put forward as the common denominator for the development of a visual prosthesis. He made it very clear that for each blind person there was a different set of requirements for some sort of prosthetic device; but he said, "You know, what I really want is something that makes me totally independent, and the only way I can get this is to have something which will give me some information that one gets visually."

PROSCIA: Wouldn't a device of that type, by the definition just stated, undermine the implant project, because it would not make you totally independent? It may allow you to read, according to the statements made here, but it would not allow you to drive a car, or to do things as other sighted people do.

BERING: John Dupress was not so keen on driving, although he did drive a car. He had a special Jeep with radar on it which he drove on his own place. So, this did not bother him. What he wanted to do was get around, go in and out of the bathroom, get food in a place where he had never been previously, when no one else was there. What he meant by "independent" was simply taking care of himself all alone.

INGHAM: Would the prosthesis do this?

BERING: This was his definition of what he wanted from a prosthesis.

POLLACK: I would like to raise a point which may attenuate one of these issues. We have been referring to an available population of blind people, some fraction of whom would benefit from this prosthesis, and we have been talking in terms of the prosthetic as a competing alternative.

It could, however, be argued that once an effective prosthetic is available it would be available to a population of blind individuals at some time before such competition tends to build up, so that this tendency for competing alternatives may be substantially reduced. It would be introduced at the earliest possible stage, so there would no longer be a question of its competing. It would be competing with nothing, in a sense.

MINSKY: It is interesting to hear these different positions. There is a taboo that I might call the "stimulation taboo." This is a matter of history: In the first half of the 20th century, the neurophysiologists decided that it was inconceivable that stimulation of the brain could directly lead to anything interesting. You all know the history of attempts to localize functions in the cortex, which fell into disrepute, especially in the period of Lashley.

It was generally concluded that the brain acts as a whole; that it does not work as a mechanistic system; that memories do not occur at particular sites. This atmosphere is present today in the enthusiasm for searching for chemicals that transmit learning from one animal to another, and in the popularity of holographic theories of memory.

Now we are gathered here for two distinct purposes. The neurosurgeons, by and large, say that they are here for building a sensory prosthetic. The blind people say they are here, if for anything, because they are interested in brain physiology, and even possibly participating in experiments that would find out more about how the brain functions.

I think that the "stimulation taboo" is about to disappear with the confirmation of the fact that phosphenes exist. Those of you who were here at the last prosthesis meeting may have noticed that the majority of the neurophysiologists did not believe that stimulation of the cortex would lead to discrete points of subjective illumination. I think that was a reflection of their commitment to the Lashley Thesis.

If a visual prosthesis can be built, I think we all see but do not want to talk about the idea that there might be a memory prosthesis.

It is not impossible that a set of finely placed electrodes on a temporal lobe, with a suitable computer, could be connected to an information storage area and lead to the subjective acquisition and use of memory data, and new experiences about which nobody knows.

Just as the first astronauts were willing to risk their lives to simply go into orbit and not step on the moon at all, we are on the verge of an era where this kind of experimenting will happen; and I think we are gathered here together to wonder together whether that time has started.

STERLING: The fact is, however, that when we see a simple way of developing useful information, for instance, having the computer produce Braille, a sudden difference is made in the lives of a large number of blind individuals. I have encountered similar taboos before and I am sure that to most of you here who are in the business of dragging your colleagues into the 17th, 18th, 19th, and sometimes even into the 20th century, these remarks will come as no shock.

VAUGHAN: I would like to address myself to a question which has been in the background of a good deal of the discussion: How good is a visual prosthesis likely to be?

I think that this is the crux about which Dr. Hallenbeck is concerned and is implicit in many of the comments that have been made here. How will this approach stack up against other known and conceivable alternatives?

It is probably unwise to consider visual prosthesis as a sensory aid for all cases of blindness. There are a large number of blind people not suitable for this approach, such as persons of advanced age. There will be others for whom this approach may become suitable over a period of years, as we gain more knowledge, for example, the congenitally blind.

I have no idea whether this can be eliminated from consideration a priori; but in terms of system development it would be unwise to select a congenitally blind person as a participant because of the possibility that there might be significant changes in visual physiology which could cause the device to fail. It would be very unfortunate for early attempts to fail because of an inappropriate selection of blind participants, or other factors which are irrelevant to the question—"Can it work?"

These are quantitative issues that we are discussing, and until we talk in terms of quantity rather than in terms of impressions as to whether a visual prosthetic would be superior to a particular adjustment which an individual has now achieved, we are merely expressing our own particular prejudices and feelings.

First of all, a visual prosthesis could be a general-purpose device. I am not at all sure that it is justifiable to pursue this approach if the visual prosthetic, that is, an implanted stimulating system, will be useful as a mobility aid, or as a reading device, but not as both.

Once you make this requirement for general purposes—and this relates to the diverse functional needs of the blind— certainly as a bare minimum you have to be able to read, and you have to be able to get around the environment.

We are also hung up on another taboo: the issue of "artificial vision." We are not talking about restoring normal vision. We are talking about transferring a significant quantity of information through a channel of the nervous system which is already specialized for visual perception. As Dr. Minsky has pointed out, it is quite possible that there may be very severe limitations on it; nevertheless, we do know already from Dr. Doty's experiments, and Dr. Bach-y-Rita's work, as well as from a number of earlier psychological studies, that learning is likely to improve the discriminability of almost any pattern input to the nervous system.

When we stimulate the visual cortex, we are really at a very early stage of the visual system. This is something neurophysiologists do not like to think about, but this is just the first of the areas of the brain that we know to be concerned with the organization of visual information. The thalamus, the frontal lobe, etc. are all involved in the very complex system of visual information processing.

Therefore, I think it very likely that the information delivered to the striate cortex is subject to very extensive reorganization later on in the brain, under the combined influence of previously learned information about space and the associations which occur between other avenues of sensory information and visual input, even if artificial.

We know that the association between kinesthetic and visual information is essential to the original learning of visual space. It is important in the formation of the body image as well as in learning about the configuration of objects in external space.

It is not at all unlikely, therefore, that with a visual prosthesis, regardless of the fact that the information it provides the cortex may be quite unsatisfactory in terms of the normal input to the visual system, a blind person would actually learn through kinesthetic information, in fact, to perceive various objects, even though this kind of stimulation to the visual system is not normally there.

JOHNSON: I just want to lend some emphasis to the points of Dr. Bering. When John Dupress said he wanted "independence," he was not talking about sitting still as a passive observer, being able to name the things around him, and to verbalize about what was his experience. He was talking about the use of visual space to increase the resolution of what he was doing.

SCHIMMEL: We have to distinguish between two stages here. One is the experimental stage; the second is one where the prosthesis is widely available, assuming it will work. Of course, the experimental stage, and who cooperates among the blind, is a matter of individual choice and attitude.

I also see, however, and with some understanding, that those who are blind do not welcome this kind of development, because what is at first an option in life very quickly, as it is widely available, no longer becomes optional. In other words, if there is a working prosthesis that is equivalent, let us say, to 10,000 points of normal vision, the options begin to disappear for the blind as to have or not have such a prosthesis, even though they have made an adjustment without one. I think deep down the blind speaking here are concerned over the kinds of pressures we have in our society, individually, if we are forced to modify our way of life by new developments of this kind. I do not think they apply only to the blind. It is a part of the concern we, all of us, have as to the nature of our technological society.

I think that those who have already made some adjustment were not looking forward to this kind of pressure. For example, although I just about manage to get by, I am very often under pressure from intimates to wear a hearing aid. I tried it, and I did not make a good adjustment the first time around. I will try it again when the situation gets rougher. The pressure is there and if we have a good working prosthesis five years from now, the pressure will be on the very blind individuals sitting here to adopt it.

INGHAM: The issue of brain research, and all the rest of it, as propounded by Minsky, Vaughan, etc. is one issue; and if people want to do this sort of thing, fine!

The other issue, and I think the one before this conference, is what are the functional solutions for the problem of blindness which would make the blind independent, or whatever? I think the conference is on the right track when it begins to assess the possibilities inherent in the visual prosthesis, and compares these with the solutions of the other sort, such as the reading machine, the cane, and so on.

The major question in my mind is that given a large base of research going on in the various institutions now, some of which is really quite promising, would you not tap off and divert funds which would be better spent in bringing these solutions to actual implementation and delivery to blind people? This effort in visual implantation is going to be a large and costly one, and it is going to take time.

These other solutions, I maintain as a research, are available now. They should be endorsed. They should be financed. They should be provided to the blind. It is a functional solution we want.

I should hope that at some time we address ourselves to these questions that are related to at least one of the visual prostheses about which you are talking.

HALLENBECK: We have heard a great deal about the functional aspects of visual prosthesis and what can reasonably be expected from it; I would like to point out that this is not the only thing to be thinking about in terms of visual prosthesis.

In Dr. Brodey's and Dr. Johnson's paper I think they make some very fine points about the incorporation of any prosthetic device into the body image of the user, which, as you know, has a history of its own. I take it to refer to the incorporation of a device into one's self-concept. It has to be defined as a part of one's self so it is not used as something external or separate.

In that respect there is another point, in addition to what the thing does, and that is what it looks like. In addition to the functional aspect of prosthesis, the prosthesis does have a "social stimulus value," as it is called, and this needs to be considered.

The skullcap of Dr. Brindley's patient is an obvious problem from this standpoint. I am sure there are many sensible things that blind persons could do to enhance their informational access, but which perhaps they do not do because of the social stimulus value. This may be a trivial point, but it needs to be considered.

BERING: The cosmetic or "social stimulus value" has been pointed out by others. Anything which tends to call public attention to a handicap is not popular with potential users, and unless the device is absolutely essential it may be rejected on this basis.

STERLING: I think there are two very important points that have been raised. One of them is that when Dr. Vaughan spoke about the limitation of a visual prosthesis, he fell, to some extent, into a trap (which I will not call a "conservative trap" because it would be silly in this group to talk about a "conservative" to "radical" scales). This is a "trap" in which we rely very heavily upon what the nervous system can do naturally on its own. As Dr. Hallenbeck has pointed out, why do we have to present data in the structure to which we are accustomed? Why do we have to rely on the nervous system to learn what these points really mean? I think we can go beyond this question, and here I am not arguing with Dr. Vaughan at all. He is right. Learning and the kinesthetic sensations mixed in with the stimulation of some sort of a punctate matrix are very important. But in addition the nervous system has to learn what sensory impressions from an ashtray or from a glass might be. These sense impressions may be some sort of a mishmash. Somehow the nervous system has to reorder that mishmash and make some comprehensible signal out of it. This is a task which we must keep in mind at all times. We can rely on the nervous system to learn or we can build digital logic to interpret sense impressions for us. For this purpose such portable hardware can be built now. Therefore, I think when we talk about the limitations of a visual prosthesis we must consider them not only in terms of what we can recognize, and learn to recognize, but also what we can make that thing produce for us in terms of data structure. Some of us are in administrative positions and have to answer the question of why to invest money in visual prostheses. Why not invest it in the sort of work which we know will pay off?

Dr. Ingham raised this point, and I have heard it often. But where do we stop in this choice? Could we not say the same thing about Ingham's work? He is trying to produce speech. He is developing a probe to be put over a page which will get back a spoken report of what is contained. Now, I could say the same thing here—why not go along proven channels? Why put money into artificial speech? Why not continue to support different ways of producing Braille?

We cannot do that. I think that when a possibility presents itself, such as an opportunity to explore a new medium of information, we have to pursue it. We have to pursue it because the people who are interested will want to pursue it; and, because if we limit this type of research we really start going back and begin to limit other types of research, until only staunch conservatism prevails.

DOTY: Although I have a very large investment (or commitment) to electrical stimulation of the brain, I must say immediately that I do not think it is yet clear as to whether it is more advisable to develop a prosthesis to be put onto the skin or into the head. Much more knowledge is required before making such a decision and at the moment I think it is a tossup.

In considering why one might go into the brain, there are two possible advantages over a device using stimulation of the skin.

First, there is the inherent spatial organization of the visual system, linked automatically to the reflex control of body orientation. There is probably a significant difference here from what one would get from stimulation applied to the skin. In other words, when a point in the visual cortex is stimulated it commands the individual's attention to a particular point in space. This is built into the system. That conceivably could have considerable advantage in orientation.

There is a second consideration which might be labeled "esthetics." Although the blind at this meeting have rather dismissed this, Djourno and Eyries'[1] in Paris with the first prosthetic device in which the auditory nerve was stimulated in deaf individuals, found that the mere fact of auditory perception was extremely fascinating for an individual who had experienced long-term deprivation. It is conceivable that similarly even crude visual experience could be attractive, were it properly developed, and more attractive to the blind I would imagine than would be an equal amount of information put into the skin.

INGHAM: What emotional upsets are these people likely to experience? Dr. Brindley's patient was newly blinded.

POLLACK: This becomes part of the adjustment process. It addresses itself to a population that has not had the opportunity to adjust to some alternative, so we are not talking about a person who is adjusted, and how it fits into his adjustment.

INGHAM: You talk as though the device is going to replace a purveyor or provider of visual experience. It is not. All of your adjustment problems are going to be there, manifold.

POLLACK: It is not a new set of adjustment problems. It is *another* set of adjustment problems, over and above what the person had to adjust to in the first place.

SIMMONS: No one has any idea of what the limits of such a prosthesis would be in terms of perceptions. It seems to me until we have at least a reasonable idea of what these are, arguing this question seems to be irrelevant.

BRODY: I, simply as a free man, wanted to put in an image as I see it of the larger picture, because as one closes a conference of this type, the larger picture is quite fascinating.

Dr. Hallenbeck has said that the blind do not need a device of the sort that we are planning for them. Now we have new tools. We want to use them. We will inevitably use them—new tools that arrive on the scene such as the

[1] Djourno, Y., and Eyries, U., *Presse Med.* **65**, 141F.

strength of the present computers; such as the strength of the knowledge that we have derived from them already, which will inevitably be used there. There is no way out of it.

So, people will want to do their own thing by enhancing their own perceptions.

Here we shall find that some people, as with some blind people, will want these devices. Some sighted people will want to enhance their own skill, their own perception, using devices of this nature.

They may wish to enhance the number of loops with which they can experience such things as the microscopic world. There are new experiences in the offing that are as strange as if we had said to a blind person a few years back, "Look, we are going to give you a visual screen so you will have visual phenomena of some sort." They would have laughed.

I remember not too long ago when I was with a blind person and said, "Don't be too discouraged. You know, with technology going as it is, it won't be too long before something has been developed." And something is developed now that was not there before.

The direction that we are headed is toward a high-information environment, much higher than we have ever had previously, and an information environment where we can play with the world around us in a much richer way than we have previously; and where some people at least will be very much looking for enhancing their children so that the children will not go through the kind of programming that has been the case up to the present time.

I am saying that in this device here, in the laboratories we have built, we are moving into this broader picture of the future. And this, to my mind, is the breadth, the richness of the approach that has been presented here in terms of the blind, because we need, in some way, an excuse, but it has a much richer kind of value toward the future.

APPENDIX A

A Summary of
The First Conference On Visual Prosthesis
December 2–4, 1966
Endicott House
MIT
Cambridge, Massachusetts

INTRODUCTION TO APPENDIX A

The first conference attempted to establish, within the boundaries of free scientific inquiry, whether the data, and opinions based on them, indicated that an artificial visual device could be conceived. To be sure, many "facts" presented with great conviction were proven to be irrelevant or untrue by Brindley's subsequent experiment. It is still likely that many of the objections that were raised to the development of a visual prosthesis may yet prove to be correct. For all of us who participated in it, and for the reader, there may be lessons in the sparse records of this conference. These are important not only because they reflect the different steps within the historical progression of science but because they also mirror the human substance of which science is constructed.

INTRODUCTION TO
THE 1966 CONFERENCE SUMMARY

A meaningful discussion about the possibilities of building a visual prosthesis is beclouded not only by phenomenal engineering, physiological and psychological difficulties, but also by a reluctance even to give this topic serious consideration. Nevertheless, a burgeoning technology forces an evaluation, in a very critical fashion to be sure, of some of the more imaginative approaches and alternatives that become possible now. For this purpose an informal exploratory conference was held December 2–4, 1966, at MIT Endicott House.

At no time was it intended to suggest principles for building a visual prosthetic device. The object was to see whether there were areas of investigation which, after satisfactory solution of attendant problems, could possibly open the doors for research designed specifically to gather technical information useful for developing a sensory prosthesis. The participants in the conference had been selected for their ability to take a very sober look at such imaginative possibilities as well as for their grasp of present achievements. It was hoped that, after a modest amount of preparation, three days of shop talk would suffice for a fruitful exchange of knowledge and also stimulate new constructive ideas. The format of the conference was designed to instigate and provoke thought rather than report on recent work. Conferees participated in one or more of six panel discussions. Each panel discussion had a leader and a group of conferees who were responsible for illuminating a number of integrated topics. Each conferee was asked to provide the panel with a short and concise statement of his position on a particular relevant topic or issue. All of these statements were summarized by the panel leader and circulated among all members of the conference prior to the meeting. Since the subject matter of each panel was familiar to most conferees, no more than a concise description of the major points of controversy was really required.

The conference proceeded through a logical sequence of discussions for which each panel was held responsible in its turn. During each of these discussions the panel members could take the privilege of summing up or commenting briefly on their already circulated position. Discussion was then thrown open to the whole group.

There were no prepared papers, no tape recorders, stenographers, or note takers, so that the conference took place in an informal and relaxed atmosphere. A remarkably effective dialog was established among the 30 participants. Because of the free atmosphere, participants were willing to speculate more and to extrapolate results further than if they would have been "on the record."

It would be difficult, because of the format, to give a justifiable summary of conference content. Two participants had been asked to develop from their memories and personal notes, as best they could, a review of the crucial points of discussion. This challenging task was made even more difficult because of the spirited conversations that took place during late evening hours or at dinner. Nevertheless, a record of some of the more important exchanges ought to exist if for no other purpose than to offer a base for comparison with subsequent events.

It would be correct to say that this summary is an aggregation of connected descriptions of statements which were made by panel members and discussants in the course of a three-day dialog. Although the statements ascribed to various panel members were checked by them for accuracy of content, no such summary could capture the total meaning of the give and take that occurred on various topics. Readers who are conversant with the subject matter might gain some of the flavor of the discussion. It might be fitting, therefore, to attempt to sum up the points of view expressed at the confernce.

Perhaps the single most important finding of the conference was that there is not a single point of view. There is a good bit of dogma, to be sure, and some of it may be based on scientifically sound experimental information. There is also hearsay, presumption, allusion, and simple faith and belief in certain points of view. Some positions, strongly held and defended with vigor, turned out to be not necessarily internally consistent or free from contradiction by external evidence. There was no agreement among participants on either a completely positive or negative attitude toward a visual prosthetic device. By this lack of consensus, the conference may have contributed considerably toward reopening many experimental issues which had been considered closed.

It should not be concluded from this disagreement that any of the problems under discussion lead to a simple solution. In fact, one might almost say that if there exists a problem with a simple solution, it was not mentioned during the conference.

One of the most overwhelming impressions was that there is simply not enough known about the visual system for anyone to say with certainty what would happen if the optical-to-cortical pattern was stimulated with an array of electrodes over a long perod of time. There appears to be little doubt that attempts to implant electrodes into cortical tissue will occur in the next few years. In fact the consensus was that such experiments ought to occur even if they will only serve as a reinforcement toward what might now be prejudices about their negative outcomes. The technical feasibility for optical-to-cortical pattern stimulation is certainly not the sort of problem about which one can be sanguine at this time. There are a large number of difficulties facing any proposal to place a film array of electrodes on the visual cortex. Not only are the engineering problems themselves extremely difficult, but we must question whether there is a topological map of visual field and if so, what is it? This matter is made even worse because the visual systems of those individuals who would be the most likely subjects for such experiments may be atrophied with disuse or damaged as a cause of blindness. But even if such individuals were used, what is the "language" in which one could address their visual system? Can such a language be reproduced even if it were known? Furthermore, the quality of stimulation from implanted electrodes may change unpredictably with time. There is the danger of producing an epileptic focus. Cells, which are themselves involved in formulating percepts, may not be in physical proximity to the areas which can be reached by film electrodes. Thus, the visual cortex may not even be the right place in which to inject information. Finally, there are questions concerning the intensity of stimulation because at impulse levels needed to excite the small cells, large cells may be simply overwhelmed.

These difficulties are indeed severe and their list is certainly not exhausted here. While problems in these areas ought to be attacked with vigor for the largest payoff and long-term gains, other intermediate work along parallel lines should be encouraged. It would be most reasonable to develop useful prosthesis through other sense modalities. Certainly tactile senses offer the best possibilities for transmitting and translating visual information. What appears to be needed is a concentration of research on how tactile information can be made more meaningful.

Yet, even if the problems of physiological display were resolved, whether by direct implantation into the nervous system or through mediation via substitute sense modalities, a large and so far untouched issue remains concerning the automatic "perception" of the environment through instrumentation and its preprocessing to a format that will make it acceptable to the intervening nervous tissue. The problems of making a machine "see" are perhaps as difficult as those of building a visual prosthetic device. Yet, because of the enthusiasm with which these problems are constantly attacked, it is likely that solutions for automatic perception will precede those for sensory substitution. Many important insights may be gained through automatic vision. One interesting conclusion was that blind persons should be taught to interact effectively with large computing systems as a valuable way to take advantage of whatever new advances in pattern recognition have been achieved. Translated through proper instrumentation, such advances may well lend themselves to provide better "perceptions" of the environment. This requires a constant and alert contact between the blind and computing, supported by concentrated training efforts.

Thus, we see at least four major lines of work which ought to be pursued in the future. Attempts to implant large arrays of electrodes and then test the reaction of the nervous system to them may be viewed as the sort of investment that simply must be made to see what is in it for the blind as well as for the sighted. Developments of prosthetic devices using sensory substitution offer many promises for the near future if properly pursued. New ideas for automatic machine perception are sorely needed and a manifold increase of work in this area must be brought about. This is a young, difficult area which is little understood so far. Much value may also stem from having the blind individual keep close to developments in computer science.

The sponsorship of the conference came from the Association for Computing Machinery. It seems fitting that this young and vigorous discipline is attempting to integrate one of the most complex areas of human endeavor. The conference closed with an expression of appreciation to the Association and especially to those members of the Association which have made this conference possible.

St. Louis, Missouri   Theodor D. Sterling
May, 1967   Conference Chairman

LIST OF PARTICIPANTS

H. B. Barlow
University of California, Berkeley
G. Baumgartner
Universitat Freiburg, Germany
E. A. Bering, Jr.
National Institutes of Health
E. Bizzi
Massachusetts Institute of Technology
J. C. Bliss
Stanford Research Institute
W. M. Brodey
Massachusetts Institute of Technology
R. W. Doty
University of Rochester
J. K. Dupress
Massachusetts Institute of Technology
M. Gleser
Albert Einstein College of Medicine
R. L. Gregory
University of Cambridge, England
O. J. Grusser
Universitat Berlin, Germany
R. Held
Massachusetts Institute of Technology
E. R. John
New York Medical College
B. Julesz
Bell Telephone Laboratories
J. Y. Lettvin
Massachusetts Institute of Technology

J. C. Lickliker
IBM Corporation
T. L. Lincoln
National Institutes of Health
L. E. Lipkin
National Institutes of Health
D. MacFarland
Vocational Rehabilitation Administration
D. M. MacKay
University of Keele, England
W. S. McCulloch
Massachusetts Institute of Technology
M. L. Mendelsohn
Hospital of the University of Pennsylvania
M. Minsky
Massachusetts Institute of Technology
R. Pritchard
McCaster University, Canada
W. Richards
University of Illinois
A. H. Riesen
University of California, Riverside
L. Stark
University of Illinois
T. D. Sterling
Washington University
H. L. Teuber
Massachusetts Institute of Technology
H. Vaughan, Jr.
Albert Einstein College of Medicine

Panel I *NEUROPHYSIOLOGICAL ASPECTS OF VISUAL CODING*

PANEL LEADER

J. Y. Lettvin

PANEL MEMBERS

H. B. Barlow   J. C. Bliss
G. Baumgartner   O. J. Grusser
H. Vaughan, Jr.

Lettvin introduced the problem of a visual prosthesis and described what he considered to be the two main approaches: (1) the use of the nervous system itself as a coder by presenting information to another sense modality and (2) by-passing natural sensory coders by coupling directly into the visual system at some still intact point. He felt that the main subject of this conference was the second approach. (Sterling remarked that he had not intended to limit it to any topic.) Lettvin made it clear that he felt that those proposing to put a large array of electrodes on a human's cortex were doing so only to obtain government funds to build up their departments. He also thought that the conference should give thought to the idea that there is a topological map in the visual cortex in which real space is isomorphic with cortical space (an assumption of the proponents of the second appoach). Barlow was asked to summarize what is known about the organization of the visual cortex.

Barlow briefly reviewed the physiology of the retina and the presently accepted belief as to how the visual stimulus is transformed into the nerve impulse. He discussed the limits of visual interpretation, which he put at 5 sec of an arc or less. It was pointed out that the signals going to the brain, while still arranged spatially in relation to the retina in the optic pathway to the cortex, do contain information about the wavelength (color) and intensity of the visual object. Does the eye speak to the brain in a language already organized to be interpreted, or is the brain organized to interpret its input? Is the structure of the retina such that the ganglion cells fire as if they can discriminate? In fact, it is believed that some receptors may respond only to certain stimuli. He briefly described and reviewed the types of cells in the retina, pointing out that the conventional "all or none" responses of action potential, known to be the basic response of cells connecting the peripheral and central nervous system, have only been recorded from retinal ganglion cells.

He went on to review the visual pathways and their projection on the cortex, paying particular attention to the work of Hubel and Weisel. The receptive fields of the lateral geniculate cell are more or less circular overlapping fields which converge on single cells in the visual cortex. Receptive fields of the visual cortical cells are oblong, characterized by a sensitivity to slits of light and enormously sensitive to the direction or orientation of the slit. Such cells are classified as simple. Complex cells respond vigorously to movement in the opposite direction. The cells are arranged in vertical columns in the visual cortex with receptive fields having similar orientations. Adjacent columns have receptive fields arranged in slightly different orientations. In Areas 18 and 19, simple cells are no longer found and complex cells are more numerous. Two varieties of hypercomplex cells now appear. *Lower order* hypercomplex cells respond to oriented lines which are terminated within the receptive fields (corner detector). These behave as though they had received inputs from two complex cells, one exciting and the other inhibiting. However, hypercomplex cells respond to lines in either of two orientations 90° apart as though they had received inputs from large numbers of low-order hypercomplex cells. It was also pointed out that in the optic nerves the visual pathway is at its narrowest and in the primary cortex it is probably at its widest.

Baumgartner continued the discussion, bringing up the problem relating to optic nerve degeneration and pathological changes if it was ever stimulated electrically over protracted periods. He also pointed out that functional training was required for the cortex to handle visual inputs. This was related not only to the input through the optic nerve from the retina, but also to a great many nerve fibers which go from cortex to retina and to the function of these fibers. However, the existence of such cortico-fugal fibers or their exclusive importance was not universally agreed on.

A vigorous discussion took place at this time, bringing in many participants. Teuber described some cataract cases and how they could see images produced by x-rays through lead foil with holes in it. Brodey pointed out that there are many adventitious blind people so that the question of whether a congenital blind person could see again if his visual apparatus was restored should not preclude the development of a visual prosthesis. Lettvin stated that there were possibilities in using the tactile sense for visual information but that he had many cautions regarding the second approach, including the lack of a topological map of visual space in the cortex and the fact that we do not know how to "speak the language" of the visual system. Dupress asserted that if we cannot specify the visual code, we still cannot say the second approach would not work. Lettvin suggested the discussion be halted until the rest of the panel members had made a statement.

Bliss, the next panel member, pointed out that Morrell and Chow have found that some cells in the lateral geniculate and Area 19 of the visual cortex respond to auditory and tactile stimuli as well as the appropriate visual stimulus. Moreover, their response patterns to visual stimuli are modifiable by auditory or tactile "conditioning." This result suggests that it might be possible to transmit information to the visual cortex by means of auditory or tactile stimuli. Bliss stated that, based on engineering considerations, he felt that the first approach was the only practical one at this time.

The question of stimulating the brain with chemically implanted electrodes came up for considerable discussion, especially with regard to pathological problems that would be involved. The tolerance requirements in terms of biological reactions to electrodes and the heat generated by repetitive stimulation were both mentioned as problem areas. John pointed out that electrodes could be implanted in the brain permanently and kept functioning for years, as demonstrated by his experiments and those of Doty.

Grusser then mentioned that he had implanted 60 electrodes in the brain for recording purposes and had found that in some cases local epileptic discharges were produced. He felt that, in addition to the unpredictable threshold problem with implanted electrodes, there is also a real danger of producing an epileptic focus.

Lettvin agreed and said that epileptic foci could also be produced by a process as simple as putting alumina cream on the cortex and then rubbing it off. Vaughan agreed that this problem of induced epilepsy indeed needs to be solved and that more data on electrodes are needed, but he also pointed out that a considerable amount is known from a wide variety of sources. This information could be brought together to help resolve problems of implantation. Licklider summed up the discussion by maintaining that none of the difficulties mentioned by this discussion could not yield to technological developments.

Vaughan then reviewed the technical problems of implanting electrodes. He described the Raytheon proposal for a film array of 300μ electrodes on 1-mm centers as an example of what electronic technology can offer. He said that acceptable tissue damage may be possible with this type of electrode. He felt this left the question of whether or not it is necessary to know all the preceding visual transformations before inserting signals into a higher center. His conclusion was that the existing data in man are sufficient to answer this question.

Vaughan then reviewed the Button and Putman [1] experiments as the only example of a visual prosthesis previously being tried. He pointed out that some of their descriptions, if trustworthy, were certainly suggestive of very primitive visual responses. He also revealed that his colleague Dr. Schimmel, had visited Dr. del Campo in Mexico. His impression was that del Campo's work offered little promise.

A discussion followed in which Lettvin again described the locally holographic nature of the visual system and Dupress pointed out the key question was to what extent the system could be trained.

Julesz suggested that if one could stimulate a single edge detector cell in the visual cortex, the resulting perception would not be of an edge. His point was that unless the cells that reported local brightness, contrast and all the other properties of the edge were simultaneously stimulated the information would be insufficient for the subject to "see" an edge. He also argued that each of these groups of feature detectors, such as edges, slits, brightness, movement, etc., must have its own "private wire" to higher centers. MacKay pointed out that this information may never come together at the same location again. The implication was that indiscriminate stimulation would cause cells to respond with contradictory reports. This would be particularly likely since cells that report all the consistent features of a natural percept need not be in close physical proximity in the cortex. The percept resulting from stimulation of cells that give contradictory reports would be unusual, and perhaps not even a visual experience.

[1] Button, J., and Putman, T., Visual responses to cortical stimulation in the blind, *J. Iowa Med. Soc.* **52**, 17 (1962).

John divided the second approach, that of stimulating the visual system at some point beyond the retina, into two approaches: (a) supplying the information by means of an arbitrary code with the hope that this would be useful even though it did not result in natural visual percepts and (b) mimicking the by-passed natural visual system so that the stimulation code would be the same as in a natural system. He felt that the second approach was much less practical, particularly since feature extractors change.

Sterling then suggested that the position on visual mechanisms proposed by Lettvin and Barlow (also Hubbel and Wiesel) and defended with such vigor were not necessarily free from internal contradiction or conflicting evidence. He expressed on opinion (which he acknowledged as his own) that a good deal of "dogma" existed where skepticism was called for. He then suggeseted that since all that had been heard up to now was the negative side, Vaughan be given the floor after dinner to present the positive side for visual prosthetic possibilities.

Vaughan began by reviewing the objectives of prosthesis for the mobility and language areas. He said that another sense modality could be used for the language problem. However, he implied that direct linkage to the visual nervous system would be required for form perception of any quality. The key question was whether the visual system is sufficiently plastic and adaptable to be able to make use of the kind of stimulation that is technically feasible. He felt that the data on this point were not conclusive.

Lettvin again pointed out that real space may not be mapped into cortical space. He suggested that what is needed for a prosthesis is a "general purpose" input and that other sense modalities offer some possibilities along these lines.

Bering concluded that sights should be set higher and not limited to talking about transducers. He called for more optimism and more impetus to start work and try. He also suggested that stimulation of the optic nerve or the intact retina in partially sighted subjects might be a more feasible place to start.

Discussion continued in small groups late into the night and formally resumed the next morning after breakfast. Lettvin called on Bliss to present the case for the first approach, that of using another sense modality to present visual information.

Bliss began by challenging the implication, made the previous evening, that the tactile sense was inadequate for supplying form information of the quality required. He pointed out that the rates achieved by Braille readers and the speech comprehension attained by blind-deaf persons using the vibration method indicate that the tactile sense has sufficient information capacity. He then illustrated the capability of tactile form perception by showing a movie in which a subject had 96 phototransistors. The phototransistor array was hand-held and the subject could point it around a room while simultaneously feeling the resulting tactile image on his fingers. The objectives of the experiments were to evaluate the technical feasibility of this type of prosthesis and to investigate the importance of the proprioceptive feedback inherent in the hand-held feature. Also illustrated were two types of pattern transformations called an "edger mode" and a "movement only" mode. The subject in the film performed a number of tasks, such as finding an object, scanning a large square, distinguishing a square from a triangle, performing an acuity test, and locating on object in depth. The conclusions were that the subject's performance was limited by the equipment in its present form, not by the tactile channel, and that a great deal was possible, even with this relatively crude display.

After the film Bliss discussed some basic tactile psychological experiments including a tactile experiment analogous to Sterling's experiment in vision. This tactile experiment indicated that, with training, the tactile channel provides a "buffer" with remarkable short-term capacity and operates similar to Sterling's model for visual memory tasks.

Lettvin asked about drawing images on the skin rather than simultaneous presentation of all the points of a pattern. Bliss explained that while they had not experimented extensively with this, attempts to do so produced several illusions, such as losing corners, apparent motion phenomena, and other image distortions.

Panel II *CURRENT CONCEPTS*
OF PERCEPTUAL MECHANISMS

PANEL LEADER

H. L. Teuber

PANEL MEMBERS

E. Bizzi   *W. S. McCulloch*
D. M. MacKay   *R. Pritchard*
W. Richards

Teuber opened the panel by characterizing the second approach as the "science fiction version." He then called on Dupress to discuss his "visual" sensations.

Dupress gave a very interesting account of how he had visual imagery in his dreams for about a year after his eyes were enucleated. His "visual" field now consists of a gray volume in front of him which moves with his head movements. He likes to center sounds and objects in this volume. If he knows by touch that an object is in this phantom visual field, he does not have a visual image of the object, but rather an expectation that the object is there.

Teuber brought up two questions: (1) If certain visual systems are bypassed and the signals are injected into a latter stage of the system, can the feature extraction mechanisms modify themselves to accommodate this new input code? (2) How important is the fact that some units send information downstream as well as upstream? He also suggested the feature extraction mechanisms may not be really detrimental to visual prosthesis. Teuber concluded by raising the problem of what happens in the visual cortex when a vertical line in the visual field is tilted.

MacKay went over the following questions:

(1) How detailed is the topographical representation of the retina on the occipital cortex? If perception is regarded as the updating of the cerebral organizing system in matching response to clues extracted from the sensory input, it can be argued that even the fine performance level attained in visual acuity tests can be accounted for without demanding a corresponding sharpness in the occipital "neutral image." If this is so, then even if punctuate stimulation of the primary occipital cortex were feasible it would not yield sharp perceptual images. The question of the kind of stimulation that *would* do so may be worth discussing, especially in the light of current evidence of "feature-filtering" in the visual system.

(2) How far might temporal structuring of stimulation be used to supplement spatial structuring? It would seem important to gather and systematize available evidence on the time–rhythm–sensitivity of visual signaling and analyzing mechanisms. Phenomena such as Benham–Fechner colors, and some recently discovered illusions of motion and pattern evoked by uneven temporal rhythms of optical stimulation, may be relevant.

(3) A third question of potential importance concerns the requirement for stability of the perceived world as mediated by visual prosthesis. Shall we need compensatory cancellation of the effect of exploratory movements upon the signals we supply (as with a radar display on board ship)?

He then described an alternative to a "cancellation theory" for the effect of tilt of a vertical.

McCulloch, the next panel member, began by revealing that he had been an eidetica until he was 21. He convinced himself that this pictorial storage was not in the eye. Then he began to lose portions of this memory field until it was completely gone. Beginning in 1929 he began to have scotomata of migraine and he recently began recording the blind regions of the field as a function of time. While these blind regions have a remarkable resemblance to the "edge detector" receptive fields of Hubel and Wiesel's cats, McCulloch felt that the visual cortex was the wrong place for the source of the difficulty. This was partly because the pattern of blind regions always started at the center of the field and progressed outward and that visual cortex is too homogeneous for this. He suggested the superior colliculus as the location of the trouble and described the phenomena as "backfiring," He implied that the visual cortex may be the wrong place of insertion of prosthetic signals and suggested stimulation of superior colliculus instead.

He indicated also that during the scintillating scotoma there were no changes in the EEG, but during the hallucination there was considerable activity. McCulloch also said that the flicker rate in the scintillating scotoma was 5–10/sec. Doty pointed out that the developing hemianopsia suggested spreading depression.

Pritchard began by defining what he meant by a percept as contrasted to a sensation. He reviewed his work on percept decomposition in stabilized images, saying that he had found seven ways to cause fragmentation of the visual field including reducing contrast ratio, producing partial stabilization, limiting illumination, shortening stimulus duration, and defocusing. The point was that, by perturbing the visual system sufficiently, the image begins to fragment and this fragmentation reveals certain cells, or small groups of cells that operate as "feature detectors," receiving insufficient stimulation. Thus the fragmentation process produces information about the characteristics of the "feature detectors."

Pritchard described a model for attention emphasizing the importance of the effects of the efferents. He suggested that the receptive fields found by Hubel and Wiesel may be feature detection for the purpose of commanding eye movements to bring the object of interest into the view of the fibers of the foveola, which in turn scan to perform pattern recognition.

Bizzi described his work on the direct influence of the ocular motor nuclei on the visual pathways and the input into the lateral geniculate body from the ocular motor nuclei. The question was raised as to whether the modification of events occurring at the geniculate body would have any effect on the design of a prosthesis.

Richards asked whether events occurring in the body might be used. The visual system handles a lot of information and complete understanding of relay stations like the geniculate body might help to solve the coupling problems. The topic of feedback to the eye and retina were again raised at this time.

Licklider explained a model for perception generally held in audition. According to this view, what is perceived is the winning hypothesis based on information from the senses and/or internal criteria. He compared the visual application of this model to a hardware system contaning a slide projector, millions of slides stored in memory and a televison camera connected to a computer. The computer continually analyzes the output from the camera and selects the slide most consistent with the results of this analysis. The projection of this slide is then what is perceived. It was generally agreed that this model for visual perception was all right if the hypothesis testing could be done in a local area instead of on the whole slide.

Bizzi presented some interesting experiments in which he simultaneously recorded eye position and activity in the lateral geniculate. He recorded both single cell activity and gross evoked potentials in the lateral geniculate. It was clear that eye movements occurring at certain times with respect to a visual stimulus significantly modify both the single cell and gross potential responses. For example, if a light is flashed during movement, the response is reduced.

Doty described some data that also indicated that other inputs can tend to turn activity on or off in the lateral geniculate.

Panel III   *CAPABILITY OF THE VISUAL MECHANISM TO ADAPT TO DISTORTION*

Panel Leader

R. Held

Panel Members

R. L. Gregory	*D. M. MacKay*
B. Julesz	*H. L. Teuber*

Held suggested that as a major question, the panel consider the extent to which the visual system can adapt to disordered input.

MacKay made a distinction between types for adaptation. In the first type, distorted forms cease to be seen distorted and in the second type, the motor system compensates for the distortion.

Julesz showed some slides of his computer-generated random stereoscopic patterns and then showed a movie of dynamic noise which could also be seen in depth. He reviewed his work with Derek Fender on binocular disparity and related this work to the question of plasticity.

Teuber revealed that he had been informed during lunch that, regardless of what the participants in this meeting thought, someone was going to put an array of electrodes on the visual cortex of a human. In view of this information, he felt the discussion should be directed to the question of what experiments should be done with this patient. He suggested that at least we might be able to find out something about the visual system. He then reviewed a number of results from experiments with brain lesions and discussed the possibility that visual images might be produced by stimulation of some other modality or by drugs. He suggested that the visual cortex may not be the appropriate place for an array of electrodes for a visual prosthesis.

The problem of visual motor coordination was brought up next. What was discussed particularly was that one has to work to recover from anything that distorts the visual motor coordination. If there is a delay in the visual input, the motor coordination breaks down. This same thing is true of other sensory inputs, such as hearing. Speech becomes garbled with a delay in auditory feedback, and one cannot understand it. Presumably there are some training factors that could work here as in singers who are able to sing in groups quite distinctly from one another, although they cannot hear themselves. This is related to what should be presented to the cortex and to discontinuities in reading where scotoma exists. It was pointed out that an adaptation to prismatic spectacles is ruined in the presence of frontal lobe lesions. This exemplifies the problem of diffuse representation for coordination of all visual information into the performance of an individual.

Again, the problem of electrodes came up and the alternatives to electrical stimulation were suggested. There was further discussion on spatial differentiation at the cortical level and the technical difficulties this presented in terms of a practical coupling device.

The question of hallucinogenic drugs and their effect on the blind was brought up and there apparently is no sound body of pertinent data.

Gregory reported on the return of vision after surgery as an example of how physiologists are willing to get minimal information. Much of this knowledge appears to be based on a German Ph.D. thesis, done entirely in the library. Though often quoted, it does not represent original observations by the author and many of the theories put forward are not necessarily fact.

Panel IV   *PSYCHOLOGICAL AND PHYSIOLOGICAL IMPLICATIONS OF BLINDNESS FOR VISUAL PROSTHESIS*

PANEL LEADER

R. L. Gregory

PANEL MEMBERS

J. K. Dupress   R. Held
A. H. Riesen

Gregory introduced Riesen who reviewed the results from experiments with animals reared in darkness. He pointed out that these animals "go wild" if vision is introduced to them suddenly. After a year with vision some of these animals appear normal. He felt that, if a visual prosthesis could be built, it would be important to introduce the new stimulation gradually, rather than all at once.

Held reviewed his results from deprivation of motor action in a monkey and cat.

MacFarland was asked what kind of prosthesis a blind person wants. For example, what objection would he have against wearing "cat whiskers" to protect his head. MacFarland explained how the prosthesis depended on the individual involved, that is, one blind person may wish to be able to view his surroundings, a blind artist would like to be able to appreciate the aesthetics of a painting, and a blind businessman may wish to be able to read any document. MacFarland considered the auditory outputs of existing reading aids as their principal shortcomings. He thought "cat whiskers" were undesirable because they protected a region which is already well protected by "facial" vision. Besides, "cat whiskers" would appear ridiculous.

McCulloch spoke about blind people's needs, which are as varied as the people themseves. Some would like to read, some would like to see art, some would like to be able to travel, some would like to drive, some would simply like to just take care of themselves. So the needs are quite different, and because of this, it was concluded that any effort should include a blind person in the planning, so that the developers could relate to the actual needs of a sightless person.

After the problem of the seeing eye dog was raised, consideration was given to utilizing the output from an animal's eye, and in some way, taking the information that was being sent through the optic pathway of the animal and transferring this to the human for interpretation. This would require a special pickup device as well as a special input coupling device.

Panel V *PSYCHOPHYSIOLOGICAL ASPECTS*
OF ARTIFICIAL INPUT TO THE VISUAL SYSTEM

PANEL LEADER

E. R. John

PANEL MEMBERS

W. M. Brodey   *B. Julesz*
R. W. Doty   *W. S. McCulloch*
R. Held   *L. Stark*
H. Vaughan, Jr.

John introduced this panel by saying that the members would relate what has been found by introducing information directly into the nervous system.

Doty began by reviewing the purposes of a prosthesis for a blind person. He considered the reading problem as not being the province of this meeting. For mobility he felt that a wide angle field of view was needed with depth or range information. He listed the stimulus dimensions that could be used for coding information as spatial locus, frequency, and intensity, considering these to be the only practical dimensions regardless of whether the brain or the skin is used. He said that because of his background he would particularly like to stimulate the brain, but he felt we are not ready for this. He pointed out the skin has the same information-bearing parameters available as the brain, but a visual experience would not result.

Doty felt that this reduces the question to the desirability of a visual experience. However, he concluded from Lettvin and Barlow's remarks that even with cortical stimulation we will never be able to obtain a prosthetic device that will give a complex visual experience. Stark asked whether Lettvin and Barlow had really said this and Lettvin verified that they had. Doty's conclusion was that brain stimulation is an unattractive approach for a visual prosthesis since the skin offers as much promise and is technically much easier to stimulate.

Doty further pointed out that, when most cortical points in man are stimulated, nothing happens. This is not true in monkeys and the significant difference is that of training. He then described the adaptability of the responses and how by paired stimulation a flexor point could be converted into an extensor point. If three electrodes, A, B, and C, are put into the visual cortex of a monkey, he can be trained to respond to point A, differently to point B, and he can react is if he could tell whether point C is more like point A or point B.

Doty discussed other stimulation problems important to the visual prosthesis attempt. One problem is that when the current is high enough to stimulate the small cells, a lot of the large cells will be overwhelmed.

In one experiment he put two pairs of electrodes in Area 19 of a monkey. The electrodes in each pair were 100μ apart and the pairs were 1 mm apart. The monkey could respond to a particular electrode. However, this experiment also works in frontal cortex. The conclusion was that in the cortex spatial discrimination was excellent but frequency discrimination was not.

Lettvin asked if the monkey could distinguish between both electrode pairs simultaneously stimulated and stimulation through either electrode pair alone and Doty did not know.

Doty described a case in which a human was stimulated in Area 18 and this resulted in her reaching out for an imaginary butterfly. He had also seen a similar response to cortical stimulation in the monkey.

Vaughan, the next panelist, suggested that the major questions regarding the organization of the visual system were whether or not there are topographical maps, whether or not there is orientation specifically, the extent of plasticity, including what factors can modify receptive fields, and how haptic experience serves to organize vision.

Held suggested that the plasticity he observed in his experiments may all be in the motor system. He felt that this location for plasticity is more reasonable than on the sensory side because the motor system must continuously adapt to the change in size of limbs resulting from growth.

McCulloch emphasized the role of efferents, which make up 10% of the optic nerve. He also described anatomical changes that occur in visual cortex with sensory deprivation.

Licklider asked if it was a fact that the bypassed part of the normal visual system could not be imitated. There was some discussion, with most participants arguing that this could not be done.

Julesz described his "pentagon" experiment in which the sides of a pentagon are illuminated one at a time either in sequential or random order. Flicker disappears at a lower frequency for the sequential order than for the random order of illumination, illustrating the importance of temporal pattern. He also brought up the possibility of visual information coming from within a person by quoting William James on hypnosis.

John said that if a subject is shown a visual stimulus a number of times and the evoked potential recorded and then if he is asked to imagine the stimulus, the resulting evoked potential has the same shape. This suggests that the evoked potential may be a good indication of visual imagery coming from within.

Stark related that some work by Marg indicates that more complicated sensations than a blob of light can be elicited by electrical stimulation. He suggested that only a small amount of electrical stimulation may be necessary to evoke an illusion.

Brodey described his work on speech recognition. He said that he was able to progress only after he made the problem easier by making use of context and redundancy and by tailoring the system to particular speakers. He suggested a similar approach to visual prosthesis. He also suggested that the sensory aid should give the subject a wealth of "noisy" information for him to organize, but that the subject should be able to process this information without a lot of conscious effort.

Lettvin then made an interesting suggestion. He first reviewed John Dupress' previous comments about his visual world and MacFarland's comments about the blind artist who would like visual imagery with the aesthetic qualities and richness of visual experience. This suggested the question: "Is there some way we can use visual cortex as association cortex?" That is, could John Dupress be hypnotized, or can drugs be used, so that when he has an expectation of an object in the gray volume that is his phantom visual field, he will actually experience a visual image of this object?

Bliss suggested that, if this were possible, an optical-to-tactile image conversion system would be even more important because the information supplied tactually by the device could cue the visual experiences.

The problem of a partially blind with some visual apparatus intact came up. How could these people be helped by a device such as was under discussion? McCulloch took an optimistic view and said with the next few years we could probably get into the brain, whether it was through the cortex or visual pathways. There might be some other way of sensory input to the visual system, but this is quite a question.

Questions were brought up as to how percepts were organized; whether by using electricity with frequency, intensity, or duration of perceptual data and visual space.

It was suggested that if the same fiber optic systems were used, all visual scenes would be scrambled in the same way and might well become meaningful, although the scenes would not be reassembled in their original form.

Held discussed the degree of accuracy needed for the artificial input to be useful. Orienting and analyzing systems, along with the coupling devices, would have to deal with these problems, but there would really be no gain if the feature detectors were such that they could not be utilized by the brain in a meaningful way. Certainly, this cannot be determined without testing.

Questions were raised about what happens in visual regions in blind persons after the eye is nucleated. It was said that some experiments show that various cells become more excitable after nucleation. This again brought up the question of how percepts were organized. Why should a person who is 20 years old stop having images and hallucinations after becoming blind?

Panel VI   *PROBLEMS OF LOGIC*

AND HARDWARE IN AUTOMATIC PREPROCESSING

OF VISUAL INFORMATION

PANEL LEADER

T. D. Sterling

PANEL MEMBERS

J .C Bliss	L. E. Lipkin
J. C. Licklider	H. L. Mendelsohn
T. L. Lincoln	M. Minsky

Sterling introduced Mendelsohn as the first panel speaker. Mendelsohn described a computer system for recognition of cells. This system scanned the pattern to be analyzed onto a 200×200 array in which the intensity at each point measured to 8 bits (64 levels). This is equivalent to 400,000 bits, or about 10,000 words of English. Mendelsohn thought that a system of comparable complexity would be needed for a visual prosthesis, and this would mean that the subject would have to carry a cartload of equipment around with him.

Lipkin thought that convenient equipment would become available but, whatever the implementation, the important thing was to make it possible for a blind person to interact effectively with a general-purpose computer. In this way the blind subject could be a member of the design team and pattern preprocessing could be developed by changing the software of the system. He also stressed the importance of the accommodation function of vision and other efferent control.

The question of electrically stimulating small cells or cell groups was again discussed. There are many problems, but there is a good deal of information available. What is needed most is information on what kind of a visual image or visual response or experience will be generated if one had a multiple array stimulator for possible use on the cortex or applied to the optic radiation.

It was conceded that if the right kind of stimulation in sequential array could be done on the retina, the visual experience would be like the real scene photo stimulated on the retina. However, the problems here are that the sequence and rate and order of kinds of firing of the cells are not really known in relation to any given image. This must be learned. There is need for knowledge about the transformation that takes place at the geniculate body in various cells and cell groups, complex and hypercomplex cells of the cortex that are oriented for shapes, edges, motion, and so on. How and what is done and how is the image reassembled for interpretation?

Minsky showed a film of a visual computer and discussed the problems of programming it to learn to see a cube and pick it up. He showed some of the manipulators that his laboratory had, including an arm built on the design of an arthopod. He pointed out that miniaturization technology is producing transistors that are getting to be the size of cells, but the coaxial cables are still too large to use these. He felt that electricity was still the best stimulating agent.

Bliss described experiments at Stanford and showed a film in which a device scanned the visual field and activated a series of tactile stimulators so that a form is punched on the skin.

The problem of cortical stimulation and conditioning was brought up; whether or not the brain could be trained in this way is difficult to say; while it is possible for use in man, there are considerable barriers.

The conference closed with a vote of appreciation to the Association for Computing Machinery for its part in sponsoring the conference.

APPENDIX B

BLINDNESS IN THE UNITED STATES

K. Trouern-Trend and E. A. Bering, Jr.

This conference was convened to consider ways and means for developing a device to stimulate the visual system of a person who has lost his sight; to give him a visual input about the world around him. Programs directed toward that purpose will involve basic research as well as instrument development and will extend over a number of years. It seems appropriate, therefore, that the magnitude of the blindness problem be reviewed.

Blindness occurs at any age and stems from many causes which may affect the visual apparatus from the cornea to the cerebral cortex. Each of the blinding lesions leaves parts of the visual apparatus intact which might be utilized if suitable image pickup and coupling devices to the visual system were available. This paper surveys this problem as background to research for the development of devices which will provide meaningful visual experiences for the blind through their remaining visual system.

Blindness has as strong an emotional impact as any disease suffered by man and has from the beginning of time affected him and his social structure. It is surprising, therefore, that the information on blindness is still as inadequate as a recent study has shown. This particular inquiry—performed for NINDS [1, 2]—represents one of the first steps in approaching the visual prosthesis problems and constitutes the source material for much of this paper.

Public concern for the welfare of the blind—as opposed to the avoidance of their destitution—appears to have emerged in about the middle of the 18th century. In 1785 Valentine Hauy opened his National Institute for the Young Blind in Paris, representing the first attempt at providing organized education for the blind, although the famous Quinze-Vingts had been opened in 1254 to provide care for blinded crusaders.

The movement for practical implementation of concern for the blind spread from France to England, where the first school for the blind was opened in 1791, and to the United States, where in 1832, the New England Asylum for the Blind was opened. This latter institution later became the now famous Perkins School for the Blind, Watertown, Massachusetts.

Enumeration of Blind Individuals

The magnitude of the blindness problem is indicated by the estimate that about 300,000 Americans have sufficient visual impairment for them to be classified as legally blind. However, the definition of "legal blindness" varies from state to state so that this figure is open to some legitimate question. There are conflicting opinions as to the most realistic and helpful method of defining blindness. In general terms one may think of it as essentially a functional disability resulting in the necessity of devising alternative techniques in order to perform efficiently activities which would normally depend on sight. For statistical purposes the definition of blindness used here is one developed by the Model Reporting Area Project of the National Eye Institute. According to that definition an individual is considered blind if his vision is 20/200 or less with the best correction in the better eye or visual acuity of 20/200 if the widest angle of vision is no greater than 20°.

Official attempts to obtain information on the number and characteristics of blind persons began with the 1830 census, continuing every 10 years up to the census of 1930. None of these attempts provided other than qualitative impressions. Accordingly, in 1930 the Committee on Statistics of the Blind formed by the National Society for the Prevention of Blindness and the American Foundation for the Blind—both of which organizations were pioneers in the field of recognizing the need for adequate data—recommended that the census enumeration of the blind be discontinued. The Committee continued to study the problem of enumeration and developed a set of practical and effective guidelines which represent the basis for a standard report form submitted by examining physicians. This form provides uniform classification of measurements of degree of vision and causes of blindness. The standards have been gradually developed to the present stage where they are in general use in the United States under the sponsorship of the National Institute of Neurological Diseases and Blindness.[1] The classification system is accepted in Canada with only minor modifications and that used in the United Kingdom is also essentially the same, although with a reduced number of categories of the degree of vision.

National Health Surveys have attempted to obtain statistics on blindness throughout the United States by means of interviews with selected households. However, the results are of limited value because no standardized definition of blindness has been used and there have been no measurements of visual acuity.

The situation has been steadily improving since 1962 as a result of the establishment of the Model Reporting Area for Blindness Statistics (MRA), organized under the sponsorship of the National Institute of Neurological Diseases and Blindness (NINDB) and now under the National Eye Institute (NEI). This is a voluntary association of individual states (now numbering 16). Each state maintains a register of persons with serious visual impairment, in accordance with rigorously prescribed standards. The member states are Connecticut, Georgia, Kansas, Louisiana, Massachusetts, New Hampshire, New Jersey, New Mexico, New York, North Carolina, Oregon, Rhode Island, South Dakota, Utah, Vermont, and Virginia, and several others are organizing their blindness registers in preparation for membership.

Projected Estimates of Blind Population

Until now, most states have estimated their likely total blind population on the basis of the prevalence rates calculated by Dr. Ralph Hurlin,

---

[1] It has now reorganized as the National Institute of Neurological Diseases and Stroke and the National Eye Institute.

who used a selection of the statistics of the general population to predict the total number of blind persons likely to be found within the population. Now that the registers of the MRA member states have become available, it is possible to make direct comparisons between these totals and those predicted on the basis of estimated prevalence rates. It has been found that the estimates are generally higher than the members appearing in the registers. As an example, the 1965 prevalence figures for 14 MRA states predict a total of 78,750 blind persons in those states, as compared with a registered total of 54,595, or about 30% less.

Using the MRA data, a new set of estimated prevalence rates has been prepared based on four statistics of the population:

(1) proportion of the population at least 65 years of age,
(2) infant mortality rates/1000,000 live births,
(3) number of physicians/1000,000 population,
(4) income per capita.

The impact of race structure has not been included as a factor in the estimation of the prevalence of blindness. While, in the MRA as a whole, the rate of blindness is higher among nonwhites than among the white population, there are indications that this difference has its origin in economic rather than physiological factors. The present estimated prevalence rates are generally lower than those made previously. Based on the rates, the total estimated blind population is about 300,000, compared with 430,000 estimated on the previous basis.

Distribution of Blind Individuals by Age

There is a relative increase in blindness with age. That is, there is a higher relative incidence of blindness (number of blind/100,000 population) among older people, but the absolute numbers are less in that group. Thus, in 12 MRA states there were 5249 blind individuals 85 years of age and over, representing 3% of that population (3136/100,000); in the 20–44 year age group there were 8319 blind individuals, representing only 0.06% of that population (60/100,000).

It is really interesting and important to examine the degree of blindness in the various age groups. Only 12% of the blind in the MRA population were absolutely blind and another 12% just had light perception, while the majority had some vision. The development of devices to help this large group with some vision should be a secondary goal as part of an overall prosthesis program.

Causes of Blindness

The causes of absolute blindness were found to distribute as follows: 23% by injuries, 12% by infectious disease, 23% by neoplasms, and about 6% for each of seven other causes. It is of considerable importance that 68% of the absolutely blind are under 65 years of age and 55% are under 45. Thus, most of the absolutely blind are in the productive age years. This is a group whose economic productive potential is high and offers a real return for the effort.

Economic Impact of Blindness

The economic impact of blindness is recognizable in two distinct areas. The first is seen in examining the costs for the blind which differ from those associated with either the corresponding standard of living or, more properly, that which would be enjoyed by a person of similar capacity, if sighted. Second, and in the reverse sense, is the potential income lost to individuals as the result of their blindness.

Living costs are generally higher for blind persons than for those who are sighted. Although many individual examples may be cited showing that skilled blind persons in appropriate professional activities earn annual incomes in access of $20,000, these represent only a minute percentage of the total blind population. It is impossible to arrive at any figure which can be considered representative of the earnings of the blind, but there is no doubt that their median income is extremly low, amounting to only a few dollars per week. The majority of the blind are condemned to exist at a level far below that which they could achieve with minimal effort, if sighted.

It is very difficult to identify, except in very general terms, costs which can be considered as being consequent upon blindness and which would not be incurred by sighted persons under the same circumstances. In the majority of cases, blind individuals, when questioned, will dismiss suggestion that additional expenses are incurred due to their blindness. This is especially so when they are employed and performing essentially the same tasks as those who are sighted. This refusal to admit to additional expenses, which has been found over a wide range of individual economic circumstances, may be attributed both to the general concern not to be regarded in any way as exceptional and to the fact that much of the additional cost of blindness must be measured in effort and in loss of personal independence, rather than in dollars. In many cases a high level of ability and motivation, which has made possible the development of the techniques required as alternatives to sight, are linked with a fierce independence of spirit which will not allow the individual to admit, even to himself, the high cost of competing with those possessing adequate vision.

In order to identify at least the categories of additional cost which blind persons are obligated to bear, an attempt has been made to follow the course of an individual through the varying phases of life, noting in each of the activities or circumstances likely to produce costs which differ from those of a sighted person.

From the general statistics related to items identified as being important, and from numerous personal interviews with blind individuals and their families by whom they are largely supported even if in receipt of aid, estimates of total costs have been made. The most likely of these appears to be about $1,700 a year. This is a mean annual support value and is applicable to the blind of all ages and to both sexes for their lifetime.

The probable validity of these figures is supported by the fact that payment under Aid to the Blind has now increased to about $1,100 per year which is variously estimated by the Public Health Service to represent about 55–75% of the total needs for direct support. If it represents 65% of needs, this corresponds closely with the value of $1,700. The estimate does not include the fairly well identified and additional equivalent costs of schooling (about $120 per year) and Services to the Blind (roughly $60 per year).

The income lost as a result of blindness may be estimated by assuming that any blind person represents an otherwise typical example of the sighted population of that particular grouping by age and sex, has the normal expectancy of life and, as time progresses, would earn the median income of his age group while employed and would have the normal probability of employment at any given age. Based on the current estimates of the total blind population and the median income earned by different age groups of the general population in 1966, the total annual income lost to blind persons is about 0.6–0.8 billion dollars. The total cost of support in the same year on the basis of $1,700 per year per person amounts to about 0.5 billion dollars.

It is possible to divide the estimated blind population into each of the recognized categories of age, degree of vision, and major etiology. Within each category we can estimate the number (total, male and female) of persons concerned, the present value of the lifetime income of those within the category, the present value of lifetime support at $1,700 per year and the total of these, representing the effective "economic value" of the particular category of blindness.

Based on this approach it can be shown that the total theoretical economic benefits of eliminating *all* blindness would have a present value, if discounted at 5%, of about 11 billion dollars. If based on the earlier estimates of the total blind population, this could amount to as much as 17 billion dollars.

The hypothetical value of providing any prosthetic device may be estimated by assuming that all those within the blindness category to which it is appropriate can be restored to adequate sight. This represents the upper limits of what is possible, but it is recognized that there will be individuals who cannot benefit from even the most generally accepted device. As an example, Table 1 provides an illustration of the economic value of prosthesis applicable to the most severe forms of blindness. The numbers of persons shown in that table are estimates of the total of those within the blindness category and of those age less than 65 years. It is unlikely that many of the older individuals would be candidates for the more heroic measures and it has seemed that this is a realistic division of the estimated blind population. The table also shows estimates of the lifetime cost of the support of those age less than

TABLE 1. Estimated Economic Impact of a Successful Visual Prosthesis

Blindness category	Total numbers in category	Median age	Number in category less than 65 yr	Cost of support	Income lost	Total cost	Cumulative cost versus blindness categories included
			Present value of lifetime costs for those less than 65 yr.[a]				
Absolute blindness	35,500	57	22,000	0.59	0.79	1.38	1.38
Light perception	36,000	61	20,000	0.53	0.66	1.19	2.57
Light projection	3000	64	1500	0.04	0.05	0.09	2.66
Acuity <5/200	49,000	66	24,000	0.60	0.76	1.36	4.02

[a] Discounted at 5% ($ billion).

65 and of the income lost to them as a result of blindness. Both these values, and their corresponding totals, are shown at present values discounted at 5%.

REFERENCES

[1]   Blindness in the United States, Final report, Contract P. H. 43-67-1463 to NINDB. Available: Clearinghouse for Federal Scientific and Technical Information, U.S. Department of Commerce, 5282 Port Royal Road, Springfield, Virginia 22151.
[2]   Exploratory Research to Develop Devices to Enable the Blind to Utilize Their Remaining Visual Apparatus, Final report, Contract P. H. 43-67-1342 to NINDS. Available: Clearinghouse for Federal Scientific and Technical Information, U.S. Department of Commerce, 5282 Port Royal Road, Springfield, Virginia 22151.

LIST OF PARTICIPANTS
AT THE
SECOND CONFERENCE ON VISUAL PROSTHESIS

Held at the Center for Continuing Education
The University of Chicago, Chicago, Illinois
June 2–4, 1969

JOHN ADAMS, M.D.
Department of Surgery
University of California
San Francisco, California

PAUL BACH-Y-RITA, M.D.
The Institute of Medical Sciences
Pacific Medical Center
San Francisco, California

BERNARD BECKER, M.D.
Department of Ophthalmology
Washington University School
*   of Medicine*
St. Louis, Missouri

MICHAEL BEDDOES, PH.D.
Department of Electrical Engineering
University of British Columbia
Vancouver, British Columbia, Canada

EDGAR A. BERING, JR., M.D.
National Institute of Neurological
*   Diseases and Stroke/DHEW*
National Institutes of Health
Bethesda, Maryland

RANDALL G. BINKS
Department of Applied Mathematics and
*   Computer Science*
Washington University
St. Louis, Missouri

JAMES C. BLISS, PH.D.
Engineering Sciences Laboratory
Stanford Research Institute
Menlo Park, California

HOWARD BOMZE
Department of Bioengineering
Irene Johnson Rehabilitation Institute
St. Louis, Missouri

WARREN M. BRODEY, M.D.
Environmental Ecology Laboratory
Boston, Massachusetts

WILLIAM BRODSKY, M.D.
Department of Ophthalmology
Mount Sinai School of Medicine of
*   the City University of New York*
New York, New York

379

RONALD M. BURDE, M.D.
Department of Ophthalmology
Washington University School of Medicine
St. Louis, Missouri

JOHN W. CARR III, PH.D.
The Moore School of Electrical Engineering
University of Pennsylvania
Philadelphia, Pennsylvania

LESLIE L. CLARK, M.A.
International Research Information Service
American Foundation for the Blind, Inc.
New York, New York

DAVID G. COGAN, M.D.
Howe Laboratory of Ophthalmology
Harvard University Medical School
Cambridge, Massachusetts

CARTER C. COLLINS, PH.D.
The Institute of Medical Sciences
Pacific Medical Center
San Francisco, California

ARMANDO DEL CAMPO, M.D.
Av. Revolución No. 1734
Mexico 20, D.F.

WILLIAM H. DOBELLE, PH.D.
Department of Surgery
University of Utah, College of Medicine
Salt Lake City, Utah

ROBERT W. DOTY, PH.D.
Center for Brain Research
River Campus Station
University of Rochester
Rochester, New York

EMERSON FOULKE, PH.D.
Department of Psychology
University of Louisville
Louisville, Kentucky

CARLOS EYZAGUIRRE, PH.D.
Department of Surgery
University of Utah, College of Medicine
Salt Lake City, Utah

KARL FRANK, PH.D.
Laboratory of Neural Control
National Institute of Neurological Diseases and Stroke/DHEW
National Institutes of Health
Bethesda, Maryland

MALCOLM A. GLESER, M.D., PH.D.
Department of Medicine
H. C. Moffitt Hospital
San Francisco, California

CHARLES E. HALLENBECK, PH.D.
Department of Psychology
University of Kansas
Lawrence, Kansas

LEON D. HARMON, PH.D.
Department of Visual Research
Bell Telephone Laboratories
Murray Hill, New Jersey

KENNETH R. INGHAM, PH.D.
Research Laboratory of Electronics
Massachusetts Institute of Technology
Cambridge, Massachusetts

AVERY R. JOHNSON, PH.D.
Environmental Ecology Laboratory
Boston, Massachusetts

KENNETH C. KNOWLTON, PH.D.
Bell Telephone Laboratories
Murray Hill, New Jersey

WEN-HSIUNG KO, PH.D.
Biomedical Electronics Laboratory
Case Western Reserve University
Cleveland, Ohio

WIKTOR KUPRIANOWICZ, ING.
Pomorska Akademia Medyczna,
Klinika Okulistyczna
Szczecin, Poland

IRVING H. LEOPOLD, M.D.
Department of Ophthalmology
Mt. Sinai School of Medicine of the City University of New York
New York, New York

GERALD E. LOEB
The Thomas C. Jenkins Department
of Biophysics
The Johns Hopkins University
Baltimore, Maryland

DOUGLAS C. MACFARLAND, PH.D.
Division of Services for the Blind
Rehabilitation Services Administration,
SRS/DHEW
Washington, D.C.

D. M. MACKAY, PH.D.
Department of Communication
University of Keele
Keele, Staffordshire, England

EDWARD F. MACNICHOL, JR., PH.D.
National Institute of Neurological
Diseases and Stroke/DHEW
National Institutes of Health
Bethesda, Maryland

ROBERT W. MANN, PH.D.
Department of Mechanical Engineering
Sensory Aids Center
Massachusetts Institute of Technology
Cambridge, Massachusetts

ELWIN MARG, PH.D.
School of Optometry
University of California
Berkeley, California

MARVIN MINSKY, PH.D.
Department of Electrical Engineering
Massachusetts Institute of Technology
Cambridge, Massachusetts

EUGENE F. MURPHY, PH.D.
Research and Development Division
Prosthetic and Sensory Aids Service
Veterans Administration
New York, New York

GEORGE B. NAGY, PH.D.
IBM Watson Research Center
Yorktown Heights, New York

PATRICK W. NYE, PH.D.
Booth Computing Center
California Institute of Technology
Pasadena, California

GERALD OSTER, PH.D.
Department of Biochemistry
Mount Sinai School of Medicine of
the City University of New York
New York, New York

LAWRENCE R. PINNEO, PH.D.
Neurophysiology Program
Stanford Research Institute
Menlo Park, California

SEYMOUR V. POLLACK, M.CH.E.
Department of Applied Mathematics and
Computer Science
Washington University
St. Louis, Missouri

VITO A. PROSCIA
Center for Sensory Aids Evaluation
and Development
Massachusetts Institute of Technology
Cambridge, Massachusetts

L. DENO REED, PH.D.
Sensory Study Section
Departments of Health, Education, and
Welfare
Washington, D.C.

ROBERT D. REINECKE
Howe Laboratory of Ophthalmology
Harvard University Medical School
Massachusetts Eye and Ear Infirmary
Boston, Massachusetts

THEODORE S. ROBERTS, M.D.
Department of Surgery
University of Utah, College of Medicine
Salt Lake City, Utah

FRANK SAUNDERS, PH.D.
The Institute of Medical Sciences
Pacific Medical Center
San Francisco, California

HERBERT SCHIMMEL, PH.D.

Department of Neurology
Albert Einstein College of Medicine
Bronx, New York

F. BLAIR SIMMONS, M.D.

Division of Otolaryngology
Stanford University School of Medicine
Stanford, California

THEODOR D. STERLING, PH.D.

Department of Applied Mathematics and
    Computer Science
Washington University
St. Louis, Missouri

THOMAS STOCKHAM, JR., PH.D.

Department of Computer Science
University of Utah
Salt Lake City, Utah

LOUIS L. SUTRO, PH.D.

Instrumentation Laboratory
Dept. of Aeronautics and Astronautics
Massachusetts Institute of Technology
Cambridge, Massachusetts

KENNETH TROUERN-TREND, M.A.

Medical Systems Division
Travelers Research Center
Hartford, Connecticut

HERBERT VAUGHAN, JR., M.D.

Department of Neurology
Albert Einstein College of Medicine
Bronx, New York

JOHN WEAVER, M.D.

Wills Eye Hospital and Research
    Institute
Philadelphia, Pennsylvania

JAMES J. WEINKAM, D.SC.

Department of Applied Mathematics and
    Computer Science
Washington University
St. Louis, Missouri

NORMAN M. YODER, PH.D.

Staff Development & Research
Sight Center
Cleveland, Ohio